Integrative
Health Care

Complementary and
Alternative Therapies
for the Whole Person

Integrative

Health Care

Complementary and Alternative Therapies for the Whole Person

Victor S. Sierpina, MD
Associate Professor
Clinic Medical Director
Department of Family Medicine
University of Texas Medical Branch
Galveston, Texas

 F. A. Davis Company
Philadelphia

F. A. Davis Company
1915 Arch Street
Philadelphia, PA 19103
www.fadavis.com

Printed in the United States of America

Last digit indicates print number: 10 9 8 7 6 5 4 3 2 1

Acquisitions Editor: Margaret M. Biblis
Developmental Editor: Bernice M. Wissler
Production Editor: Michael Schnee
Cover Designer: Louis Forgione

As new scientific information becomes available through basic and clinical research, recommended treatments and drug therapies undergo changes. The author(s) and publisher have done everything possible to make this book accurate, up to date, and in accord with accepted standards at the time of publication. The author(s), editors, and publisher are not responsible for errors or omissions or for consequences from application of the book, and make no warranty, expressed or implied, in regard to the contents of the book. Any practice described in this book should be applied by the reader in accordance with professional standards of care used in regard to the unique circumstances that may apply in each situation. The reader is advised always to check product information (package inserts) for changes and new information regarding dose and contraindications before administering any drug. Caution is especially urged when using new or infrequently ordered drugs.

Library of Congress Cataloging-in-Publication Data

Sierpina, Victor S., 1949-
    Integrative health care: complementary and alternative therapies for the whole person Victor S. Sierpina
        p. ; cm.
    Includes bibliographical references and index.
    ISBN 0-8036-0704-0 (alk. paper)
        1. Alternative medicine. 2. Integrated delivery of health care. I.
[DNLM: 1. Alternative Medicine. 2. Delivery of Health Care, Integrated. 3. Holistic
    Health. WB 890 S572I 2000]
R733.S54 2000]
615.5—dc21   00-043047
                                                                              CIP

DEDICATION

This book is dedicated to my best teachers. These are my patients and Dr. Kenneth Kessel of Countryside, Illinois. My mentor and advisor throughout medical school and family practice residency, Ken first taught me the gentle art of medicine and the skills of observing, listening, and learning from each patient.

The way he taught me to practice is based on caring deeply about my patients, listening to their stories, applying simple preventive measures, and whenever possible, using safe, natural therapies. This is the organic, holistic foundation of excellent clinical care. It is his legacy to me and to his many students over the years.

Ken, may your organic garden continue to bear a wonderful harvest of healing, joy, and professional integrity for many years to come.

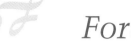 # *Foreword*

"Will medicine ever change?" This is one of the questions I am most frequently asked. It always comes from people who want to take a preventive, proactive approach to their health. They believe that conventional medicine's focus on treating established disease is short-sighted. They want more on their side than drugs and surgical procedures. They are interested in self-responsibility. My response to their question is always, "Hang on to your hat. Medicine is one of the most dynamic institutions in our society. The question is not *whether* medicine will change, but *when*." Dr. Victor S. Sierpina's *Integrative Health Care: Complementary and Alternative Therapies for the Whole Person* confirms my prediction. It is about the sweeping changes currently taking place within medicine in the area that is called integrative, complementary, or alternative medicine. As you will see, these are not small, incremental changes but colossal shifts that are shaking the foundations of modern health care. In fact, this transition is one of the most remarkable social movements of the twentieth century, now extending into the twenty-first.

Still, this field remains unfamiliar to many patients and physicians alike. Anytime we enter unknown territory, we need experts to help us find our way. A good guide does not push us along but shows the way and invites us to follow. This is what Dr. Sierpina does in this fine book. He gently instructs us each step of the way, giving us the information that we need to make intelligent choices about our own health.

Our culture has been under a powerful spell. We believed we could create an approach to healing based purely in "the physical," and that this type of medicine would answer all our needs. Now we know that this hope was an illusion, a goal that was impossible in principle. "Physical medicine" is an oxymoron, a self-contradiction, because if a system of medicine limits its attention to physical factors, it actually fosters some illnesses even as it tries to cure others. For example, studies show that a positive sense of meaning and purpose in life correlates with greater longevity and better health; that rich interpersonal relationships between people foster good health; and that the experiences of empathy, love, and compassion actually change our body in healthful ways. Other studies show that job dissatisfaction, depression, and illiteracy are correlated with heart disease, yet these issues are almost always overshadowed by our attention to physical risk factors—smoking, high blood pressure, high blood cholesterol, and so on. These physical factors are indeed important, but additional concerns must be added to the physical side of life if we are to be whole persons—issues such as values, meanings, purposes, emotions, and so on. Ignoring the importance of these factors misleads people and sets the stage for illness, because if individuals believe that they've taken care of the physical issues, they may think that they are in the clear, which is often not the case. The same problem crops up in the therapies we choose. If we expect physical measures such as drugs and surgery to do the job alone, we shall often be sorely disappointed. Other therapies, such as the integrative, complementary, or alternative measures discussed in the pages that follow, are often more effective, safer, and less expensive than the physical therapies to which we've become accustomed. The goal of this book is to describe these alternatives and how they can be integrated with the current physical therapies. The result is Dr. Sierpina's whole-person medicine—an approach that honors not only the physical body but the mind and spirit as well.

Some people fear that the trend toward whole-person health care will take medicine back to the dark ages. They say a body-mind-spirit approach dishonors science and rejects the magnificent medical advances that were the hallmarks of the twentieth century. But whole-person medicine is not the rejection of science, but its fulfillment. Whole-person medicine enriches scientific medicine by honoring, expanding, and empowering it. There is nothing far-out or fringe about whole-person medicine. Neither is whole-person medicine futuristic. It is not waiting to happen, it is happening now, as you are about to see.

As we venture into whole-person medicine, let's try to avoid the tendency to regard these approaches as somehow "higher" or "better" than drugs and surgical procedures. Each type of therapy has its place. Whether we use drugs or surgical procedures in our health care, or whether we opt for herbs, acupuncture, imagery, or prayer, we should be grateful for each of them. *Both* penicillin and prayer are blessings; both are miracles in their own domain. Whole-person medicine does not ask us to take sides; it is a both/and, not an either/or, approach.

There is an old saying: "Some people make it happen, some people watch it happen, and some people say, 'What happened?' " Amid the tumultuous changes that are enveloping medicine, which group are we in? We, as health care professionals, and our patients have a choice about how to respond to these developments. We can choose to be passive observers of the changes taking place in health care, encouraging our patients to depend on us to keep them healthy and bail them out of trouble when their health fails. Or we can help "make it happen" by applying the new integrative approaches. If we choose to do so, *Integrative Health Care* is the tool we are going to need.

André Malraux, the late French novelist and Minister of Culture of France, said, "The twenty-first century will be spiritual or it will not be at all." Similarly, I feel that twenty-first-century medicine will be spiritual or it will not be at all—at least not in any form that is fit to apply to humans. Some shy away from "the spiritual" in medicine, yet there is a deep longing on the part of millions of people to recover a sense of the spiritual that has gone missing in medicine. Whole-person medicine is sensitive to this longing. It is concerned not only with physical health but also with achieving harmony, balance, and fulfillment, and tapping the inner sources of wisdom and transformation that lie within everyone. These issues must be attended to if we are to be genuinely healthy. Can we muster the courage to make a place for these issues in our vision of healing, as healers have traditionally done? Can we envision a medicine comprehensive enough, *human* enough, to honor *all* we are? I am certain the answer is yes—and so is Dr. Victor S. Sierpina, as you are about to discover.

LARRY DOSSEY, MD
AUTHOR, *Reinventing Medicine*
EXECUTIVE EDITOR, *Alternative Therapies in Health and Medicine*

Preface

When I first began to study and practice medicine over 20 years ago, the use of alternative therapies by patients was relatively rare. The only ones integrating herbs, vitamins, mind-body techniques, and the like into their lives or into medical treatments were a small number of "health nuts." This "yogurt-granola set" did amazing things like eat low-fat diets, take vitamins regularly, meditate, and jog. It seemed as if they all lived in or came from California.

Today, the medical landscape has changed dramatically. We are rapidly moving into an era of patient-centered care. Yesterday's wellness radicals have become today's mainstream population. Studies have shown that the number of those who use alternative therapies approaches 50% in the United States and Canada. What was once an occasional inquiry about alternative therapies in medical practice is an everyday event.

More than ever before, patients are well informed, active, and responsible in seeking healthy lifestyle choices. They earnestly seek the perspective and opinion of their health care provider in sorting out various sources of information. Today's patients scan books, the lay press, and the Internet and confer with friends and alternative practitioners as they seek their own path to wholeness and well-being.

Most of the self-care therapies these patients use are incompletely or minimally covered in standard health-care curricula. Therefore, diligent practitioners must study independently and inform themselves about alternative and integrative medical practices.

It is important for us to become informed for several reasons. First, we must be able to communicate comfortably and reliably with our patients. Our ignorance creates a barrier and an information gap that decreases trust, respect, and collaboration. Second, as wise clinicians, we continually seek new and better methods to manage our patients' problems. When safe, natural methods and healthy lifestyle choices offer alternatives to drugs, surgery, or invasive procedures, we must follow the dictum of *primum non nocere* ("first do no harm") and offer the treatment that has the least potential to do harm. Finally, as seasoned clinicians and health care practitioners with a broad perspective on the human condition in health and disease, we must protect our patients against dangerous, expensive, and unproven therapies. To do this, we must build an atmosphere of trust based on our being prepared with reliable knowledge and the willingness to communicate with our patients, including our willingness to admit ignorance in certain areas.

In addition, our professional curricula pay little attention to the health of the health care provider. Healthy eating habits, exercise, and sleep are generally neglected or taken for granted during training. Practices that would be helpful for personal wellness, such as stress management, mind-body medicine, healthy relationships, and spirituality issues are covered minimally, if at all. Future practitioners paradoxically are encouraged to teach healthy lifestyles that they themselves are not practicing.

The issues include not only our own health, but also our role as a model for patients and our credibility in communicating with them. The nurse uncomfortable with his or her own mortality, the respiratory therapist who smokes, the obese physician, the sedentary physical therapist, and the physician assistant who is secretly an alcoholic will be less effective in their daily work. When dealing with the dying patient or attempting to encourage behavioral change in patients with health risk factors such as substance abuse, obesity, and inactivity, can they be credible? Can they, with their own imperfections, addictions, and lifestyle issues, be good motivators for patient change?

The answer is both yes and no. All of us have unhealed elements. In fact, the "wounded healer" and the awareness of our incompleteness and imperfections are often the very things that lead us into the helping professions. Yet, so far as we are able, we must practice what we preach and attempt to become our personal best—whole in mind, body, and spirit. In this book, I hope to create awareness about the importance of self-care for health care providers and to offer some tools to increase our choices of healthy lifestyles.

Our patients have always been, and will always be, our best teachers. Be willing to collaborate with them, counsel them, and learn from them. Be willing to model and reflect healthy behaviors in return. You will become a better clinician as well as a more whole person.

This book provides the tools for the treatment of the whole person. As much as possible, I have chosen useful references and evidence-based citations to support therapies that are often still out of the mainstream of medical education and practice. Spend some time with the literature so that you gain the knowledge base to add these helpful practices to your methods of treating and counseling patients as well as adding them to your own life. I trust you will enjoy the healthy and healing journey.

Victor S. Sierpina, MD
Galveston, Texas

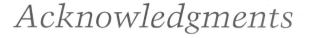

Acknowledgments

A work like this takes a lot of inspiration, perspiration, and persistence. I am especially thankful to Dennis Blessing, who suggested to Sandy Reinhardt, then senior medical editor of F. A. Davis, that I author such a work. Sandy enthusiastically promoted this project and worked tirelessly to explore ways of bringing the content to the Web and generally making the book available to as wide an audience as possible. My constant companion by e-mail, fax, and phone for the past several months, Bernice Wissler, the developmental editor, has been a superb partner in ensuring the consistency, readability, and quality of this book. Thanks to you, Bernice.

I also wish to thank my many students whose energy and imagination have fired my interest in creating a useable book for their introduction to complementary and alternative medicine (CAM) therapies and integrative medicine. Thanks too to my patients over the decades who have trusted their health to my care. They have contributed greatly by bringing me lots of real-life experiences, new therapies I had never heard of, and the opportunity to develop skills in integrative care.

The guiding lights of this field who have really helped and inspired me through their books, lectures, teaching, and personal and professional contacts are Larry and Barbie Dossey, Andy Weil, Marc Micozzi, Joe Helms, Mary Fenton, Chuck Moss, Dave Eisenberg, Wayne Jonas, Sam Benjamin, Doris Milton, Don Counts, Robbie Lee, Russ Greenfield, Ben Kligler, Woodie Merrell, and Mary Ann Richardson. I am also thankful to our wonderful Chairman of Family Medicine, Barbara Thompson, and my many colleagues at the University of Texas Medical Branch who have supported these efforts.

I particularly want to credit the intense scholarly research and review of the CAM literature done by Edzard Ernst, Steven Wirth, Michael Murray, Joe Pizzorno, Alan Gaby, Jonathan Wright, Steve Austin, Don Brown, Schuyler Lininger and his team at Healthnotes Inc., and Kirk Hamilton's *Clinical Pearls* newsletter. I referenced their work heavily in preparing the tables, evidence criteria, and treatments.

And finally, thanks to my children, Geoff, Todd, Suzi, and Dave, and my wife, Michelle, who have supported me through this project though it often meant I had less time to spend with them. You all are the reason I go on.

May God bless you all.

 *Contributors*

CONTRIBUTING AUTHORS

Linda L. Blakemore RN, BSN, BA
Reiki Master
Friendswood, Texas

J. Dennis Blessing, PhD, PA-C
Associate Professor and Chair
Department of Physician Assistant Studies
Executive Director, Center for Allied Health Research
School of Allied Health Sciences
University of Texas Health Science Center at San Antonio
San Antonio, Texas

Daniel Blodgett, MD
Assistant Professor and Inpatient Director
Department of Family Medicine
University of Texas Medical Branch
Galveston, Texas

Michelle L. Edwards, MSN, RNCS, FNP
Family Nurse Practitioner
Department of Family Medicine
University of Texas Medical Branch
Galveston, Texas

Mary Anne Hanley, RN, MA
Coordinator, Center for Healing Practices in Nursing
Assistant Clinical Professor
School of Nursing
University of Texas Medical Branch
Galveston, Texas

Lew Huff, DC
Associate Professor
Clinical Rotations Coordinator
Texas Chiropractic College Health Centers
Pasadena, Texas

Lisa R. Nash, DO
Assistant Professor and Curriculum Coordinator for Obstetrics
Department of Family Medicine
University of Texas Medical Branch
Galveston, Texas

Connie Silva, RN, PhD, HNC, CHTP
Associate Professor
School of Nursing
University of Texas Medical Branch
Galveston, Texas

DESIGN AND PREPARATION OF TABLES

Sonia Carolina Salas-Robazetti, MD
Research Fellow, Obstetrics and Gynecology
University of Texas Medical Branch
Galveston, Texas

RESEARCH, RESOURCES, AND REFERENCES

Michelle Sierpina, MS
Health Care Writer and Consultant
Tiki Island, Texas

Contents

Section

I

Introduction

If a man empties his purse into his head, no one can take it away from him. An investment in knowledge always pays the best interest.
—Benjamin Franklin

There is need of a sprightly and vigilant soul to discern and lay hold on favorable junctures.
—Pierre Charron

In Chapter 1, I introduce the core principles, vocabulary, history, driving forces, social context, and controversy related to integrative health care. I define terminology, such as *alternative, complementary,* and *integrative,* and describe changing professional and public attitudes and relationships in this new era of whole-person health care.

Chapter 2 gives the student and practitioner some practical tools for working with patients who prefer alternative therapy. I offer an "ABCDE" approach to integrative care, explaining the importance of skills such as asking the right questions, being willing to listen and learn, communicating and collaborating, diagnosing accurately and meaningfully, and explaining and exploring preferences.

Chapter 1

What Is Integrative Health Care?

Life belongs to the living, and he who lives must be prepared for changes.
　　　　　　　　　　　　　　　　—Goethe

Have no fear of change as such and, on the other hand, no liking for it merely for its own sake.
　　　　　　　　　　　　　　—Robert Moses

The term *integrative* does not refer to a new field of medicine, nursing, or health care. It refers to a *process* and *method* of care that uses both conventional diagnostic and treatment methods and alternative therapies. It also represents a worldview, a paradigm shift in the model of delivering health care. In addition to the compassionate, caring, and competent care that is expected of every health care worker, the integrative health care model utilizes the following key ingredients:

1. *Patient- or client-centered care*
2. Encouragement of *self-care* and personal responsibility for health
3. The joining of *mind, body,* and *spirit,* which are mutually essential to the healing of whole persons
4. A goal of *promoting* vibrant *health, wellness,* and the highest *potential* for human beings, not just treating disease
5. *Collaborative partnerships* involving interdisciplinary teams of health-care providers and the patient
6. Openness to using *alternative or complementary therapies* that have a record of safety and efficacy but are outside of the conventional biomedical model
7. Application of *evidence-based, critical thinking skills* when integrating alternative therapies with conventional therapies
8. Using *natural, less invasive approaches* whenever possible
9. Accepting that *health and healing are individually determined* and may be different for each person, so a person may be "healed" without being cured

10. *A change to a different view of health care,* often requiring a *paradigm shift* for the health care provider and perhaps for the patient

▬▬▬ DEFINITION OF TERMS: COMPLEMENTARY, ALTERNATIVE, INTEGRATIVE—WHAT'S WHAT?

Before we progress with the tour, perhaps an introductory language course will prepare us for the land into which we are traveling. You noticed the term *integrative* in the title of this book and in the Preface. No doubt, you also have heard the terms *complementary* and *alternative.* Other terms you may encounter as you study nonconventional therapies are *holistic* (or *wholistic*), *natural medicine, rational medicine, whole-person care, traditional medicine, nontraditional therapies, wellness promotion,* and so forth. From the dark side of the force you'll hear less cheerful terms such as *quack medicine, irrational medicine, unproved therapies,* and even *health care fraud.*

To make matters more interesting, other cultures use different terminology. The Germans use the term *Nichtschulmedizin* (medicine not taught in school). A traditional Chinese physician thinks of acupuncture as "traditional" and Western medicine, to some degree, as "alternative." To an African or other Third World society that cannot afford expensive pharmaceuticals, its historic herbal remedies are not "alternative" but mainstream. In Europe, herbs are not only commonly prescribed by physicians but are reimbursed under health care plans. *Conventional? Unconventional? Alternative? Traditional? Complementary?* Which is the correct term?

By fiat, Congress has defined language and thinking in the United States. By establishing the Office of Alternative Medicine (OAM) and recently by redefining it as the National Center for Complementary and Alternative Medicine (NCCAM), we at least have name recognition. The deep thinkers in this field are dissatisfied with both terms, however. *Alternative* has a bit of a confrontational tone to it. It implies, "Use my medicine or treatment *instead of* another treatment." Those who proposed the term *complementary* were trying to accommodate to the fact that people usually use nonconventional therapy *along with* standard medical treatment. One problem with this term is that many people spell it wrong. Instead of *complementary,* it is often written *complimentary,* which makes it sound like saying something nice. The other concern about *complementary* is that it seems like something that is extra, added-on, and nonessential. Instead of being the main course, it is like the parsley garnishing the plate. This removes *complementary* therapy from being an equal partner in a collaborative balance of various healing systems and techniques.

Enter Dr. Andrew Weil, guru-in-chief of the natural-healing movement. Our bewhiskered friend introduced the term *integrative* medicine, which he defines as the blending of the best of conventional and nonconventional therapies. Andy is a great gourmet cook of healthy, natural foods, so it is only natural (no pun intended) that he use a term like *integrative*. To really benefit from both nonconventional and conventional therapy, it is best to blend them, just as in fine cooking.

Another term I like is *rational* medicine. Michael Murray, ND, a highly respected naturopathic physician, discussed rational medicine at a conference I attended. By this term he meant using our minds, our science, and our literature to determine the appropriate approach to a patient and his or her problem. Rational medicine means selecting the best option for each individual patient based on condition, preference, and the state of known science, rather than relying on arbitrary definitions of *conventional, alternative,* or *complementary.*

To add to the mix, Larry Dossey, MD, impishly coined another phrase recently: *accommodative* medicine. This indicates yet another twist in this labyrinthine semantic jungle. It reflects the fact that medical care ought to accommodate different cultures, beliefs, and techniques. No single system has all the answers, so it makes sense to accommodate a blend of therapies in our approach.

For the purpose of this introductory handbook, I will primarily stick with *integrative* to identify this model of care, which often involves the use of nonconventional or "alternative" therapies. *Alternative* will be used when referring to the therapies themselves or to systems of therapy and when discussing well-known publications that have used this term. Because the distinction between *integrative* and *alternative* is somewhat fluid (it even befuddled my editor and me at times), both terms will often be used somewhat interchangeably.

▬▬▬ USE OF ALTERNATIVE THERAPIES: A CHANGING WORLD, A CHANGING CULTURE

No reference to the place of alternative therapies in our contemporary culture would be complete without reference to the landmark work of David Eisenberg, MD, of Harvard. In 1993, Dr. Eisenberg published in the *New England Journal of Medicine* the results of a survey about the use of integrative therapies in the United States (Eisenberg et al 1993). His study revealed that over one-third of the adult population was using some form of alternative therapy—yielding over 450 million visits annually to alternative practitioners, compared to about 400 million visits to primary care medical doctors.

By and large, patients did not discuss their use of these therapies with their physicians and paid for these services out of pocket, with an estimated expense of $13 billion, more than they spent annually for all physician services. Clearly, a huge sector of the health care market had been invisible and out of the mainstream of medical care.

But Dr. Eisenberg and his colleagues did not stop their study there. In 1998 they published a follow-up study in the *Journal of the American Medical Association*, in which they reported the changes between their earlier study and a newer survey, which was completed in 1997 (Eisenberg et al 1998). The proportion of users of alternative therapies had expanded dramatically to over 42% of the U.S. public, with especially rapid growth in the use of herbs, massage, megavitamins, self-help groups, folk remedies, energy healing, and homeopathy. By the 1997 survey, estimated visits to alternative providers numbered 629 million, vastly exceeding visits to all primary care physicians (386 million). Expenditures for these therapies were conservatively estimated at $27 billion, comparable to the projected out-of-pocket expenditure for all physician services.

Clearly, from the two data points in these surveys, not only are alternative therapies here to stay, but they are being used at an increasing rate. The highest use of alternative therapies was in the baby boomer age group, 35 to 49 years of age. In this large group, 50% used these therapies. As the baby boomers age, we can expect their use of these therapies to increase even more. A study in Canada showed increasing use of integrative therapies with age, with up to 70% of those ages 65 and older using some form of alternative therapy. This is not too surprising, because the elderly have more medical conditions and would be expected to use more therapies of all kinds.

Most of the time, these therapies are integrated with conventional treatment, rather than substituting for it. Several studies in the United States and abroad have shown that 70% to 90% of those using alternative therapies are using them for a condition they have already discussed with their regular doctor. They usually do not discuss the alternative therapy with their doctor, however. We will examine some of the possible reasons for this reluctance later.

THE NATIONAL CENTER FOR COMPLEMENTARY AND ALTERNATIVE MEDICINE: GATHERING EVIDENCE

The charge of the original OAM, now the NCCAM, was to encourage the study of the wide variety of alternative and complementary therapies and start to separate fact from fallacy, evidence from chicanery, and then to present this information to the public, professional communities, and policy makers.

When it started work in 1993, the OAM had a budget of only $2 million dollars, 0.0025% of the $80 billion budget of the National Institutes of Health (NIH), a truly "homeopathic" dose of funding. Nonetheless, as in the practice of homeopathy, a little bit goes a long way. Over the next several years, about a dozen OAM Centers were established around the country to study alternative therapies. Prestigious schools such as Harvard, Stanford, Columbia, the University of Texas, the University of Arizona, and Bastyr University (a naturopathic medical school in Seattle) were given grants and other support to establish research programs in complementary and alternative therapy. Topics included back pain, cancer, HIV infection, aging, women's health, and pediatric care.

By 1999, the OAM had been upgraded to the NCCAM and given a budget of $50 million and its own authority to grant funding for projects within its mother organization, the NIH. This has had the effect of stimulating scholarly research and inquiry into a wide array of alternative therapies. The resulting knowledge is increasingly vital in this age of over-choice, so that health care providers and patients alike can make choices based on quality information.

To clarify and organize the field of inquiry and discussion, the OAM set out the following seven categories (covered later in this book) as the areas of study (Workshop on Alternative Medicine 1992):

1. Alternative systems of medical practice
2. Bioelectromagnetic therapies
3. Diet and nutrition
4. Herbal medicine
5. Manual healing methods
6. Mind-body medicine
7. Pharmacological and biological treatments

These categories recently were modified slightly, but we will continue to use them.

▬▬ VIEW OF ALTERNATIVE THERAPIES: QUACKS, QUACK-BUSTERS, AND SKEPTICS

While studying this field, you will find the kind of turmoil and debate that the NCCAM was established to address and that it tries to clarify with an objective, scientific viewpoint. As in Chinese medicine, you will discover two polarities that nevertheless share some similarities. On one extreme are those practitioners, often well-intentioned, who believe that the treatment they practice is a panacea that requires no scientific evidence or theory to explain it; they generally make excessive claims of efficacy. These folks usually can be identified by their bias against all allopathic care. They say such things as, "Surgery, drugs, chemotherapy, and those other things your doctor recommends are all bad for you." These are the "quacks."

On the other side there waddles another group, the "quack-busters," who are equally fervent in their opposition to all systems of healing outside the allopathic, conventional medical model. This group is equally implausible both scientifically and psychologically. "Quack-busters" believe that any integrative or nonconventional therapy is health care fraud or some other kind of nefarious scheme foisted on an ignorant public. They classify as "unproven" therapies that have been used for hundreds of generations by thousands of cultures—including prayer, imagery and relaxation, diet, acupuncture, herbs, meditation, and Oriental exercise regimens like tai chi and yoga. Ignoring adequate clinical trials of these therapies, they pride themselves on being defenders of the scientific status quo, refusing to accept evidence contrary to their highly rationalistic worldview.

Frankly, I am a bit suspicious of radicals at either extreme, although they help to refresh and strengthen the "radical center," which is a healthy and honest place to live, breathe, and think. Lao Tsu, the ancient Chinese sage, said that approaching the universe should be done like cooking a small fish—that is, gently. The wise person, according to this ancient philosopher, should recognize the virtue in both good and evil, acknowledging their mutual strengths and weaknesses. Thus, the polarity of quacks and quack-busters, though distracting at times, actually enlivens the discussions around nonconventional therapies.

I recommend counseling and a transformative experience of some kind for members of both groups. No doubt, each has a kernel of truth, which is encrusted in a dogmatism and rigidity that may have grown out of individual pain. I like, encourage, and respect a bona fide skeptic who is a true scientist, sifting carefully through fact and fantasy for the truth. But those who are intolerant of others' ideas and culture without studying the evidence are guilty of bigotry as surely as those who are intolerant of another's race. As professionals, we must look at both positive and negative evidence for any therapy, consider the limits of our understanding and even our science, and above all, seek the best, safest, and most cost-effective care for our patients.

WHY THE POPULARITY OF ALTERNATIVE AND INTEGRATIVE APPROACHES TO HEALTH CARE?

Perhaps the biggest question is why these therapies are now so popular. Why is their use so widespread across a broad range of ages? The answer to this multifactorial cultural phenomenon can be broken down into the following factors:

- The desire for personal autonomy in health care choices
- The cost of care
- Perceived safety issues between alternative and conventional therapies
- Legislative and insurance regulation changes
- Changes in the therapeutic relationship between patients and their health care providers

The Desire for Personal Autonomy in Health Care Choices

The traditional medical model has focused on the authority, knowledge, and influence of the health care provider. The ill patient, suffering, confused, and unsure of what to do, has gratefully accepted advice, orders, prescriptions, or surgery from the physician or other health care expert.

We baby boomers—flower children of the 60s—and our children have developed a cultural distrust of authority, however. I am reminded of some graffiti I saw on my son's college campus: "Question all authority!" Some wag had scrawled beneath this brief manifesto, "Says who?" At any rate, a couple of generations have now grown up without attachment to authority figures and a patriarchal model. We want to make up our own minds rather than having them made up for us, especially about things as important to us as our health.

Another powerful cultural force that has encouraged this autonomy in health care choices is the wellness or fitness movement. Jogging, cycling, eating low-fat diets, quitting smoking, meditating, praying, doing aerobics, drinking bottles of spring water, and so on have become culturally accepted and encouraged. People are increasingly aware that they must take responsibility for their own health. The choices they make in their lifestyle have much to do with their health outcomes. In fact, several studies have estimated that lifestyle change alone could shave hundreds of millions of dollars from the U.S. health care budget annually. People who take the time to exercise, meditate, and eat right are well aware of the health value of these choices. No longer do they depend on the medical system to "provide" health in the old consumer model. Health just isn't something one can buy off the shelf in a doctor's clinic, pharmacy, or even a health food store (although sometimes we try!).

As people make choices about health, they have developed an insatiable appetite for high-quality information about health, fitness, nutrition, and the prevention or treatment of various illnesses. In the past, most of this information was available only to professionals who took years of training, read certain specialty books and journals, and practiced daily in the health care area. No longer is this the case. The World Wide Web, giant bookstores, magazines at grocery checkout lines, and radio and television programs are all brimming with information about health and health care. People want to know what they can do to stay healthy, become healthier, lose weight, manage stress, have better sex lives or relationships, eat better, and so on. Though the quality of information available through these sources varies tremendously, these informed people are trying to sort through the information and misinformation.

Because people may feel they are drowning in an overload of information, they seek help from the health care professional in a new and different way. Patients are likely to come to the clinic with an article, a sheaf of printouts from the Internet, or a book. They are more likely to ask their health care provider's opinion about this outside information than to depend solely on the professional's knowledge and expertise for advice on what to do. A well-informed professional can give patients clinical and scientific perspectives, helping them choose wisely, sorting beneficial from harmful treatments for them.

An exercise I require of my students when they study integrative health care is to spend some time in a health food store. The variety of products, their many claims for efficacy, the information resources, the salesclerks' opinions—all these are part of the complexity our patients face when making choices about vitamins, herbs, supplements, and other health-related products and activities. I also encourage the students to look on the Internet for the diversity of health-related topics in conventional and alternative care. This experience again gives a taste of the barrage of information, misinformation, advertising claims, testimonials, and sometimes questionable science that our patients must sort through.

Our patients' desire for increased autonomy and personal responsibility for their health is something we should encourage in helping them "be all they can be." The simpler time when health professionals were unquestioned authorities is long over. We must learn to work collaboratively with our patients in a role that is more like mentoring, counseling, and guiding.

The Cost of Care

Another driver in the modern world of health care is the cost of care. At the beginning of the 1900s, medical care was inexpensive because few therapies were available. At the beginning of the 2000s, technology rules. The many technological advances have improved our longevity and overall health in many ways, but the cost of care has risen astronomically. Insurance is needed to pay for both advanced and basic care. Many do not have access even to basic medical coverage because the insurance premiums are rising so rapidly to keep pace with costly advances in technology that insurance has become unaffordable for many families.

To get around these costs, many seek inexpensive alternatives to conventional care. If the latest arthritis drug costs $80 a month but an over-the-counter arthritis product like glucosamine sulfate is available for less than $30, an elderly person on a fixed income has a clear choice. For many, this choice can mean the difference between being able to afford adequate food and other necessities or going without. This choice becomes especially important for the many elderly patients who take a half dozen or more prescription medications, which together may cost several hundred dollars a month. Added to the cost issue is the potential risk for complex and unpredictable drug interactions. If lifestyle change, dietary modification, mind-body techniques, vitamins, minerals, or herbs can help a person's medical conditions safely and cheaply, these then become the desired alternatives.

The traditional use of alternative therapies was thought to be among the poor, for whom a strong cultural or familial belief system often supported the use of convenient, inexpensive remedies supplied by a folk healer (for example, the Hispanic *curandera*), an herbalist, or even one's grandmother. But although the poor often use traditional and home remedies because they lack access to conventional medical care, the use of these therapies is not limited to them. Several studies have shown that the use of alternative therapies in the United States is growing most quickly among those with a college education and those in the upper socioeconomic categories (Astin 1998). Clearly, cost is only one aspect of the decision to use integrative therapies.

Indeed, by integrating an alternative therapy with conventional therapy, the total cost of care in the short run may actually be increased. Studies have shown that using a chiropractor for an acute back injury might save money and reduce time off from work. But if the person also goes to an orthopedist, who prescribes an expensive (though unnecessary) MRI, the costs become additive.

Will cost continue to affect people's choices in this area? Absolutely. However, as these huge sums are spent, the need for high-quality research into outcomes and studies of the safety, efficacy, and proper use of alternative therapies (whether taken alone or integrated with conventional therapy) is increasingly evident. A few dollars saved by a person employing the wrong therapy may end up costing them and the medical system thousands more in unnecessary hospital costs because effective treatment is delayed. Good attention to whole-person care, including lifestyle and preventive issues at the primary care level, is critical. The wise use of an integrated blend of conventional and alternative therapies may offer the best chance to reduce the burdensome and increasing cost of medical care.

Perceived Safety Issues between Alternative and Conventional Therapies

One of the most frequent concerns patients raise about treatment is the risk of conventional therapy. A recent study showed that over 100,000 people had died in U.S. hospitals in the past year due to adverse reactions to medication alone (Lazarou et al 1998). Medical mistakes were recently reported in the general newspapers to cause as many as 80,000 deaths per year. Many millions of drug side effects affecting outpatients substantially burden both patients and the health care system. For instance, the use of over-the-counter nonsteroidal anti-inflammatory drugs (NSAIDs) like ibuprofen or naproxen accounts yearly for thousands of hospital admissions for gastrointestinal bleeding and many deaths.

So-called natural products are by no means entirely safe, of course. Several documented reports of heavy metal toxicity resulting from treatment with Hispanic and Chinese herbs indicate the risks of these products. Many Chinese patent medicines include prescription drugs such as steroids, antibiotics, and anti-inflammatories, which may cause side effects, allergic reactions, or drug interactions in patients unaware of their contents.

I recall clearly an enthused patient who came back from Mexico clutching a jar of "herbal" pills, which had markedly improved her asthma. Fortunately I could read Spanish and was able to decipher the list of ingredients for her. To my surprise, I found a powerful steroid among the constituents. I told her that as much as I hated to deflate her joy about this miracle "natural" cure, I could have given her $5 worth of prednisone and gotten a similar effect. She had not wanted to move to the more powerful prescription drug, but when it came disguised as an herbal remedy, it was more palatable to her. She stopped taking it and we managed her asthma conventionally by optimizing her inhaled steroid dosage, a much safer approach.

However, we commonly integrate the use of conventional drugs, with their powerful immediate effects, and alternative products, with their milder, longer-term effects. Given immediately after a myocardial infarction, for instance, beta blockers clearly reduce the risk of cardiac death. Prophylactic aspirin also reduces myocardial risk. Whether to routinely add antioxidants like vitamin C and E and beta carotene to this regimen for heart patients has been studied and continues to be investigated. Thus far, these antioxidants have not provided these patients the degree of protection given by the more powerful drugs, which do have greater potential side effects. So safety becomes a matter of clinical judgment. Using the antioxidants is safe, but their efficacy for heart patients has not been demonstrated as clearly as the efficacy of beta blockers and aspirin.

This example again illustrates the value of integrative care. The informed patient (consumer) can work with a cooperative, collaborative health-care provider to plan an optimal treatment that is based on the best of known science. In this case, using the prescription beta blocker and aspirin plus the antioxidants is the most rational care.

One of my favorite areas of study and practice over the years has been herbal therapy (see Chap. 10). Many societies have a long tradition of using herbs, which are considered safe by most patients. Yet make no mistake about it: *herbs are drugs.* Their effects are exerted through a wide variety of biologically active compounds, which can and do interact with other medications and have the potential for side effects of their own. Some, like coltsfoot, comfrey, and chaparral, are toxic.

By and large, however, herbs are a gentle form of medicine. In many cases they act gradually, more like a food than a drug. In a German study comparing St. John's wort, an herb used for depression, with the then-standard pharmacological agent, the dropout rate because of side effects was under 2% for the herbal arm of the study but nearly 30% for the drug. Herbs are well tolerated by most people and are generally quite safe. The informed provider of health care must be aware, however, that herbs and supplements can interact with certain drugs. For example, warfarin, a blood-thinning drug, has a wide range of interactions not only with many other drugs but also with foods like green leafy vegetables, which contain vitamin K and can decrease warfarin's effect, and garlic, ginkgo, and vitamin E, which increase its effect.

If a drug is unsatisfactory to a patient because it has unacceptable side effects, doesn't work, or is too expensive, it is often helpful to offer an alternative product with a better safety profile. I teach my students the value of having one more thing "in your back pocket" to offer patients who need therapy but won't or can't take a conventional medication. So the patient who wants protection from heart disease but cannot tolerate aspirin because of gastrointestinal bleeding or other side effects may get a similar benefit from using garlic, vitamin E, or ginkgo. Another person may wish to use inositol hexaniacinate or a product derived from Chinese red yeast (Cholestin) to lower cholesterol instead of the potentially hepatotoxic HMG-CoA reductase inhibitors.

Having options that are safe, useful, and inexpensive is core to the way I practice. Using these options along with potent conventional therapies that have a higher level of scientific evidence of efficacy but are often more expensive and have more potential side effects is essential to the art and science of integrative care.

Legislative and Insurance Regulation Changes

The type of legislation that created the NCCAM has created a new role for integrative medicine on the U.S. health scene, stimulating scholarly discussion and research. Some states, such as Washington, Oregon, Alaska, and California, have made provisions in their laws to encourage or require health care insurers and HMOs to cover integrative therapies in their plans. Several large insurers, such as Prudential, Aetna, Oxford, Blue Shield, and Kaiser, offer some type of benefit for complementary and alternative medicine (CAM). Varieties of coverage include premium-added options, discount certificates to providers of alternative care, referral arrangements with alternative practitioners, and even networks of credentialed alternative providers, such as naturopaths or chiropractors, who are designated as primary care practitioners.

Besides legislative requirements, insurance companies have started to pay attention to marketing and coverage in this area because of high market demand and the potential for cost savings and improved patient outcomes and satisfaction. Much research remains to be done to verify claims about this kind of potential. But insurance companies also have found that patients who use integrative therapies tend to be more health-attentive and therefore at lower risk, so they are more desirable as clients under any health care reimbursement strategy.

Changes in reimbursement policies have also encouraged dozens of groups, including hospitals and physician organizations, to start "integrative," "holistic," or "alternative and complementary" medical clinics. They hope that these centers will offer a new context for patient care and a new model of interdisciplinary, whole-person care. Whether these centers will remain financially viable is open to question. Many of them accept only self-pay, fee-for-service arrangements with patients. Though this is helpful for initial start-up and immediate financial stability, the long-term generalizability of this arrangement to broader, less affluent populations has been questioned.

Politics, power, and capital undoubtedly will move integrative therapies to a more central role in the health care market. What is now "alternative" may become mainstream if research shows improved outcomes and costs. Today's professionals must prepare to face this new world of health care because it will be practiced in the years ahead, with knowledge of both conventional and alternative care options. As Pope Pius XI said, "We must therefore take account of this changeable nature of things and of human institutions, and prepare for them with enlightened foresight."

Changes in the Therapeutic Relationship between Patients and Their Health-Care Providers

Gladys McGarey, MD, one of the founding members of the American Holistic Medical Association, described her life in the late 1940s as a country doctor in a small town in Ohio. It was a very different world—slower paced, rural, with a sense of community and intimacy rarely found in our contemporary scene. She was available around the clock for routine and emergency problems. She had to sneak out of town to go to a movie, and even this attempt was frustrated one time when the local police tracked her down to answer a phone call from the anxious mother of a constipated baby. They had found her car parked a couple of blocks from her brother-in-law's home, where she had hoped it would escape notice. They then noticed that his car was missing from his garage and alerted nearby town constables to look out for his license plate. When they found it in the parking lot of a theater 30 miles away, the jig was up!

In that time before pagers, cell phones, faxes, and computers, patients paid for their own medical care. An office call was $5, a house call $10, a delivery $25, a home delivery $75. There was no Medicare, no HMOs, no health insurance. Payment was usually cash but not always. I used to practice in a town of 63 people in the mountains of Colorado, the only full-time doctor in a 3500-square-mile county. Those who needed medical care but could not pay cash might perform services such as chopping firewood, training a colt, or running a backhoe, or might give gifts like sacks of potatoes, homegrown rabbits, cleaned trout, or homemade artwork. Like Dr. McGarey 40 years before, life for me meant being on duty at odd hours. Many a time I sewed up a laceration or looked down a sore throat over my own kitchen table. But in this setting, the doctor was a member of the community, well known to all, who learned from friends, neighbors, and other patients just what was happening to everyone and what the latest community scandal was. The psychosocial history thus often evolved not only from the patient but also from the community itself, so the doctor had a deeper and more whole view of what was going on in the patient's life, not only physically but also in the context of family, school, work, and town.

By contrast, the average physician visit today is often 7 to 10 minutes, owing to the constraints of managed care contracts, decreasing reimbursements, and productivity demands. In this context, the opportunity to know a patient deeply is limited. The health care professional in an urban or suburban setting may have no knowledge of the patient's life and situation beyond what can be revealed in 7 minutes, so the professional is often an unfamiliar face treating an anonymous person.

This lack of time and context has been another impetus driving patients' search for alternative therapies and methods of health care delivery, as they look for something deeper and more meaningful in the therapeutic relationship. The patient finds a homeopathic practitioner, an herbalist, a massage therapist, or a chiropractor who spends more time, seems more interested, and makes a more human connection than the hurried clinician in a conventional setting. In addition to a proper diagnosis and treatment plan, patients deeply desire understanding, caring, courtesy, and respect. If these are not found, the therapeutic power of the relationship between healer and the person seeking healing does not evolve. The healing force of trust and placebo is excluded.

Of course, time constraints need not win out. Many health professionals succeed in achieving a close encounter in a short time. Some solutions to the problem of time constraints will be discussed in Chapter 5, which addresses relationship-centered care.

◼◼◼◼ CONCLUSION

Health care culture and the world in which it exists are changing dramatically. From the authoritarian model of the past has evolved a new model: the informed, consumer/activist patient, eager to take responsibility for his or her health. These patients relish making their own health-related decisions, yet seek the advice, counsel, and support of their health care professional. The transaction cost for patients to learn everything about their particular conditions is often too high in terms of time and effort. Though patients may read up on a condition in some depth, they still look to the health care professional for the perspective that can come only from years of study and clinical experience.

Being an excellent provider of health care in the coming era means being an information master, a communication specialist, and a creative problem solver who seeks solutions for patient problems from both conventional and nonconventional sources. To be technically competent requires more than school or book learning. It requires an awareness of broad public movements in health and a willingness to work with patients in the context of these changes.

An example of the power of the attitudes of the public to change behaviors is seen in the tobacco smoking problem. When it was no longer seen as romantic and sophisticated to smoke, when restaurants, offices, and many public places developed policies limiting or forbidding smoking, the rates of tobacco use began to drop for the first time in decades. What health professionals had been campaigning for one-on-one with patients was greatly amplified and reinforced by public policy, attitude, and awareness. Public pressure to provide health insurance for vulnerable populations such as children, the elderly, and low-paid workers will likewise amplify the ability of professionals to improve society's health.

The public is using alternative therapies on a broad basis. To best serve them, health care professionals must learn the good and bad points of these therapies. Enlightened professionals will work with informed patients to integrate the most useful and proven therapies into their standard practice. In such a setting, patient satisfaction is bound to increase. By applying scientific rigor in evaluating the alternative therapies, we will protect our patients while offering them the best of care: the integrative care model.

Chapter 2

How to Talk to Patients about Integrative Care

The great secret of succeeding in conversation is to . . . hear much.

—Benjamin Franklin

The opposite of talking isn't listening. The opposite of talking is waiting.

—Fran Lebowitz

With thee conversing I forget all time.

—John Milton

> **The ABC Approach: Guidelines for Advising Patients Who Seek Alternative Therapies**
>
> 1. **A**sk, don't tell.
> 2. **B**e willing to listen and learn.
> 3. **C**ommunicate, **C**ollaborate.
> 4. **D**iagnose.
> 5. **E**xplain and **E**xplore options and preferences.

When patients come to your office, whether for the first time or the 50th, how do you discuss integrating an alternative therapy into their treatment plan? If you wait for the patient to bring up the topic, you may find, as Dr. Eisenberg's studies showed, that two-thirds of the time it will not happen. You need to take the initiative, using the ABCDE approach summarized in the box. An excellent discussion in this area is another paper by Eisenberg that details a step-by-step approach to advising patients in the use of alternative therapies (Eisenberg 1997).

ASK, DON'T TELL

Health care workers must inquire about patients' use of alternative therapies. These therapies may be helpful or they may be useless. They may even be contraindicated for certain patients or conditions or may interact in a harmful way with other treatments. Even if the alternative therapies are not actually harmful, patients who rely on them may delay their acceptance of other proven therapies, with effects that can be disastrous.

Reasons given for patients' reluctance to discuss alternative therapies with health care professionals are many. Essentially, they are worried about being thought foolish, being made to feel ashamed, or even losing the relationship. Even if they have read and studied a good deal to find a therapy that fits them, they feel vulnerable before an "expert" who may dismiss their conclusions as irrelevant or silly.

My conviction is that most patients are intuitively aware of both what is wrong with them and what they need to remedy the problem. Therefore, health care providers would do well to ask about patients' opinions and what therapies they may have tried already. This can be done easily while taking the history, either the history of the present illness or the medication list. For instance, you might say,

> "Besides ginseng, what else have you used or considered for your sexual problem?"

> "Have you tried any over-the-counter products for this condition?"

> "Have you heard about any other therapies for this problem that you would like to try?"

> "Do you have any questions about any other possible therapies?"

If you as the "expert" introduce the topic of alternative therapies, the patient feels much less vulnerable. Your openness to the subject is likely to elicit the most accurate and honest response the patient can give. This mutual openness will be helpful in the next phase of the process—listening and learning.

■■■■■■ BE WILLING TO LISTEN AND LEARN

Patients will bring you a wealth of information (and misinformation!) about their alternative therapies. Try to suspend judgment initially and just listen. Patients report that a large part of their satisfaction with many alternative practitioners comes from the willingness of those practitioners to *listen*.

Have you ever had anyone listen to you—*really* listen? This kind of listening can move mountains. A person looks you in the eye and pays total attention to what you have to say, as if you are the most important person in the world. This person doesn't interrupt, interject his or her own judgments, or seem to have anything else to do or anywhere else to go.

In this kind of timeless encounter, you feel totally respected, appreciated, even loved. Such empathy and attentiveness are essential to a really excellent patient-provider encounter. The skill of listening to your patients is essential not only to getting good information about alternative therapies. It is essential also to their satisfaction with you and to your satisfaction with your work.

One thing I have learned over years of practice is that patients *want* to collaborate with you. They want to be involved in their own health care choices, and when you are willing to listen, they will bring a wealth of information to you. It's like having a few thousand librarians looking for better ways to improve their health, except that these librarians are doing it for very personal reasons. It is, after all, *their* health.

From your patients, you will quickly accumulate journals, magazines, clippings, tapes, books, videos, and downloads from the Internet. Your willingness to learn from your patients' reading, research, and recollections of conversations with friends and family will provide a rich source of lifelong learning. They don't read the latest medical journals, but they do watch the news and continually scan many information sources.

True, they will come in with an amazing array of folk medicine and curious practices that may seem outrageous. Just because you haven't heard about a certain therapy, no matter how outlandish it seems, *suspend judgment* initially. Nothing cuts off communication from a patient more quickly than an incredulous snort, subtly raised eyebrow, or dismissive wave of the hand from a trusted health care practitioner. Once you have judged the content of a patient's presentation negatively, this patient is unlikely to share anything else with you.

Instead, be curious, objective, and accepting. If something doesn't make sense to you, realize that it at least holds psychological value for the person telling you about it. It reveals something about this person's thinking, inner values and beliefs, and what he needs or she thinks she needs. For example, a patient might ask you your opinion about going to Mexico to take an unconventional treatment for breast cancer. She really may want you to reinforce her decision not to go, despite the advice of well-meaning friends. Still, she is revealing her interest in trying a different approach, to keep fighting the condition. Your response can be reassuring. You can say you disagree with the over-the-border treatment, but use her question as an opportunity to inquire about what else the patient may have discovered about alternative therapies for her problem. You may learn something new from listening to her response while building good communication with her.

The first day you went to college, you didn't claim to know all about chemistry, math, or Spanish. It was your willingness to admit ignorance about these subjects (plus the need to get enough credits to graduate) that allowed you to pursue these studies successfully. Now you are a successful member of a respected profession because you were willing to admit your ignorance. Somewhere along the way, however, some professionals get a "God complex." Out of fear, limited thinking, or hurry, they erroneously conclude that they know it all. At this point, their education ends and a slow death by true ignorance occurs. Their patients suffer because these professionals no longer are learning new and better ways to help them get healthier. The professionals themselves become burned-out. Instead of getting satisfaction from the glorious calling of healing, they may become depressed or turn instead to drugs, alcohol, or other addictions for satisfaction in life.

Patients often report that their satisfaction with alternative practitioners stems from their willingness to listen. When you are willing to listen and hear what your patients are saying, you will learn all about them. Not only will they often give you the diagnosis by the details in their stories, but often they will give you the treatment as well. Be silent, be receptive, be willing to listen and to learn. You and your patients will both be happier.

■■■■■ COMMUNICATE AND COLLABORATE

Communicate

Besides listening to your patients with an open and receptive attitude, you must be willing both to communicate your concerns or lack of knowledge and to share with patients the information you possess about the safety, efficacy, cost, and other aspects of alternative and conventional therapies. Remain humble in the face of the mysteries of life, health, and the human experience. Avoid the arrogance into which some professionals retreat when faced with a situation that is unknown, uncomfortable, or just plain puzzling to them. The poet T.S. Eliot once wrote, "In order to arrive at what you do not know / You must go by a way which is the way of ignorance."

I am reminded of a story from Larry Dossey's wonderful book, *Reinventing Medicine* (1999), in which a woman was miraculously cured of crippling multiple sclerosis through prayer. Her neurologist was decidedly not humble in the face of this amazing event. Instead, he became angry, claimed that there was no such thing as a miracle, and denounced her as a fake and a fraud. Although the woman was now happy and restored, whatever therapeutic relationship she had had with the neurologist was immediately dissolved.

Of course having an open mind is not the same as totally accepting everything patients share with you. Patients will often bring questions about herbs, supplements, or other therapies just because they do want your opinion. If you are open and receptive, patiently hearing them through, then they are more likely to listen to your ideas and opinions in return. Just as you shouldn't say "no" to every idea or alternative therapy that patients bring, you need not say "yes" to every one either. If you have concerns about safety, efficacy, drug interactions, cost, toxicity, or lack of solid scientific evidence about a therapy, express them. This advice is what the patients came to you for. While I was in Colorado, I saw a woman of 33 years who had just moved there from Canada. She had come there to die, but it could have been prevented. Like many patients these days, Amy was interested in treating her health conditions with the simplest, safest, and least invasive or toxic approach. On discovering a small lump in her breast, she visited her doctor in Canada, who advised her to have it removed immediately. She asked him whether there were alternative approaches, including watching it with serial mammography, treating it with diet, taking supplements, meditating, and so on. He became angry and dismissive when she questioned his recommendation. Rather than engaging her beliefs, that doctor alienated his patient.

She chose not to seek further care for the lump at that time, a choice that was precipitated by her distress at the "nonhealing" encounter with her physician. Unfortunately, hers was one of the unusual cases in younger women in which an aggressive malignancy developed. By the time she had the courage to venture into the medical arena again, it had spread to her lymph nodes, lungs, and bones. It was probably incurable at this stage. She was unwilling to risk a bone marrow transplant—an invasive, highly dangerous, though sometimes helpful procedure using high-dose chemotherapy.

Had her original doctor taken the time to understand her concerns and elicited her trust to follow up on the necessary surgical biopsy, her life might have been spared. As a health care professional, you must develop sufficient rapport and trust with your patients to be able to evaluate them thoroughly and completely. If a patient refuses a test or recommendation, be willing to refer that patient to someone else, or examine why the interaction did not go as expected.

When you are open and receptive, willing to admit ignorance and to share your knowledge, trust develops within the therapeutic relationship. This trust will bring rich rewards in terms of healing and improved patient care for years ahead.

Collaborate

As you learn to communicate with your patients, you not only will be able to engage them in a collaborative, mutually respectful way, but also will learn to develop new colleagues in the healing arts—the alternative practitioners outside of mainstream medical care. Communicating and collaborating with our colleagues who provide alternative therapies is essential to a complete integrative approach. No matter how interested you are in integrative care, no matter how much you read and study, no matter how open-minded you are, you can never know all there is to know about every therapy. Establish a network of reliable, preferably licensed, alternative providers. Communicate with them in the same way you would with any other consultant, such as a cardiologist or pediatrician. Discuss patient problems and treatment issues with them (with the patients' permission, of course). Then you should be able to offer your patients in-depth, flexible, and individualized approaches to their problems.

As an acupuncturist, for example, I often treat low back pain. Many of my patients are also working with a chiropractor, Rolf therapist, or massage therapist. In difficult cases, I've found that patients get more benefit from the needle session if they are relaxed, so we devise a plan in which they get a massage or an adjustment before they visit me. Speaking with the alternative practitioner can yield a new perspective on a patient's problem, help in designing a collaborative treatment plan, and lead to the forging of a consulting relationship based on mutual trust and respect. You will learn from your alternative therapy consultants, and they from you.

Keep in mind that your patients value their relationship with you. If you refer them to another practitioner, schedule regular follow-up visits every month or so to keep in touch. As you collaborate, continue to communicate. These visits allow you to review their progress and their satisfaction with their care. The additional information is helpful if you wish to discuss the treatment plan with the alternative practitioners in your network.

This collaborative relationship can work both ways, with the alternative practitioner consulting you and sending referrals your way. When I was practicing in the mountains of Colorado, I often referred my patients to one of several excellent chiropractors in the same valley. One sent me a referral that I will always remember. It was a 48-year-old woman who had visited the chiropractor for treatment of sciatica, a common condition in which irritation of the nerves in the spine causes pain along the leg. She was not responding as expected to chiropractic adjustment, so after a few sessions I was asked to see her, possibly for acupuncture.

I began by taking a thorough history and performing a physical exam. Her symptoms did not seem particularly intense or in any way out of the ordinary, but my internal alarms went off when she told me that she had been successfully treated for breast cancer about 5 years before. I gave her a couple of acupuncture treatments, which relieved some of her pain, but I also ordered some laboratory tests and a bone scan, integrating an alternative system of healing with conventional practice. Which brings us to our next section, making a proper diagnosis.

▰▰▰ DIAGNOSE

No matter which model of care you use, making a complete and accurate conventional diagnosis is essential to ethical, competent treatment of the patient. As it turned out, this woman had a more serious problem than sciatica. The blood tests and bone scan verified the suspicion that the chiropractor and I shared: she had metastatic bone cancer, a recurrence of the breast cancer. I could have relieved her symptoms with acupuncture for some months or she could have continued chiropractic treatment. Although either approach might have reduced her pain, it would have ignored the real problem. But by collaborating and blending the alternative and conventional approaches, the chiropractor and I could properly identify the serious underlying cause of her pain. Had it remained undetected, she could have suffered a malignant fracture of her spine with possible paralysis, incontinence, or worse while under our care. Although her prognosis was poor, she was grateful that we were thorough in evaluating what had seemed to be a bothersome but uncomplicated complaint.

If a patient requests a therapy for a vague and uncertain complaint, you must do your best to establish a diagnosis in the most reasonable way possible before referring the patient to someone else or recommending any therapy, alternative or conventional. One helpful way to start the process of diagnosis is to have patients with chronic problems start a symptom diary. They should list the degree of pain or disability, perhaps using a rating scale like 1 to 10, with 10 being the worst pain and 1 being a minimal amount. They can keep track of how often an episode occurs, how much medication it took to control it, and how much it affected their lives.

Functional assessments are very important. For instance, were they in bed all day, missing school or work because of their migraine, or did it go away when they took a couple of aspirins? The diary will be important in the treatment phase because it will give you and the patient a baseline of how the condition acts before any treatment. This information is important both in making the diagnosis and in selecting therapy.

▰▰▰ EXPLAIN AND EXPLORE

Sometimes patients seek alternative therapies before they are willing to try conventional methods. They may just prefer an alternative approach. But sometimes they don't understand or know of the standard therapy. Although in fact it may be safe, proven, inexpensive, quick, and the most direct solution to their problem, they may fear it as dangerous or ineffective.

Explain and explore all treatment options thoroughly so the patient understands them well. When conventional therapies have failed or have been refused, discussion and initiation of alternative therapies is appropriate. It is also appropriate to begin discussing the integration of conventional and alternative therapies early on if there is a reasonable chance that the two may be synergistic.

For instance, patients often come to me requesting acupuncture for simple injuries such as tendinitis, which often responds quite nicely to rest, ice, and immobilization rather than a series of acupuncture visits. Although both may work, in this case the conventional treatment is cheaper and more convenient.

A medical journal recently reported a case in which the parents of a child with a brain tumor declined radiation therapy, which was highly effective for that particular tumor type (Coppes 1998). They elected to follow an unproven dietary supplement plan. By the time they realized the child was getting much worse, it was too late for the proven therapy to work.

In a similar story, I had another woman as a patient who chose unproven nutritional therapies instead of surgical treatment for her breast cancer. She owned a health food store and strongly believed that drugs, surgery, chemotherapy, radiation, and other oncology treatments were uniformly bad. What was truly bad was that when she came to see me for support in her "natural treatment" plan, the tumor had been growing for over 2 years and was the size of my fist. It was about to ulcerate through the skin and she already had hard, matted lymph nodes in the axilla. Although she was in a very advanced stage of cancer, she was still fixed in her belief that conventional medicine could not help. At that stage, she was right. Earlier, the story would have been different.

Perhaps the greatest danger of alternative medicine is the delay of proven and effective therapy in favor of that which is yet unproved. Michael Lerner, in his extraordinary book about alternative treatments for cancer, *Choices in Healing*, makes a strong point: *There is no proven cure in alternative therapies for cancer* (Lerner 1994). Alternative therapies may help to support the immune system, promote the person's psychological strength, help deal with pain, help manage a crisis in meaning, address spiritual issues, and have other important effects. But no major trials of alternative therapies have proven to statistical significance that they are curative. (In fact, if such trial results are published, that "alternative" therapy will then become conventional and mainstream.)

Dr. Andrew Weil's successful program in Integrative Medicine at the University of Arizona ran into the problem of delay with cancer patients. Once they were diagnosed, they reasonably sought advice at his clinic for integrative care, but because of the clinic's popularity, there was a long waiting list. By the time a patient waited 6 months or so for an appointment, the cancer already may have spread. Quickly recognizing the problem, Dr. Weil and his colleagues reached an agreement with the oncology department to fast-track these patients rather than delay their treatment.

Until alternative therapies are proven curative, the best solution for serious problems such as cancer and heart disease—as well as for less life-threatening problems—is to integrate the best of known conventional treatments with supportive alternative therapies. To follow this strategy, the patient and the health care professional need to share and explore their knowledge, preferences, and experience, and consider the availability of competent professionals to whom the patient can be referred.

Concerns about safety, efficacy, toxicity, and delay in therapy are high in the minds of health care professionals when dealing with alternative therapies. If we have some knowledge of these areas, we can give our patients the quality counsel that they deserve. Exploring and explaining patient and provider preference will help guide choices for therapy.

■■■ CONCLUSION

The importance of communication cannot be stressed too strongly. Patients' health can be seriously damaged if they cannot communicate well with a trusted, informed health care provider. Helping patients to make wise choices requires sensitivity to their particular needs and beliefs. It also requires that we as practitioners develop skills, knowledge, and attitudes about these therapies that will enable us to counsel, treat, and refer our patients with wisdom, accuracy, and compassion.

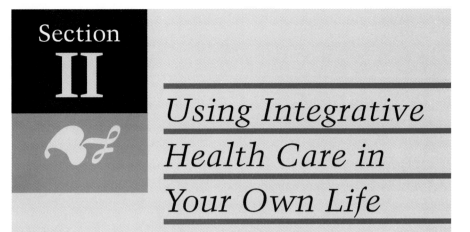

Using Integrative Health Care in Your Own Life

Be really whole, and all things will come to you.
—Lao Tsu

A humble knowledge of oneself is a surer road to God than a deep searching of the sciences.
—Thomas à Kempis

Whole-person care involves much more than merely caring for people who are sick. In Chapter 3, I introduce the vital concepts of *wellness, self-care, role modeling*, and *balance*. Learning to be an outstanding health care professional requires awareness and commitment to one's own health in many areas: physical, mental, spiritual, social and relational, and environmental. We professionals must keep ourselves healthy if we are to encourage healthy lifestyles in our patients.

Because I believe we are spiritual beings having a human experience, I devote Chapter 4 to *spirituality*, describing data, clinical tools, real patient stories, and some key metaphysics related to spiritual belief and practice in the health care setting. To my mind, one's spiritual path, wisdom, awareness of deep feelings, and compassion all come from a consciousness as well as a willingness to grow in the area of spirit. This chapter is about finding one's own path to discovering truth, rather than a particular religion or belief system. It describes how being on that path allows one to go beyond being a mere health care technician to becoming a healer of the whole person.

Chapter 3

Being Well, Being a Role Model

The best doctors are Doctor Diet, Doctor Quiet, and Doctor Merryman.

—Jonathan Swift

He who would be well taken care of must take care of himself.

—William Graham Sumner

As a first-year medical student, one of my greatest joys was exercise. I had lifted weights, played tennis, jogged, and cycled since childhood. My newfound knowledge of anatomy and physiology moved these familiar exercises to a new level. As I ran, I felt the major muscles of my legs, hips, and buttocks coordinated with the marvelous processes of respiration and cardiac contractility. I understood my exercise movements and processes in a new way. This was a peak experience combining the scientific with the deeply personal and the almost mystical. Leonardo da Vinci's diagrams of human anatomy became animated in me as I took new joy in the normal, healthy functioning of my body.

As I progressed in my medical training, I learned how the body reacted to disease: with dysfunction, adaptation, and deterioration. Though I never forgot those halcyon days when my body, my breathing, my motion all integrated with a new level of awareness, disease and disability came more and more to the forefront of my consciousness as an evolving health care professional.

By the time I was an intern, I realized that much of my work would be centered on the chronic diseases, organ failure, and irreversible terminal illnesses of my patients. I was often fatigued from spending 36 hours in a row caring for patients whose return visits were either an inevitable part of their chronic disease or the result of their own renewed attacks on their physiological reserves. Smoking, alcohol excess, overeating, lack of exercise, and substance abuse were again and again implicated in my nightly rounds in the emergency room. The chronic lung patient, the patient with cirrhosis, the out-of-control diabetic patient, the inactive and overweight heart patient, the strung-out speed freak: all these persons were the daily and nightly work of a tired and increasingly disillusioned intern.

The grand drama I had anticipated that medicine would become, the joyful celebration of the body's healthy functioning, had become lost in the very real exigencies of caring for patients whose health problems were often a result of their lifestyles—choices that had caused their illnesses. It became easy and adaptive to joke and become callous about the pain and suffering we interns faced daily. Yet I could not become hard-hearted to the plight of our patients.

I felt there was more to medicine, more to health, than merely caring for those whose prognosis was poor, whose motivation to be healthy was based only on their current suffering, and whose choices had inevitably led to their state of disease. My thoughts started to move from those sickly bodies and crushed spirits who haunted our emergency room and hospital beds to the world outside the hospital. I thought of the healthy children I saw in my office practice and in the local park every day. I thought of healthy young women who conceived in joy and delivered wonderful new infants in the fullness of their lives. I thought of my 97-year-old patient with faculties still well intact who lived as an inspiration to us all. I thought about myself and the lack of exercise, lack of sleep, and poor diet pressed upon me by the long hours of internship.

▰▰▰ WHAT IS WELLNESS?

As I reflected on these things, a new idea of health care emerged in my mind. The questions occurred to me for the first time: "What is wellness? What is health?" Clearly the answers lay outside of the disease model in which I had been so carefully and thoroughly trained. Dr. Don Ardell provided illumination to this question by describing wellness, health, and disease as a continuum (Table 3–1). As a second-year family practice resident, I also began a research project to determine an answer to these questions about wellness and health. We surveyed those attending a local health fair and patients in our family practice clinic, asking about attitudes and beliefs regarding the components of well-being. We found that the ordinary folk of our community and our patients knew the answers. They recognized that wellness and health are vibrant states of life that are *not merely the absence of disease* resulting from lifestyle choices and practices. Healthy eating and exercise patterns, positive mental attitudes, and active and deep spiritual practice all are the birthing ground of the healthy individual, family, and community. Our community survey showed that even in the early 1980s people were well aware that promoting wellness meant avoiding known detrimental behaviors: excess alcohol, tobacco, a high-fat diet, and inactivity.

Table 3–1   THE CONTINUUM OF LIFESTYLE CHOICES

HIGH-LEVEL WELLNESS

Whole-Person Excellence or Superhealth

Orientation to positive payoffs
Personal responsibility to health
Development of supportive environment
Integrated and balanced lifestyle
High self-esteem
Conscious commitment to excellence
Implementation of a personal wellness plan

INTERMEDIATE-LEVEL OMNIBUS TINKERING WITH HEALTH

Sporadic Efforts toward Better Health

Nonsystematic health initiatives
Cyclical efforts to change
Rhythm method of girth control
Short-term resolutions
Illness-avoidance motivations

MIDDLE-LEVEL MEDIOCRITY

Equating Not Being Sick with Health

Listlessness
Low energy levels
Lack of commitment
Poor self-image
Unawareness of negative norms

LOW-LEVEL WORSENESS

Health-Robbing Choices or Minimal Functioning

Lack of exercise
Alcohol abuse
Use of nicotine
Reliance on caffeine
Obesity
Casual acceptance of tranquilizers/other medications
Unrealistic expectations regarding medical system
Low self-esteem

Source: Ardell DB. 1999. *14 Days to Wellness: The Easy, Effective, and Fun Way to Optimum Health.* Novato, CA: New World Library, p 8 (used with permission).

What we found confirmed the beliefs we had about healthy behaviors and their contribution to a long and healthy life, but our findings also mystified us. Why did people who *knew* that certain behaviors caused illness and disease continue in these very same self-destructive patterns? Why, despite their knowledge of healthy activities, diet, and exercise, did they avoid them even though they recognized the potential negative outcomes?

Understanding motivation became a key issue for me. "How do we motivate healthier behaviors in those we serve?" I asked. Information alone does not motivate people. Something else is required.

Answers seemed to come from areas outside medicine. Education, the business world, human relations, psychology, and other areas peripheral to clinical medicine provided clues to the motivation of the patient. As Bernie Siegel says, "People need *inspiration* so that they can undergo a *transformation* which allows them to use the *information* they have to choose healthy behaviors." How then would I as a health professional motivate my patients to change their lifestyles and become healthier people?

▬▬ THE PERSONAL SELF-CARE PLAN

While doing this research, I encountered the work of Don Ardell and others who were engaged in defining the term *wellness* and developing tools and methods to motivate people to achieve "high-level wellness and improved self-care" (Ardell 1977, 1982, 1999; Ardell & Tager 1982; Ferguson 1980). Again, wellness was defined not as the absence of the signs and symptoms of disease but as the balanced and happy state of living in which a person lives fully extended. Social, spiritual, physical, emotional, relational, and environmental factors all are in a state of healthy balance and allow people to potentially become "all that they can be."

As I worked with this information, I attained a personal inspiration to transformation from a clear concept: *I could only motivate others to change if I myself was engaged in my personal best health-related behaviors.* This delighted and disturbed me. Though less than perfect, I felt I had always maintained a reasonably healthy lifestyle. My youth, genetics, spiritual practices, exercise and diet patterns, and the wise advice and modeling of my parents had all conspired to keep me robust and healthy. However, I realized that many of my patients had not had these advantages. I also came to see that certain tools I had learned, such as stress management, aerobic exercise, use of a low-fat diet, smoking abstinence, and meditation and prayer, could be useful to my patients. Encouraging them to participate in these healthy behaviors required me to continue to grow and learn about these practices myself. If I had too much to eat or drink the night before, it was difficult to look a patient in the eye and say, "You know, you really need to reduce your calories and cut the amount of beer you consume." The journey to improving my care of patients had to begin with improving my care of myself. Studying imagery, relaxation, and stress management allowed me to teach these techniques to my patients in a credible way. If I exercised daily with tai chi, walked regularly, and worshiped in an uplifting setting, I could readily share these human activities and their value to health with my patients.

▰▰▰ DEVELOPING A SELF-CARE PLAN

Thus, I realized that to be the best health care professional I could be, I must, to some degree, model healthy behavior to my patients. My early work with home birthing, for example, encouraged my spouse and me to eat well and exercise regularly to ensure healthy children. This strengthened my ability to encourage my pregnant patients to avoid drugs, eat well, take their vitamins, and breast-feed their infants.

For many of my patients, stress was a large part of their lives and a major contributor to their illnesses. Simple programs like Benson's "relaxation response" were helpful to me when I was tired, burned out, or stressed out (Benson 1975, 1984; Benson & Stuart 1992). Once I had learned the simple techniques of deep breathing, quieting the mind and body, and relaxing deeply, it became easier and easier to work them into my practice.

Periodic fasting or abstaining from meat heightened my awareness of the hidden sources of fat and unnecessary calories in my lifestyle. Now I could talk to my patients more credibly about the benefits of a low-fat or even a semi-vegetarian diet in relation to my own experience.

Efforts at regular exercise at home or at the gym, racquetball or tennis court, tai chi studio, aerobics class, and swimming pool all paid off for me personally and also for my patients. I could empathize with the difficulties many experienced with long work days, poor child-care coverage, lack of motivation, and the problem of just "one more thing to do" in an already busy schedule. Yet, as I valued these activities in my life and did them, I became a more effective exponent of change for my patients. No longer did I merely say, "You should do such and such. . . ." I was able to say, "What I do for my personal health is this. These are the hurdles I met and this is how I overcame them. I acknowledge your challenges to doing healthier behaviors and can suggest how to handle them because I have done so."

Being a role model for good health became an awareness of balance in life. Though this can be very different for individuals at different times in their lives, there are some general and lasting principles. Those suggested by the elders of the Seneca Nation are reflected in "A Question of Balance."

A QUESTION OF BALANCE

The elders of the Seneca Nation traditionally encouraged their people to reflect on four essential questions to determine if they were living in balance with their world. As you read each of these four questions, pause to reflect and honestly answer each one:

1. Are you happy living how you are living and doing what you are doing?
2. Is what you are doing adding to the confusion?
3. What are you doing to further peace and contentment in your own life and in the world?
4. How will you be remembered after you are gone—either in absence or in death?

If on reflection you find that you could be doing more to bring greater peace and contentment into your life, listen deeply for what a step in that direction might be for you. Is greater balance for you to be found in taking more time alone, or in spending more quality time with your loved ones and friends, or helping others in your community? Is balance for you at this time in your life to be found in taking on more activity, or creating more quiet time? Listen deeply, pray, reflect, do whatever it takes for you to know what your next step is!

Compare how you would like to be remembered with the realities of the legacy that you have created thus far. Ask yourself, "If I were to die next week, what would I be most proud of? What wounds would I most like to heal or forgive? What words do I need to speak, and what actions most need to be taken for me to leave this world, or this job, or to complete my watch at this station of my life with integrity, dignity, and balance, as a true pilgrim on the path of wholeness?"

These compelling and poignant reminders call our attention to how much there is to learn from people who for centuries lived in harmony with one another and with the whole of Nature in all of its beauty. On the journey, according to the elders of the Seneca tribe:

- Self-knowledge is the need.
- Self-understanding is the desire.
- Self-discipline is the way.
- Self-realization is the goal.

Take some time to ponder these ideas . . . to take them to heart . . . and see how these simple but profound principles can help you to live in greater balance.

Source: Levey J, and Levey M. 1998. *Living in Balance: A Dynamic Approach for Creating Harmony and Wholeness in a Chaotic World.* Berkeley, CA: Conari Press. Cited in IONS, *Noetic Sciences Review* April–July 1999:53.

▬▬▬ HOW TO GET STARTED

A balanced plan for personal well-being and change must include several key factors:

1. *Physical health*, including a healthy diet and personally suitable exercise program
2. *Mental health*, including stress management and healthy emotional processes
3. *Spiritual health* and well-being, including an awareness of the sacred in everyday life, a proper relationship with your true values, and a commitment to a deeper understanding of your spiritual nature
4. *Social and relational health*, including an awareness of the value of a supportive community of friends and family and deeper relationships with a spouse, children, and significant others
5. *Environmental health*, including the choice to live and work in a place that supports your healthy choices and that is free of pollutants and unsafe or violent situations, and that encourages personal creativity and self-expression

By setting goals in each of these areas, you can start to develop a personalized plan for improving your well-being. Your goals should be both achievable and measurable. Several excellent books and workbooks are available to help you structure your personal wellness plan. These offer helpful suggestions based on the best scientific data about what constitutes a healthy lifestyle. Dr. Andrew Weil has written a book, *Eight Weeks to Optimal Health* (1997), which follows in the genre of such earlier books such as Don Ardell's *14 Days to a Wellness Lifestyle* (1982, 1999). I prescribe these books to my patients *after* using them myself and applying their principles to my own lifestyle.

Our medical school offers an elective course, "Integrative and Alternative Medicine" for medical students and residents. We always require the students to develop a personal wellness plan. Examples of these plans are reprinted in the chapter appendix, beginning on page 41. These plans show that a self-care plan can be as individualized as you are yourself. It can be a life-transforming process or a minor tune-up. It can help you reconnect with your values and identify areas that are out of balance or aspects that you would like to improve, restart, get rid of, or in other ways change.

Whether encouraging my students to change their lifestyle choices or attempting to do so myself, one principle immediately emerges:

change is a gradual process and is best done incrementally. Both Weil and Ardell recognize this important fact and encourage change in small and digestible steps. Yet how often have we told a patient, "Eat less fat, quit smoking, start exercising, and learn to relax"? Only when we have attempted even one lifestyle change of our own can we appreciate how overwhelming such a prescription is to a patient. As Mark Twain once said, "Habit is habit, not to be thrown out the window by any man but rather coaxed down the stairs, one step at a time."

This wise humorist has hit on a key factor in human behavior and motivation: change in behavior occurs slowly and gradually. I contend that if we are to expect our patients to change, we must inspire them to do so by role modeling. We can teach only what we know ourselves. As we practice better self-care habits, we can not only be convincing to those we seek to motivate to change, but we can also be realistically aware of the barriers to change.

■■■■■ MOTIVATING YOURSELF

Physical Health

Move!

As Lao Tsu, the ancient Chinese philosopher, said, "A journey of a thousand miles begins with one step." *Today* is the day to start your new commitment to a healthier you, to become a role model for your patients, your family, your peers. If you haven't exercised today, *lay down this book* and take a 10-minute walk. The book will be here when you come back.

There, wasn't that easy? Wasn't it a bit liberating? OK, admit it, you walked to the refrigerator and back, didn't you? Well, it's a start!

Eat!

Speaking of the refrigerator, nutrition is the key to good health. Although we cover this topic in depth in Chapter 11, let me encourage you now to look at your own dietary pattern as it is today. First, look at the fats in your daily diet. Don't be compulsive about it but simply start gradually to substitute fruits, vegetables, and grains. Good nutrition is as essential to our own health as it is to the health of our patients. Pay attention to what goes in your mouth. Is it wholesome, nourishing food or some high-fat, sugary, and yucky form of fast food?

Another easy way to modify your diet is by using supplements. A good multiple vitamin with an antioxidant formula, which includes at least vitamins C and E and beta carotene, has been correlated in many studies with improved health outcomes. The use of vitamins is an easy and inexpensive way to start learning about the wide world of nutritional medicine. Spend some time in the health food store and if you are not sure what to buy, at least spend some time educating yourself about what is there. By the time you have finished this book, you'll be much better informed.

And be sure to drink lots of water or fresh fruit and vegetable juice daily. Most experts recommend at least six to eight glasses of water, preferably unchlorinated, as an important element in a healthy diet. This water helps flush toxins, nourish cells, facilitate transport of nutrients and fuel for important biochemical processes, and keep major organ systems adequately hydrated.

Mental Health

Relax!

And how about a short course on stress management? The very next time you feel stressed out, anxious, or burned out, try the following relaxation exercise, described as the "relaxation response" by Harvard cardiologist and stress researcher Dr. Herbert Benson (1975, 1984):

> Sit comfortably and quietly where you won't be disturbed for at least 10 minutes.
>
> Breathe deeply, slowly, into your lower abdomen, noticing the flow of the breath in and out.
>
> Relax your muscles.
>
> Focus on a word such as "one" or "ocean" as you breathe.
>
> Take a passive attitude toward your thoughts, including any that intrude or distract.
>
> Let go of thoughts that arise by returning to your focus word and paying attention to your breathing.

This technique, practiced regularly, has profound physiological effects. It reduces stress hormones like epinephrine and corticosteroids, helps settle the mind, removes tension from the body, and refreshes the spirit. We will discuss the relaxation response further in Chapter 15, but for now, just add this simple practice to your daily routine. You will find that you handle stress better, feel clearer mentally, and are more mindful of your surroundings.

As with other aspects of self-care, learning this simple technique allows you to be effective in teaching it to patients. Many of our patients and colleagues are afflicted with stress-related conditions. The practice of the relaxation response is a simple, low-cost remedy.

Biofeedback 101

A fun and really cool little biofeedback trick I learned from Dr. Benson was the use of the Biodot (Biodot International, Indianapolis).* This is a little colored dot about the diameter of a pencil eraser. It changes color according to skin temperature. It you are "uptight," the effects of the vasoconstricting stress hormones like epinephrine and norepinephrine will cause your skin temperature to be cooler; when you are relaxed, the blood vessels in the extremities tend to be dilated. If you stick a Biodot onto the back of your hand, its color change will give moment-to-moment feedback about your level of relaxation. Order some Biodots. They are only about a dime apiece and well worth it for the education and fun!

Spiritual Health

Spirituality is the awareness within each of us of the Absolute, of something within and without that is transcendent, eternal, and sacred. Like sexuality, spirituality is something powerful and deep within each of us. It drives our behavior at the deepest levels of motivation, values, and choices. It is not limited to a specific belief system, religion, denomination, or sect. Without an awareness of our own spirituality, we cannot connect in a meaningful way with this essential human aspect of our patients. The best thinking about integrative medicine emphasizes that our success as healers depends as much on our own inner healing, our own lifelong spiritual growth, as on the technical competencies we achieve in our profession. Larry Dossey, in his landmark book, *Healing Words* (1993), has documented the wide array of clinical and laboratory studies that validate the power of belief, prayer, and positive intentionality on the healing process. He goes as far as to state that with the strong evidence of the health benefits of prayer, it ought to be considered malpractice for a health professional *not* to pray for his or her patients.

Despite abundant epidemiological evidence and hundreds of studies showing that people's religious beliefs and practices have a beneficial effect on longevity and morbidity, this area is just beginning to be taught in professional health care programs. Historically, nursing schools have been more tuned to this spiritual dimension than medical or allied health programs. At the University of Texas Medical Branch, the medical and nursing schools initiated a joint program entitled "Spirituality and Clinical Care." This innovative program has been well received by faculty and students alike as they have discussed both their

---

* Biodot International, P.O. Box 2245, Indianapolis, IN 46206. Telephone 1-800-272-2340.

own beliefs and clinically relevant case studies addressing spirituality issues.

The healer's art, indeed the profession of healing, has always been a profoundly spiritual path. Consider the ancient Greek Aesculapian temples, the Lakotah Sioux medicine man, the rabbinical priesthood's dietary and health proscriptions, the ministrations and mysticism of Florence Nightingale, and the healing ministry of Jesus. The path to healing has been intimately and inextricably bound to the spiritual within us. The next chapter discusses this aspect more fully.

Meditate or Pray

Be willing to reflect, meditate, pray, and seek guidance within the great spiritual traditions or within your own personal belief system. Reconnect with your deepest values. Recognize and acknowledge the value of clarifying questions about values, pain, suffering, meaning, hope, hopelessness, and beliefs in your life and the lives of your patients. This will put you on the spiritual path to finding the answers you will need.

Social and Relational Health

Look at your relationships. By and large, are they healthy, supportive, and empowering? Or are they toxic, conflictual, and unhappy? A wide body of literature encourages us to optimize our relationships, to forgive, and to deal with anger creatively not only to be happier but also to improve our health. Just realize that a poor relationship detracts from one's health in the long term. As with spiritual involvement, study after study has shown the beneficial effect on health of positive relationships and social support. Decreased length of hospital stay, improved postoperative outcomes, and reduction in morbidity have all been demonstrated in those with robust social networks and support, especially compared to those not reporting such involvement (Berkman 1979).

Realizing the two-sidedness of every relationship and that we ourselves must often change to improve our relationships calls out deep and often difficult emotional challenges. This work can be done within the relationship by maintaining truth and honesty in communications, forgiveness, and compassion for each other. At times, professional guidance is needed.

In addition to personal relationships, having the support and involvement of a community of persons is known to be conducive to good health. Do you have a supportive community, be it a church, a club, an activist organization, family, or another support group? It is clear, as in the studies cited previously, that without this kind of support, health suffers. Volunteer, join, network, get involved—just for the health of it.

Environmental Health

Now, let me offer a few words about environment. Some years back I found a wonderful book called *The Art of Life* by Edith Schaeffer (1987). This fascinating woman had found the way to make her home, her environment, her daily mundane experiences a form of art. With a wildflower in a bud vase on a tray rather than a hastily poured cup slid across the kitchen counter, a cup of tea became an artistic event. The presence of soothing music, carefully selected artwork, and other beautiful though sometimes humble objects made her family's living space a gracious and re-energizing place to live and visit.

With our workplaces and cities filled with noise, hurry, pollutants, stress, and other negative energies, it is pressingly important to make our home environment as healing a space as possible. We need a place that provides love, beauty, harmony, and peace to recover and to re-create for the day ahead.

Healing starts at home but spreads from there. Be willing to be involved in advocating social justice and righting the ills caused by poverty, ignorance, and illiteracy. These actions will help heal you and your world. Working with our communities to reduce violence, racism, pollution, and other forms of ugliness is a powerful healing event. Michael Lerner's work with the greening of our medical spaces by reducing toxic effluents such as dioxin and mercury in our hospitals is an example of how we broaden our influence from personal wellness to community wellness.

■■■■■ CONCLUSION

To integrate the best of conventional and nonconventional care, a clear balance is required in our own lives. Healthy diet and exercise patterns, stress management, spiritual vitality, empowering social and personal relationships, and a clean and positive environment are all well documented in the literature as key elements in wellness, health, and longevity. They are as important to us as practitioners of this new model of integrative care as they are to our patients.

Walk the path you prescribe to others.

Appendix

Self-Care Plans

Student and Resident Examples*

FL (Chinese family medicine resident)

1. Exercise: continue exercise including walking, jogging, swimming, etc.
2. Stress management and relaxation: I will learn this method to deal with relatively high level of stress during residency to maintain my health.
3. I will learn Qi Gong or Taiji if possible to balance the five elements in my body (gold, wood, water, fire, and earth).
4. I believe I have a relatively high level of Yang (fire) in my body. I am using some Chinese herbs to cool it down. I feel good with it and I will continue this therapy.

SS (fourth-year pregnant medical student)

1. Prayer and scripture reading: 15 min each morning.
2. Relaxation with breathing: 5 min each morning.
3. Stretching: 10 min each morning.
4. Start walking 3 d/wk: 20 min.
5. Aerobics once per week: after baby born.
6. Strength training with husband (weights) 2–3×/wk—after baby born.
7. Eat 3 servings/d of vegetables.
8. Limit fat intake to 25 g/d.
9. When hurried at traffic/red lights, take deep breath and relax with "mini" (moment of relaxation—see Chapter 15).
10. Practice walking with head up, shoulders back, and smile at others passing.

DW (surgical intern)

I do not know exactly when it started, but as I child I do remember loving to eat. As I became a young woman and not allowed to do many

---

*Actual end-of-elective assignments done by students of the Alternative and Integrative Medicine elective at the University of Texas Medical Branch, from 1998 to 1999.

"adventurous" activities, I often found solace in food. I don't know why I did not have a weight problem then, but as I grow older this seems to be the only area in my life in which I don't have control. I have started several exercise programs in the past and actually enjoyed them, but as my schedule grew more hectic, I would gently push it to the side as my food intake remained the same or slightly increased. In the last weeks, I have really tried to envision the purpose of food in my life and have decided that I really don't need that much to be a healthy young woman. More important, I needed to correct the time and the things I ate. I decided that a salad or soup should constitute one of my daily meals and that I should have bigger helpings of vegetables on my evening meals. I know this might sound easy to do but it is a big step for me just to put this into words. I have also decided to restart my exercise routine and also increase the variety to avoid boredom or quitting. This is my third week and I have scheduled myself to work out 3–5×/wk.

Although physical appearances are very important in our society, personal health also involves the spirit. I know many people practice meditation or yoga as a form of relaxation and somehow "feed" their spirit. I find that working on my relationship with God and his Son Jesus Christ is the best form to feed my spirit, and that is what I will continue to do. As a wife, mother, and future doctor I also need to relieve stress and spend time alone. Massages help me relax and are a great way to spend time attending to my needs.

KA (medical student and bride-to-be)

Diet

Over the past 6 months, I have lost 24 pounds on the Weight Watchers plan. In spite of this I still do not believe that my diet is as healthy as it should be. For one thing, I rarely get the five servings of fruit and vegetables suggested. This is the one area I would most like to improve on. I am very good at buying produce, but it usually rots in my refrigerator (also a waste of money!). I could improve this by learning more ways to incorporate fruit and vegetables into meals. Also, I do not cook much, and eat a lot of prepackaged meals that are high in sodium and preservatives. I would like to learn to make a few basic healthy dishes that can be frozen and eaten during the week. I realize that this will be a challenge during internship, but it is essential for me to maintain my weight loss. Additional changes that I need to work on include decreasing my caffeine intake and increasing my water intake. I feel like I am fairly good at avoiding too many fats and sweets.

Stress Management

This is another area that could use some serious improvement. My main problem is that I am a procrastinator, which adds unnecessary stress to my life. I also tend to react very strongly when things do not go the way I planned, which has been a real problem during the planning of my wedding. I want to learn stress management techniques such as meditation and deep breathing that can help me through these "acute" stress episodes. Once I get past them, I am usually okay when I realize that some things are just beyond my control. I know what I need to do to improve my time-management problems, and I have a feeling these skills will make or break my intern year.

Spirituality

This is an area of my adult life that I have really neglected. I was raised in the Unitarian church, where beliefs are very individualized and nonspecific. As a result, I felt very lost as a child and didn't know what to believe. As a teenager, I joined a Lutheran church, which was very much the opposite—very strict and inflexible in its belief system. Now I feel a desire to rejoin a spiritual community, though I am not sure which one. Hopefully I will be able to find a church where I am comfortable. If not, I pledge at least to concentrate more on the spiritual aspects of my life, with meditation and prayer. This will be especially important when dealing with the losses I will inevitably encounter as an intern.

Exercise

I do get a fair amount of exercise as a result of my weight-loss efforts. I run approximately 15 miles per week, with some strength training. To improve in this area, I would like to add more variety to my exercise program. I usually run on the treadmill in the gym, and I would like to make an effort to exercise more outside (especially in the summer months). Additionally, I would like to add a stretching program to my workout—at this point I can't even touch my toes! Yoga would be a good way to achieve this goal.

Supplements

During this month I have started taking a multivitamin for women and an additional B-complex vitamin every day. I am also going to start taking vitamin C, because it seems to help most ailments!

AL (fourth-year medical student and mother of two)

1. Try to laugh more often with J & S.
2. Think positive, not negative, thoughts.
3. Pray every night, thanking God for five things that day.

4. Concentrate on maintaining good posture.

5. Concentrate on breathing more deeply.

6. Give and receive a massage each week.

7. Start using a treadmill or bicycle once we move.

8. Use the stairs instead of elevators whenever possible (e.g., when not pushing a stroller).

9. Park farther away from the entrance so I have to walk farther.

10. Start taking a multivitamin and additional antioxidant every day.

11. Drink at least 2 L/d of water.

12. Eat fish at least 1×/wk.

13. Change diet to follow the suggestions of *Encyclopedia of Natural Health:* vegetables—6 servings/d; fruit—3 servings/d; bread, cereal, or starchy vegetables—15 servings/d; legumes—2 servings/d; fats—7 servings/d; meat, fish, cheese, eggs—3 servings/d.

BB (third-year family medicine resident, avid hunter)

1. Drink green tea instead of coffee in mornings or green iced tea instead of black tea.

2. Take multivitamin including antioxidants and minerals.

3. Continue with 1 h/d of exercise.

4. Take echinacea and zinc if I get a cold.

MW (fourth-year medical student)

It is somewhat ironic that medical school students are some of the most unhealthy people I know. This includes myself. During my first 3 years, I neglected my mind, body, and spirit. I felt hypocritical telling patients to exercise and eat right. My exercise regimen consisted of walking to school. Vegetables were a rare item in my diet. I should have had an IV of Coke. I would never have recommended my lifestyle to anybody else. It is only during fourth year (when I have a little more time to reflect), that I have tried to concentrate on making myself a healthier person.

My Spirit

I consider neglect of the spirit to be the most dangerous. I tried to go to church whenever I could. My presence at church was worthless because of lack of sleep. Instead of praying, I would be dozing in the pews. Most days, I neither started nor ended the day with God. My plan:

1. Start and end each day with a prayer.

2. Set aside time to read the Bible instead of just articles and textbooks.
3. Go to sleep early the night before church.
4. Put more energy into faith rather than worry.
5. Deal with issues as they happen.
6. Family and friends are for support, not abuse.

My Mind

Most people would be surprised that I feel that my mind has been neglected. True, medical school has challenged my brain; that challenge was met by the left side. In college, I used to devour novels. Now, all reading is devoted to medicine. I have not touched my violin since college. Currently, my only connection with music is the car radio. On a more practical level, I no longer keep up with current events. Wars could be raging and I would have no idea.

1. Read a news magazine or watch the daily news.
2. Choose a novel to do some leisure reading.
3. Get violin fixed and play some on the weekends.
4. Go to museums, plays, something besides movies.

My Body

I have truly come to appreciate the importance of exercise in maintaining a happy lifestyle. My energy is markedly decreased when I do not exercise. In addition, I believe that one is more susceptible to depression. When the body feels bad, the rest of you feels bad. I constantly feel tension in my shoulders and neck.

1. Exercise at least 30 min/d.
2. Devote time to stretching various parts of the body.
3. Do more outside exercise instead of just the gym.
4. Try to get a massage (at least every 3 mo).

VT (fourth-year medical student)

1. Learn to take responsibility for myself and my health.
2. Make appointment with physician for health maintenance checkups.
3. Exercise consistently, not in spurts.
4. Drink less alcohol.
5. Learn better stress management.
6. Eat more frequently (e.g., not skip meals) and in lesser quantities; add more fresh fruits and vegetables to my diet. Avoid indulging "sweet tooth." Drink plenty of water.

7. Regulate sleep.

8. Take the time to not neglect self and make excuses for it.

9. Try to maintain more harmony in my life by living more in moderation and acknowledging my limits.

10. Not exhaust my resources by trying to juggle too many things at the same time (e.g., studies, relationships, and other people's problems).

11. Let go of the need to control certain situations. Be patient in traffic or difficult encounters.

12. Perform "mini" relaxation exercise (learned at Mind-Body Institute).

13. Integrate yoga and/or meditation into daily life. BREATHE!

14. Remain focused on my goals and stay centered emotionally.

15. Take time to "smell the roses" and enjoy the simple things in life.

16. More walks on the beach. Soak in nature.

17. Give myself credit for accomplishments rather than feel I always have to reach for more.

18. Get together with various friends more often for casual, relaxed conversation over tea.

19. Release those imaginary pressures.

20. Read a book that has nothing to do with medicine from time to time.

21. Play the piano again.

22. Forgive self and others.

23. Laugh.

CM (fourth-year medical student and husband)

Physical

1. Exercise—run at least 3×/wk, stretch well 5×/wk.

2. Diet—cut out red meat, substitute with more fish, increase fiber intake, cut out fried foods as much as possible, eat at least two raw fruits or vegetables every day, supplement daily diet with vitamins C and E, substitute green tea for teas I drink now.

3. Get monthly massage.

4. Continue to learn about herbs and supplements in order to implement them in my daily health.

Emotional

1. Continue to practice relaxation and stress reduction techniques learned at the Mind-Body Institute.
2. Make an effort to spend some time outside every day—it helps me relax.
3. Spend more time having fun with my wife.
4. Practice mini-relaxation techniques throughout the day.
5. Always be careful performing procedures on patients (to avoid stress of dealing with a needle stick, etc.).
6. Spend some time every week playing guitar (a relaxing activity for even a few minutes).

Spiritual

1. Visit Tibet.
2. Read more Tolstoy.
3. Listen to more John Coltrane.

AH (third-year family medicine resident)

1. Get dental surgery scheduled and not be afraid to use sick days regardless of schedule/administration.
2. Go to dentist and eye doctor (will do while on vacation).
3. Take brisk walks 3×/wk.
4. Read and attempt *8 Weeks to Optimal Health* program.
5. Decrease caffeine, processed food, fatty (junk food) intake.
6. Call in sick several days so I can sleep—I am exhausted.
7. Save money to afford acupuncture/hypnotherapy to stop dipping Skoal.
8. Attend 12-step meetings.
9. Pray on a daily basis.
10. Attempt to be aware of stress-induced eating pattern (feeding emotions; overeating to experience well-being).
11. Attempt on a daily basis that every time I have a negative or self-effacing thought, to consciously counteract with two positive thoughts.
12. Shave head (obviously leads to enlightenment), put on beads, earring, and skirt, and sit in front of a restaurant. Let people rub my tummy for good luck and collect tips.—The Happy Buddha!

Chapter 4

Mind, Body, and Now . . . Spirit

Great men are they who see the spiritual is stronger than material force, that thoughts rule the world.
—Ralph Waldo Emerson

God enters by a private door into every individual.
—Ralph Waldo Emerson

▰▰▰ A CASE OF FAITH

Recently, a patient with a suspected recurrence of lung cancer and I were having a talk. As an informed consumer, he was trying to decide between the opinions of two sets of radiologists and surgeons at two highly respected cancer centers. One group felt he should have a biopsy of a suspicious lesion in his left lung. The other group said no, the left lung looked fine and he should have a biopsy of the right lung, which had been pronounced benign by the other team of doctors. What should he do?

I said, "John, what do you want to do, since we have such conflicting opinions?"

His answer surprised me. "Doc, you know I have been praying about this and believe the right thing to do is just to wait and do nothing for now."

Ever since his recovery from alcoholism 17 years ago, John has been an active member of Alcoholics Anonymous and takes prayer and faith seriously in his day-to-day life and decisions. After all, he knows that the Higher Power, which he learned about in AA, already saved his life once from the deadly effects of alcoholism.

"I've had a full life," John went on, "and I really don't want more surgery. If it is my time to go, I am totally at peace about it. In fact, I go to Mass now every morning, attend AA meetings at least twice a week, and really feel that this cancer has furthered my spiritual growth."

That was 3 years ago. I continue to see John regularly, and the CT scans of his chest have shown both suspicious areas to be unchanged. He feels well, has lectured to our medical and nursing school classes on spirituality and health, and even comes in regularly for acupuncture to improve his macular degeneration, an eye disease leading to vision loss.

Just what is the story with John? Miracle? Coincidence? Denial? Depression? Psychosis? Religious delusion? Spontaneous cure?

He is of a sound mind. At age 78, he continues to do highly technical consulting engineering work. He has no signs of depression. Nor do his beliefs that God can help him work through his problems have any of the delusional content associated with psychotic, disordered thinking. In other words, John has faith, an operant faith that helps sustain him in the face of a life-threatening illness.

■■■■ EVIDENCE FOR THE BENEFIT OF SPIRITUALITY IN HEALTH

John is by no means an exception when it comes to the importance of the spiritual dimension in health. Several hundred studies have documented improved outcomes, longevity, quality of life, and other medical parameters that are influenced by patients' religious beliefs, practices, and the social support they obtain in their communities of faith (Matthews 1998). Conditions such as cancer, heart disease, hypertension, depression, and substance abuse have all been subjected to clinical scientific analysis to scrutinize the benefits of spirituality.

In addition to clinical studies, basic science research is also revealing. Effects of prayer, nonlocal consciousness, and positive intentionality have all been documented on nonhuman systems such as cells in tissue culture, biochemical reactions, and bacterial and fungal cultures. The ideas that the mind can heal at a distance, that prayer and thought affect living organisms, and that nonhuman systems such as bacteria are presumably not susceptible to the placebo effect are well described in Larry Dossey's work (1993, 1999).

Perhaps the best known study was done by Randolph Byrd, a cardiologist, who studied the effect of prayer on patients admitted with chest pain to an intensive care unit (1988). Approximately 400 patients were randomized into two groups, both of which received standard medical therapy, but one of which was prayed for by a volunteer group from several churches. The patients did not know whether they were randomized into the prayer group or the nonprayer group. In the prayer group, the patient's first name and general condition were passed out to a group of prayer volunteers. The prayer group had significantly less need for endotracheal intubation or antibiotics and a nonsignificant but noticeable trend to fewer deaths.

This illustrates one of the difficulties of study design in this area. How does one quantify prayer? Is there a dose effect? Are some types of prayers more effective than others? Are some religions more likely to

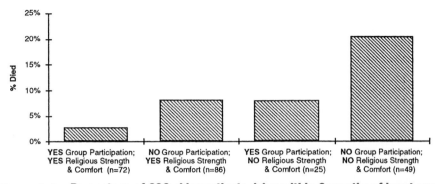

Figure 4–1 **Percentage of 232 older patients dying within 6 months of heart surgery by levels of lack of group participation and absence of strength and comfort from religion. (From Oxman, TE, et al: Lack of social participation or religious strength and comfort as risk factors for death after cardiac surgery in the elderly.** *Psychosomatic Medicine,* **1995;57:5–15, p 11, with permission.)**

receive answers to prayer than others? Of course both groups in Byrd's study could have had and probably did have friends, relatives, and others praying for them because of the seriousness of their conditions. It would be impossible, and probably unethical, to ask either the control or treatment group not to have any extraneous prayers offered for them.

A prospective, randomized, controlled trial by Oxman of 232 elderly cardiac patients is also widely cited (1995). In this study, patients reporting religious belief and social support or a social network were found to recover faster and survive longer than patients not reporting these two variables. The interesting thing was that religious belief and social support were additive variables—that is, each was a positive predictor of improved outcome but together, the outcomes were even better (Figure 4–1).

▬▬ LIFE AND DEATH—THE CALL FOR MEANING AND SPIRITUAL SOLUTIONS

Death of a Child

At times of crisis, especially crisis surrounding issues of death and dying, spirituality takes center stage. Perhaps no greater crisis can occur in a family than the death of a child. It seems out of the natural order for a child to die. The question parents and others always ask is, "Why, God?" This always creates a spiritual crisis in families. Divorce rates are very high after the death of a child, up to 70% in some studies. After the suicide of a child, divorce rates have been reported as high as 90%.

What can I tell grieving parents such as Terry and Tony, whose angelic 8-year-old daughter Lee died of renal cancer? What can really be said that will matter, that will relieve their pain, that will provide a sense of meaning? Though there is no easy answer to such a profound event, what those dealing with the death of child really are asking for is to find some meaning in what is seen as a tragic event. A colleague of mine experienced such a crisis when his 2-year-old wandered into a swimming pool during a party and drowned. As we attempted to comfort him and his family, we discovered that there are networks of parental support groups such as Compassionate Friends and Helping Hands, which are made up of other parents who also have lost a child. What these parents have come to realize is that meaning is possible, life goes on, and that they learn and grow through the pain and suffering (Frankl 1984; Lewis 1944). I share with my patients the view taught to me by Helping Hands parents, who have had to deal with this problem. It is that each soul comes to the world with a purpose, a task. When that task is accomplished, whether it takes 8 years or 80, the soul is called home. Its job being done, the soul happily returns to God, even though those left behind may not understand the timing.

Through this perspective, evolved out of the suffering of parents who have lost their beloved children, some meaning can be seen in an otherwise senseless and tragic event. Although such a concept cannot and will not remove the grieving process, it allows those going through such a tragedy to know that meaning is possible, that others have gone through the same thing and survived, and that life (and death) is a mystery after all. These thoughts can act as a balm to the pained hearts of these parents.

Death of an Old Person

Though great spiritual strength is called for in the death of a child, death at the other extreme of life can be equally trying, a learning process, a time of grief, as well as a time of joy. A person like Bill, an old cowboy, dying at home with advanced lung cancer, surrounded by his family, attended to by hospice, and visited by his family doctor, presents a unique but familiar opportunity for spiritual growth for all involved.

When Bill came to my office with yet another occurrence of cough, fever, and shortness of breath, his family and I felt it was more than just an exacerbation of his emphysema and asthma, brought on by years of smoking. A pulmonologist in a major medical center 3 hours from my little country practice confirmed these suspicions. Bill had extensive cancer of the lung, a small-cell type, which accounted for his weight loss, cough, fatigue, and hemoptysis.

For more than a year, Bill traveled the long road through the Colorado mountains, even in winter blizzards, to undergo his chemotherapy. When he was too weak to travel, we began giving the treatments in my office. Finally, Bill, his family, the oncologist, and I all agreed that his body was losing the battle against the cancer. The chemotherapy was no longer working, though it had prolonged his life for a while. To continue it now would only prolong his death, lessen his quality of life because of side effects, and produce unnecessary expense and discomfort.

Bill, an old cowboy and rancher, was tough. He continued to drive his battered old pickup to the office, on his own, for 2 or 3 more months after we stopped chemo. Sometimes, in the privacy of the exam room, he would break down and cry. But he had a strength in dealing with his illness that came from deep within him. He was a believer, active in his local church, and had a deep faith in God.

When he became too weak to drive, his wife Ramona and I worked together with hospice, his daughters, his pastor, and his community of friends to support Bill in his dying months. Simple things like mouth care, pain control, nausea control, managing his diet, bed care and toilet needs, oxygen for severe shortness of breath, and antibiotics for the episodic obstructive pneumonia all were humane, compassionate, and caring things we did as we watched his life slowly ebb.

Often, Ramona and I would pray with Bill at his bedside. At those times, the gnarled old cowboy's hands gripped my hand like an eagle's claw, tightly, not wanting to let go. When he passed away, I was there. It was a peaceful, quiet death, surrounded by his loved ones. The funeral reception and the community's support for Bill's family unfolded in a gentle, loving orchestration.

I continued to visit with Ramona for several months to support her in her grief, the loss of a husband of almost 50 years. She was often tearful, lonely, sad, and depressed, but like Bill, she counted on her church, her community, and her faith to carry her through this difficult time.

Such is the value of faith in such a time. A health care professional not in touch with the power of a patient's faith, unable or unwilling to acknowledge his or her own mortality, or somehow otherwise not comfortable with the power and momentous opportunity of life's great transition to death might not function optimally in this kind of situation. There is an urge, a tendency, to abandon the patient. After all, we aren't "treating" him anymore.

Nothing could be further from the truth. Even though we are not providing medical therapy, we must always care for and support the patient and family in end-of-life settings. Pain control and physical and social support remain as important roles. But nowhere else in medical practice is the power of the spiritual dimension so apparent as in the end-of-life period.

Some Useful Questions at the End of Life

Something I learned recently from a palliative care specialist seems very useful, so I am including it for your use: many people do not fear dying so much as they fear having "unfinished business." Part of compassionate care, in addition to the pragmatic therapeutic interventions just discussed, may include asking your dying patient the following five questions:

1. Is there anyone you wish to forgive?
2. Is there anyone you wish to ask for forgiveness?
3. Is there anyone you want to thank?
4. Is there anyone you want to tell that you love them?
5. Is there anyone you want to say goodbye to?

Encouraging patients to deal with these issues will give them permission to finish unfinished business. This is often a great relief to the dying person and his or her family. It can prevent untold grief for those left behind, who feel they missed an opportunity to obtain closure in a deep way, a way that meets the deepest psychological, relational, and spiritual needs of all.

▬▬ TAKING A SPIRITUAL HISTORY

Like asking about sexual matters, substance abuse, or domestic violence, asking about spiritual matters may at first feel uncomfortable or awkward. Yet, in the same way we must learn to inquire nonjudgmentally and professionally about sexual orientation or risk factors for sexually transmitted diseases, we must also learn to inquire gently and discreetly about spiritual issues. One acronym that's easy to remember is **FICA:**

Faith—Is faith or spirituality an important aspect of your life?

Impact—How do your personal spiritual beliefs and practices affect your health and your choices about health?

Community—Do you have a community of people (for instance, church, synagogue, mosque) that help support you in times of need?

Assist—Is there any way I can assist you in this area?

These questions open the way for discussion and allow the patient to know that you feel it is relevant to discuss matters of spirituality. Several studies (Ellis 1999) have shown that patients often want their health-care provider to inquire in this area, but either because of training or fear of invading a patient's privacy, physicians and others have been reluctant to inquire in this area. If patients decline to discuss the matter, do not have an interest, or feel their needs are adequately met by the hospital chaplain or their own clergy, the professional will move on to other areas in the history.

A nursing colleague, Dr. Carol Kinney* (personal communication, 1999) introduced the following questions as another way of inquiring into and mobilizing a patient's spiritual resources:

What helps you get through the tough times?

Who do you turn to when you need support?

What meaning does this experience have for you? (Be specific about what experience you are asking about, such as being diagnosed with a cancer or having a myocardial infarction.)

DEEP CALLS TO DEEP—A PATH TO TRUTH

Continuing with the wellness and self-care concepts in the preceding chapters, health-care professionals should reflect on their own spiritual path, beliefs, and practices in order to become a whole person, a whole healer.

In Psalm 42, the suffering soul of man reaches to relate to the divine: "Deep calleth unto deep." When "deep calls to deep," don't be caught in the shallows. When the deepest, most profound questions of human existence such as suffering, loss, chronic illness, and ultimately death are posed, will you have the depth within your own framework of reality to respond . . . meaningfully, kindly, relevantly?

Accept, if you can, the concept of each of us as a soul with a purpose. This in itself is a life-task key to our spiritual development. To recognize, similarly, that our patients are each souls on their paths of conscious and spiritual development, is an attitude and perspective that will promote healthy and, yes, *holy* therapeutic relationships. Your work is a ministry of caring, of healing, of promoting wholeness.

---

*These questions were developed by Carol Kinney, RN, PhD, Associate Professor, The University of Texas at Galveston School of Nursing.

If you are ready to do so, acknowledge that at our core we are neither bodies nor minds. In the final analysis *we are souls,* complete and whole, extensions of the divine, deriving and coexistent with a Higher Power, however we understand the Absolute. From this field of view, we begin to operate in life and make our choices around an eternal reference point. Careers, money worries, health concerns, and problems with relationships all are viewed from a new and heightened awareness.

Each life event, each relationship, each challenge, no matter how painful, is a learning opportunity on our path to truth. And the surest way to spiritual fulfillment, to enlightenment, and to peace is simply to *speak the truth*—to yourself, about yourself, to others, and about others.

What is truth? That is a good question and the topic of many a book. The *Holy Bible,* the *Koran* (Arberyy 1955), *Tao Te Ching* (Feng 1972), *A Course in Miracles* (1975, 1985), and *Conversations with God* (Walsch 1995, 1997, 1998), to name but a few, are sources that I have found useful on my path. However, I believe that ultimately truth resides *within,* not *out there* somewhere. It dwells within our divine natures, within our perfect and complete souls. The truth is manifested and revealed to us through our feelings. Our awareness of the truth is presented to us in the form of what we, in our hearts, know to be true in the deepest levels of our beings.

Learning to listen to those feelings is the key. Experiencing life in this way brings us to reflections of Unity. In this happy view, we are all One in spirit, though our bodies and minds seem to make us separate beings. Seeing one another as part of the One makes feeling and acting totally accepting, loving, and open to our patients an easy and joyful event. This indeed is the way we ourselves would like to be treated: with acceptance, love, and respect for our own individuality, yet as part of a greater plan, as co-souls on a path together. In Oneness, we can eliminate greed, selfishness, violence, and anger. There is only learning.

Instead, we often override our feelings with thoughts, attitudes, rules, or beliefs about what our feelings *should* be. This leaves us stuck in the past or in a constricted view of reality and truth, in the re-enactment of the past rather than the joyful creation of the future. We focus on separation, on lack, and on divisiveness, all of which create unhealthy thoughts, attitudes, and behaviors.

▰▰▰ CONCLUSION

To be a *healer* in the truest sense, you must be engaged in your own spiritual journey, following your own inner path. I contend that this work (and it is work) is as essential as learning proper suturing techniques, knowing how to prescribe or administer a drug or herb, or any of the many other tasks required of a competent health care professional. Patients come to us trusting that we have their best interests at heart. And they also reasonably and legally expect that we can provide competent care.

Without that deeper path, that thoughtful, reflective, soulful quest to understand life's mysteries, you can become excellent at providing health care interventions but remain a mere technician. Without this dimension, you can provide adequate care at the level of the material, physical body, and maybe even in the mental and psychosocial dimension. *This is not enough.* It is on the spiritual journey that you will meet your patients at their deepest levels and achieve the essence of healing, within and without. Curing and healing are different. *Curing* addresses primarily physical health. *Healing* seeks the way to integrate body, mind, and spirit in a process that finds meaning, acceptance, and wholeness.

When deep calls to deep, when the suffering, the pain, the loss all come, as they will in your patients' lives or in your own, these existential challenges may not initially seem to make sense. Believe, and know that you will have a truth to share, to rely on. Your personal path, if you keep choosing the truth, will guide you to answers you didn't know you had to questions you didn't realize your patients would present. Your practice will be truly caring, compassionate, and competent in the broadest sense. You will be comfortable in and capable of treating mind, body, and spirit. You will come to the therapeutic encounter as a whole person prepared to treat the whole person.

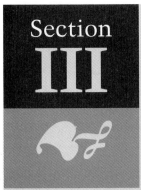

Using Integrative Health Care in Your Practice

Every man is worth just as much as the things he busies himself with.

—Marcus Aurelius

Even if you're on the right track, you'll get run over if you just sit there.

—Will Rogers

Chapter 5 describes new kinds of relationships in this era of evolving health care. Rather than the provider-centered model of old, the medicine of the future will be based on egalitarian therapeutic relationships that are patient-centered, community-based, and collaborative. This truly ecological model honors and gives voice to each member of the therapeutic process.

Working and collaborating with a *health care team,* as well as with the patient, is the topic of Chapter 6. In this era of patient-centered care, integrative practice also includes professional nurses, physician assistants, and nurse practitioners. These disciplines have their own traditions and approaches, which contribute to the care of the whole person. Blending these skills into a practice offers additional dimensions to integrative care.

Practical issues of finance, law, organization, and team building are explored in Chapter 7. This chapter gives the nuts and bolts of starting an integrative practice or bringing alternative therapies into existing practices. To provide an ideal service, it is essential to be "wise as a serpent and simple as a dove"—to be aware of the world as it is and to be willing to fly over it to reach your destination.

Continuing education is a normal part of every health care professional's life. Learning about alternative therapies is no different except that often one's formal training did not include even basic knowledge. Increasing one's skills and knowledge in these areas requires awareness of resources, initiative in self-study, and prudence in choosing the kind of training that will most benefit one's patients and practice. Chapter 8 provides advice, resources, and information on improving knowledge in integrative health care.

Chapter 5

Patient-Centered and Relationship-Centered Care

We must have infinite faith in each other.
—Henry David Thoreau

There is no exercise better for the heart than reaching down and lifting people up.
—John Andrew Holmes

In previous chapters, I have used the term *patient-centered care*. In this chapter, I will further clarify and then expand its meaning to define a philosophy of care called *relationship-centered care.*

HUMILITY

Before I go on, however, I want to introduce a term you know: *humility* (Li 1999). This single concept, this virtue, if applied to the process of caring for each other, would go far in solving all problems currently facing us as individuals, as communities, and as a world. When I approach someone with *humility*, I acknowledge that person's sacredness, entirety, and mystery. I do not claim to know his or her story or purpose. I merely am present with this individual to ask the question, "How can I serve?"

Please remember humility as you read on. If you do so, you will become a superior change agent in the lives of those you have the opportunity to serve. Discard judgment, the belief that you know. Be open; you may be ignorant of the complete situation.

PRACTITIONER-CENTERED CARE

One example of how the model of practitioner-centered care once dominated the thinking and choices of patients occurred to me while I was an intern. I was doing a preoperative exam on a man scheduled for a laparotomy for gall bladder surgery. In examining his head, I found several perfectly round indentations about an inch across and a half-inch deep. Being rather green with inexperience at the time, I naively asked what these were. Of course he told me that they were burr holes, places in the skull that had been drilled out to remove a plate of bone during brain surgery.

I naturally asked what the purpose of the surgery had been. His answer astonished me. He replied quite matter-of-factly, "I don't know. The doctor said I needed it." What I had in front of me was a man with such faith in his doctor's diagnosis and recommendation that he went through brain surgery for a condition that even then, years later, he couldn't clearly describe.

I guess you might say that anyone who would go through brain surgery without asking what the doctor expected to find and do, and what the outcome might be, needs to have his head examined! Nonetheless, as I began the study and practice of medicine, such events were relatively commonplace. Patients just did not question what their doctors recommended. The doctor was a demigod, an authority figure, someone of unquestioned reliability. Like a benevolent parent, if the doctor said to do something, it was best to do it. No questions asked—"Yes sir, yes ma'm. You said jump? How high? Cut open my brain and take something out? Go right ahead!"

▬▬▬ PATIENT-CENTERED CARE

Things have changed. Certainly it is important, even essential, to a therapeutic relationship that there be trust between the patient and the health care practitioner. But blind faith, unquestioning and meek subservience, and patient ignorance are no longer acceptable practice. The legal process in the form of "informed consent" started to break down this tradition. When the surgeon was required to begin informing the patient of the risks, benefits, and purpose of surgical intervention, patients became empowered to ask questions, to consider their options, and to inform themselves about their condition. That not all patients did so does not alter the fact that the communication model between practitioners and patients had changed. It was acceptable practice (and still is in some cultures) to conceal a life-threatening diagnosis such as cancer from a patient. Now, in our country, this is considered unethical and perhaps malpractice.

Paralleling the medicolegal requirements for informed consent were a number of social trends that increased the involvement of patients in their own care. Among these was the development of television and other media coverage of health-related topics. Newspapers, magazines, and evening news broadcasts all found high public interest in things related to health. The Internet and World Wide Web evolved as searchable sources of instant information, support groups, chat rooms, and so on for any health-related topic. Even levels of information previously restricted to a professional audience are now widely available.

Furthermore, the era of the 1960s was marked by a generation that began questioning authority—political, religious, and organizational. The willingness of the baby boomers to doubt and challenge establishment norms, to make up their own rules, and to make their own choices was a driving force in what we have described as patient-centered care.

The doctor or other health care provider was beginning to find that patients were highly informed about their conditions, treatment options, and the dangers or side effects of various drugs, treatments, and surgeries. This encouraged a mutuality of discussion, collaboration, and informed, shared decision making in health matters. This level of discussion was limited not only to direct practitioner-patient interaction but also included family members, clergy, and others in the patient's community. This social support system was often called into consultation, particularly with regard to end-of-life issues, major surgery, and treatment of life-threatening illnesses.

Out of this context, Engel and others described the "biopsychosocial" model of medicine (1977). No longer was the patient seen only as a purely biological or mechanistic entity. Emotional and psychological factors, as well as social and familial context, were acknowledged as important contributors to overall health, healing, or disease.

This patient-centered model puts the patient in the driver's seat. He or she is an active participant, not merely a consumer of health care. As in Ardell's model of the spectrum from "low-level worseness" to "high-level wellness" (see Chap. 3, Table 3–1), the patient is now the primary force in keeping himself or herself well, healthy, and whole. Rather than health somehow being doled out in bits and pieces by the health care establishment, this approach emphasizes self-care of the whole person and personal responsibility for health.

The doctor, nurse, mid-level practitioner, or other health care expert is now a consultant, guide, and mentor to patients on their own paths to well-being. Rather than being keepers of the sacred and secret records of science and health, health care providers acknowledge patients' sophistication as lifelong learners and as responsible change agents within their own lives, and gladly discuss and share decision making. This is a far cry from my brain surgery patient who went blithely into the operating room to have his head drilled open without a clear idea of why it was necessary.

Certainly, health professionals still need technological competence. We must be able to set a fracture competently, to interpret an EKG or other diagnostic test, and to make a proper diagnosis. None of this has changed. What has changed is the process of communication and shared decision making that takes place not only during the diagnostic interview and testing but also after the condition has been identified. Now, the process of deciding which of a number of therapies—alternative, conventional, or integrative—are desired or preferred by the patient and provider becomes the next and most subtle, satisfying phase of our work together.

Now, as patients make decisions about surgery, they may consult with the anesthesiologist to make sure that the physician or nurse anesthetist has the proper attitude and energy to enter that vulnerable state of sleep with them. Perhaps they will interview more than one surgeon, getting as many opinions as time allows to assure themselves that this person and this procedure is the right one. Perhaps they will consult a hypnotherapist to deal with fears about surgery, an acupuncturist to help reduce pain and stimulate immunity, a nutritionist to optimize their cellular readiness, and an exercise physiologist to improve muscle tone and decrease recovery time. In any case, patients are more in the driver's seat than ever before and have the right, perhaps even the duty, to seek out whatever resources they feel they need prior to surgery, chemotherapy, or other medical intervention.

This process may threaten the autonomy of the health care provider and may require more time and effort on our part. But remember, "Whose body is it anyway?" Clearly, the person with the highest investment in the outcome is the patient. Strengthening and encouraging the participatory process is the essence of patient-centered care.

▬▬▬ RELATIONSHIP-CENTERED CARE

Recently, the patient-centered model, which has been enormously useful in the fields of medicine, nursing, social work, psychology, pastoral care, and public health, has been transmuted by the concept of "relationship-centered care." This model emphasizes the centrality of the therapeutic relationship to the healing process. It occurs at three levels: (1) practitioner-patient, (2) practitioner-community, and (3) practitioner-practitioner. Healthy relationships, clear communications, and teamwork among all stakeholders are necessary for a holistic and complete model of care (Tresolini & Pew–Fetzer Task Force 1994). To quote from the Pew–Fetzer Foundation report on this topic:

> We . . . assert the need for a new phrase, *relationship-centered care.* In using this terminology, we affirm the centrality of relationships in contemporary health care and their importance in the context of any health care reform debate. Although always central to health care, relation-

ships that practitioners form with patients, communities, and other practitioners have not generally been explored or taught explicitly. Despite nursing's long history of emphasizing caring relationships in its practice and ethos, this focus has not become a defining force in health care. The biopsychosocial model, while helping to focus attention on the integrated nature of illness systems (i.e., that an illness incorporates biological, psychological and social aspects), ironically also invites multidimensional analysis and reductionism, further objectifying the patient and the illness experience. The patient-centered model, while promoting a more whole-person approach, does not explicitly embrace the community and interdisciplinary aspects of health care that are of such importance today. (p 10–11)

This model, then, values the *therapeutic relationship* as a primary healing factor whether it occurs between patient and practitioner, community and practitioner, or between practitioners themselves. It requires an interaction of mutual respect, of awareness of the other person or persons as whole individuals, and a willingness to reflect on and understand our own inner being. Excellent communication and listening skills, empathy, and lifelong learning are all essential components.

This need to reflect on the process of the professional encounter is a new arena in health education. "The need for the health professions to become more reflective or contemplative disciplines calls, therefore, for a profound change in professional education from a curriculum dominated by abstractions and intellectual analysis to one balanced between intellectual analysis and the depths of human experience" (Tresolini & Pew–Fetzer Task Force 1994, p 22).

▬▬▬ PRACTITIONER-PATIENT CARE: PRESENCE AND THE THERAPEUTIC RELATIONSHIP

Neither patient-centered nor relationship-centered care is any more than an abstraction without the skills and motivation of a health-care professional who brings it all together with another element, which can be described as the *therapeutic relationship*. The concept of the healer as a therapeutic force, above and beyond his or her physical ministrations, is not new. Much of the so-called placebo effect is often attributed to the trust, the desire to get well, the positive expectation that is present in the therapeutic encounter. The caring attitude of the health care practitioner further amplifies the beneficial effect of the interaction. What I am advocating is a conscious application of this approach, one that requires that we as professionals become more aware of our inner beings—the depth of our own human experience—so that we can communicate, empathize, and relate better to our patients (Table 5–1).

The work of Dr. Jon Kabat-Zinn applies to both relaxation and the concept of *presence.* He has taught techniques of self-awareness, stress

Table 5–1 AREAS OF KNOWLEDGE, SKILLS, AND VALUES FOR THE PATIENT-PRACTITIONER RELATIONSHIP

Area	Knowledge	Skills	Values
Self-awareness	Knowledge of self Understanding self as a resource to others	Reflect on self and work	Importance of self-awareness, self-care, self-growth
Patient experience of health and illness	Role of family, culture, community in development Multiple components of health Multiple threats and contributors to health as dimensions of one's reality	Recognize patient's life story and its meaning View health and illness as part of human development	Appreciation of the patient as a whole person Appreciation of the patient's life story and the meaning of the health-illness condition
Developing and maintaining caring relationships	Understanding of threats to the integrity of the relationship (e.g., power inequalities) Understanding of potential for conflict and abuse	Attend fully to the patient Accept and respond to distress in patient and self Respond to moral and ethical challenges Facilitate hope, trust, and faith	Respect for patient's dignity, uniqueness, and integrity (mind-body-spirit unity) Respect for self-determination Respect for person's own power and self-healing processes
Effective communication	Elements of effective communication	Listen Impart information Learn Facilitate the learning of others Promote and accept patient's emotions	Importance of being open and nonjudgmental

Source: From Tresolini CP, and the Pew–Fetzer Task Force. 1994. *Health Professions Education and Relationship-Centered Care.* San Francisco: Pew Health Professions Commission, p 30, with permission.

management, and situational consciousness (mindfulness) that are not only useful in the patient encounter but also practical in many life situations (Kabat-Zinn 1990).

Awareness of our own experience, thoughts, feelings, and attitudes, of our environment, and of those around us is the outcome of this process. In a Zen-like fashion, there is no "goal" per se but rather a creative process of learning that allows a fuller consciousness of our world. This is more than a "stop and smell the roses" cliché.

Kabat-Zinn emphasizes the significance of learning to meditate, to quiet our outer world and become aware of the inner. When we are in the outer world, however, we are truly *present*, which is to say we fully embrace and savor each moment, each experience, be it a flower or another person. This *presence* is a timeless place, the world of the innocent child. In this state of *presence* we do not judge, do not continuously sort right from wrong. Rather, we accept people as they are. We see them as souls on a journey to their own fulfillment, following their own paths.

Our role is not to "fix" them, but to be their helpers, guides, and facilitators as they progress from one state to another. When they are ready to change habits, lifestyles, consciousness—to move from one state of health to another—we are there to help. Like sensitive, patient gardeners, we do not force the blooms to open before their time, but do our work of watering, weeding, pruning, and so on until the moment is perfect. Then we stand by in awe as the roses open and give their sweet fragrance, or as our patients are ready to be healed and make choices we can celebrate with them at last.

The physician hurrying into an exam room and out again is an all-too-familiar example of the lack of presence. A mother brings in her 3-year-old and her 5-year-old for respiratory infections for the third time in several months. The practitioner, hurried and not really present with the situation's hidden aspects, prescribes a decongestant and perhaps an antibiotic, and moves on. Another clinician, having practiced being mindful of the immediate situation and tuning into the full biopsychosocial content of the same visit, might have noted the mother's troubled face, the unspoken word, the worry behind the child as the identified patient. After prescribing for the children, the practitioner would ask the nurse to watch the two children in the waiting room play area while she gently inquires further. Perhaps the real problem is not the children's colds but a marital problem, a distant, possibly abusive or unfaithful spouse who is creating strain in the family. Further visits could be scheduled with the mother alone or with the husband to address this deeper level of concern.

In this case, the patient encounter is seen as a "communication opportunity," which allows broader healing to take place. It requires the relationship to develop between the practitioner and the patient: here, the *family* is the patient. It also requires that the health care provider have that sense of presence, of awareness of the whole situation, thereby allowing a therapeutic relationship to evolve.

Presence can be both taught and learned. It is not necessarily a natural skill in our society, where distraction, multimedia, noise, and clamor are often the rule. It is exceptional when we find those few moments each day for stillness, quietude, and reflection.

The state of presence may be exceptional, but it is necessary. To become a gifted healer, a truly helpful health care provider, requires learning more, much more, than just the essentials of making a diagnosis and initiating a treatment plan. It requires that you become as aware of yourself as of your patients. Indeed, a failure to be aware of yourself limits how aware of your patients you can be and subsequently how helpful you are to them.

▰▰▰ PRACTITIONER-COMMUNITY CARE

An example of relationship-centered care at the level of the community is what happened at the University of Texas Medical Branch recently. Faced with cutbacks in the budget for indigent care, our Department of Family Medicine was faced with a difficult medical, social, and ethical challenge. Many of the patients with no health insurance who had attended our resident clinic for many years would not, under new rules, be able to continue being seen at our main clinic on Galveston Island. This change had the potential of leaving a gap in care for this vulnerable population. They were vulnerable because of poverty, poor health, and limited social and other resources to help them adjust to this changed situation. With creativity and determination, our department chair, residency program director, and financial officer met with the County Public Health Department over a period of months. They developed a new program with additional sources of funding, staffing, extended clinic hours, identification cards, and other essential components that provided continuing access to health care for the county's indigent population. This program allowed the patients to maintain the relationship they had had with our Family Medicine Department and the University of Texas Medical Branch, as we transferred records, personnel, and physicians to cover their care at two different county clinic sites. We developed new collaborations with mid-level practitioners, pharmacists, specialists, social workers, and other providers to strengthen the program.

In the parlance of *relationship-centered care,* this program was a solid demonstration of what communities, practitioners, and institutions can do to solve larger problems of access, community need, and maintenance of established relationships in the health care arena (Table 5–2). Expanding these county clinics as training sites will further expand services for these indigent patients without depleting a stressed university budget. Another phrase used to describe this larger concept of primary care is *community-oriented primary care (COPC).*

▬▬▬ PRACTITIONER-PRACTITIONER RELATIONSHIPS: COLLABORATION AND REFERRAL

Throughout our careers, we become used to the process of referral, consultation, and working with our colleagues in other specialties. The development of a network of alternative practitioners is a particularly challenging process, however, since it goes beyond the usual boundaries of knowledge and skills with which we have become familiar (Table 5–3).

Choosing a gifted alternative practitioner can be difficult if we know little about these practice areas. Even if we have the ability to discern, either by reputation or demonstrated clinical skill, that a clinician is qualified to care for our patients in a referral process, he or she may or may not be a team player. Sending a patient to a practitioner who will consult reciprocally with you, who reassures the patient that you are both collaborating in his or her best interest, and who maintains the highest degree of professionalism that you hold for yourself is the ideal.

Meeting such people and developing the relationships that it takes to work closely with them in the care of patients requires some effort. Visiting them in their offices or inviting them to visit you in yours, discussing difficult cases before referral, and eliciting patient feedback are instrumental to making this collaboration work. I am particularly sensitive to my patients' feedback about consultants. Whether the consultants are herbalists or oncologists, if they receive bad marks from my patients for their quality of care, communication style, or other aspects of professional care and courtesy, I pay attention. If there is a problem, I get on the phone or talk to the consultant face-to-face and try to clarify what happened. If there is no satisfactory resolution, someone else will be receiving my referrals in the future.

The key factor is more than the quality of the practitioner's competence. It is his or her ability to work together with you as a member of a team whose sole purpose is to help the patient be well. You and your patients can do without practitioners who are more interested in advocating a particular system of care than in seeking honestly what

Table 5–2 AREAS OF KNOWLEDGE, SKILLS, AND VALUES FOR THE COMMUNITY-PRACTITIONER RELATIONSHIP

Area	Knowledge	Skills	Values
Meaning of community	Various models of community Myths and misperceptions about community Perspectives from the social sciences, humanities, and systems theory Dynamic change—demographic, political, industrial	Learn continuously Participate actively in community development and dialogue	Respect for the integrity of the community Respect for cultural diversity
Multiple contributors to health within the community	History of community, land use, migration, occupations, and their effects on health Physical, social, and occupational environments and their effects on health External and internal forces influencing community health	Critically assess the relationship of health care providers to community health Assess community and environmental health Assess implications of community policy affecting health	Affirmation of relevance of all determinants of health Affirmation of the value of health policy in community services Recognition of the presence of values that are destructive to health
Developing and maintaining community relationships	History of practitioner-community relationships Isolation of the health care community from the community at large	Communicate ideas Listen openly Empower others Learn Facilitate the learning of others Participate appropriately in community development and activism	Importance of being open-minded Honesty regarding the limits of health science Responsibility to contribute health expertise
Effective community-based care	Various types of care, both formal and informal Effects of instititutional scale on care Positive effects of continuity of care	Collaborate with other individuals and organizations Work as member of a team or healing community Implement change strategies	Respect for community leadership Commitment to work for change

Source: From Tresolini CP, and the Pew–Fetzer Task Force. 1994. *Health Professions Education and Relationship-Centered Care.* San Francisco: Pew Health Professions Commission, p 34, with permission.

Table 5–3   AREAS OF KNOWLEDGE, SKILLS, AND VALUES FOR THE PRACTITIONER-PRACTITIONER RELATIONSHIP

Area	Knowledge	Skills	Values
Self-awareness	Knowledge of self	Reflect on self and needs Learn continuously	Importance of self-awareness
Traditions of knowledge in health professions	Healing approaches of various professions Healing approaches across cultures Historical power inequities across professions	Derive meaning from others' work Learn from experience within healing community	Affirmation and value of diversity
Building teams and communities	Perspectives on teambuilding from the social sciences	Communicate effectively Listen openly Learn cooperatively	Affirmation of mission Affirmation of diversity
Working dynamics of teams, groups, and organizations	Perspectives on team dynamics from the social sciences	Share responsibility responsibly Collaborate with others Work cooperatively Resolve conflicts	Openness to others' ideas Humility Mutual trust, empathy, support Capacity for grace

Source: From Tresolini CP, and the Pew–Fetzer Task Force. 1994. *Health Professions Education and Relationship-Centered Care.* San Francisco: Pew Health Professions Commission, p 36, with permission.

the patient needs most. I have inadvertently sent patients to practitioners who required the purchase of an expensive amount of their own herbs and supplements and a set number of treatments as part of the therapeutic contract. "Sorry," my patients would say, "I don't trust them. I felt they were only there to get my money." This is feedback I listen to.

Your patients are the best source of information about which alternative practitioners in the community are top quality and thus deserving of being included in your network. When possible, seek licensed providers and realize that patient needs and preferences differ, so that one person's relief may be another's poison. In larger communities, beyond looking for licensure as a guarantee of a certain amount of competence, visiting and meeting with practitioners you intend to refer to is essential. Many times, even in larger urban areas, your patients are your contacts linking you to a network of providers of alternative therapies that they already receive. This is the opportunity for you to be involved and learn to apply the principles of integrative care. By learning what resources and people are available in the community, from the well-informed health food store owner to a chiropractor with gifted hands and excellent patient rapport, you will become an expert consultant and referral ombudsman.

Whatever happens, pay close attention to the quality of the practitioner-practitioner relationship. Mutual respect; avoidance of one-upmanship; willingness to try to understand the other's therapeutic system; appreciation of differences in culture, belief, and philosophy; and a clear communication style on both sides are all aspects of creating a therapeutic alliance.

CONCLUSION

Certain skills, knowledge, and values are necessary in relationship-centered care, as summarized in the preceding tables. To understand the three dimensions of relationship-centered care clearly, it is essential to realize that they must exist in balance. Those practitioners in the matrix of personal, community, and professional relationships must interact as equal partners, each valuing the other. When this balance is achieved, all relationships are strengthened. Patients, health care professionals, and the community mutually benefit from this expanded perspective.

Chapter 6

The Role of Mid-Level Practitioners

J. Dennis Blessing, PhD, PA-C
Michelle L. Edwards, MSN, RNCS, FNP

The vocation of every man and woman is to serve other people.

—Leo Tolstoy

INTEGRATING MID-LEVEL PRACTITIONERS

J. Dennis Blessing, PhD, PA-C

To add or expand the use of alternative therapies in a practice, the expertise and skills of a nurse practitioner (NP) or physician assistant (PA) may be invaluable. Practices that already use these providers and understand their contributions to health care in the team model can work readily to expand services. Practices that have not employed a PA or NP will need to define the fit for this person in the practice. It is important that physicians and other employers understand the basis for practice of these professionals. All states have enabling legislation for NPs and all but one (Mississippi) have enabling legislation for PAs. Physicians and employers must understand the regulations that govern NP and PA practice, including the physician's responsibility in a collaborative or interdependent practice situation.

An NP or PA can be a great help in a busy practice, but physician involvement and collaboration are very important. If the PA or NP is actively supported in developing knowledge and skills desired in integrative health care, the practice and the patients will benefit and the PA's or NP's value to the practice will grow. Such an arrangement can expand the services offered by a practice without putting greater burdens on the physician's time.

The practice that already employs a PA or NP will need to define what alternative therapies will be used in the practice and who will use them. An action plan can be developed that addresses the time required for additional education for every member of the practice, the particular responsibilities of the NP and PA, the ways that alternative therapies will be applied, and the legal implications for those who apply them (see Chap. 7). Generally, PAs and NPs must practice in a setting similar to that of the physician and must provide services considered a component of the physician specialty. The physician must ensure that educational and legal requirements are met. It takes planning to ensure the successful integration of alternative modalities into a practice. The "who, what, when, where, why, and how" of the practice must be agreed on by all involved, especially if additional education or licensure is needed or when a new approach to traditional practice is considered.

There is little doubt that NPs and PAs are competent providers within the framework of their practices. The literature supports their competence and acceptance by patients. PAs and NPs can be cost-efficient in administering many alternative therapies that involve multiple patient visits or longer visits. Having these additional providers on board also enhances access, ensures continuity (because they report to the physician), and aids in any number of areas that improve the care and proficiency of the practice. Their use can be molded to fit the needs of the practice in a number of ways.

■■■■ PHYSICIAN ASSISTANTS

J. Dennis Blessing, PhD, PA-C

Physician assistants are educated and trained to practice medicine with physician supervision. The concept was developed in the mid-1960s to meet the needs of rural areas and to balance the loss of generalist physicians to specialization. With the evolution of the profession, they are now included in every medical and surgical specialty. PA practice is based on the concept of physician delegation. State requirements further define PA practice and physician responsibility, and it is the responsibility and duty of both parties to be knowledgeable of and compliant with these regulations.

On the other hand, many alternative modalities are unregulated or weakly regulated by state and federal agencies. (Exceptions are osteopathy, chiropractic, hypnosis, and acupuncture.) Therefore, the physician and PA can decide on their own approaches to applying such therapies, recognizing that the decision to use an alternative therapy, whether alone or as a complement to allopathic modalities, requires the same attentiveness to detail as the use of any other treatment or drug prescription.

For a collaborative practice to succeed, the physician must develop an appreciation for the skills and abilities of the PA. In turn, the PA must learn to practice in a manner consistent with the physician's practice. To apply new concepts of care to a practice, both the physician and the PA must be committed to the concepts. Both must become knowledgeable in the concepts and the application of the new therapy. Both must agree about when its application is appropriate and how it will fit into the practice. Ultimately, the practice should be one of interdependence, using the skills of each to maximum efficiency for the benefit of the patient. Each team of physicians and PAs must determine what their interactions will be with each other in patient care and in the use of alternative therapies, including when physician consultation is appropriate and how patient care will be reviewed by both. State statutes, rules, and regulations will affect this aspect of practice.

Certainly, the PA can become a major resource for a practice in the area of alternative therapies. It may be more economical to educate and train the PA in new modalities, rather than have the physician lose time from the practice. It also may be more economical for a PA to spend more time with patients, particularly for components of practice that generate little or no reimbursement, such as patient education. Alternative therapies often require that more time be spent on patient education than do conventional therapies.

For the practice or physician who already employs a PA, the addition of new services to be performed by the PA can be an easy transition because the abilities, skills, interests, and contributions of the PA are known. Much will depend on that person's interest, expertise, and need for additional training and education. Adding new skills will give the PA an area of "expertise" that will allow him or her to make unique contributions to the practice.

If the plan is to add a PA to a practice, recruitment plans should include expectations for the application of alternative modalities. Because PAs are educated and trained in the allopathic or osteopathic paradigms, however, the practice should expect to provide or support additional education. Initial plans should also include all legal requirements for PA practice. Whether a new graduate or an experienced PA is best for a practice is a decision that needs to be weighed against expectations.

There is no reason to believe that a practice employing a PA as well as physicians will not succeed in providing integrative health care, as long as it follows reasonable trends based on known outcomes with good patient expectations. Both professionals must be committed to quality care and to working as an interdependent team. PAs have succeeded in the breadth of medicine, and the expansion of a practice to include alternative modalities should not present an obstacle for the practice or the patients.

Case Study

Mr. J. is a 55-year-old Hispanic high school teacher. He has been a patient of Dr. S. for many years and has been seen regularly for controlled hypertension, mild obesity (20 lb overweight), and stress management. His family history is positive for coronary artery disease and diabetes. He has been fairly healthy, with his hypertension controlled by a low-dose angiotensin-converting-enzyme inhibitor. Weight loss has been difficult for him and he has gone off and on diet and exercise programs over the years. He was a high school athlete and suffered minor joint injuries on several occasions. He recently began to walk and play softball for exercise. After 2 or 3 weeks, he began to have dull, aching knee pain in both knees. He ignored it at first but had prolonged episodes of discomfort after exercise and felt that his knees were swollen on occasion. He has enjoyed playing softball and has continued his walking, but the progression of his knee pain worries him.

He was initially evaluated by Mr. B., a PA who has worked with Dr. S. for 5 years. The exam was fairly unremarkable and consistent with degenerative joint disease. Treatment consisted of ice for the knees after exercise, heat on nonsoftball days, elevation, and an over-the-counter nonsteroidal anti-inflammatory drug (NSAID) or acetaminophen, following package directions. After 3 weeks, Mr. J. reported little improvement and felt his knees "popping" at times. Mr. B. ordered x-rays of the knees, which demonstrated mild to moderate degenerative changes. It was decided to try a prescription-strength NSAID with general care. After a month, Mr. J.'s symptoms improved, but he did not want to continue long-term use of the NSAID because he feared having kidney problems, which his diabetic brother had experienced. Mr. J. had read about a number of alternative therapies in a magazine. Dr. S. and Mr. B. reviewed the x-rays and the various treatments available, and arrived at a set of combined recommendations.

They decided to suggest a course of glucosamine sulfate with a prescription-strength NSAID on a p.r.n. basis. Mr. J. was scheduled to see Mr. B. for patient education on diet, gradual exercise, leg strengthening, adjunctive care, and use of his medications, including glucosamine sulfate. Mr. J. returned 4 weeks later reporting moderate improvement in the duration and severity of his pain. His NSAID was reduced to a low-dose p.r.n., and the glucosamine sulfate was continued. Dr. S. and Mr. B. then saw Mr. J. on alternate visits for follow-up treatment.

NURSE PRACTITIONERS

Michelle L. Edwards, MSN, RNCS, FNP

Nurse practitioners (NPs) are playing a larger role in the delivery of health care, forming partnerships with physicians and other health-care professionals to provide the best in personalized and comprehensive care. Working in collaboration with the physician, the NP consistently provides high-quality, cost-effective patient care, with specific consideration for the individual patient's special needs.

Nurse practitioners are experienced registered nurses who have completed advanced academic and clinical training beyond their basic nursing training, which qualifies them to assume some diagnostic and treatment responsibilities that were traditionally reserved for physicians. NPs are prepared to manage most common complaints and many chronic illnesses. Their additional education and training, with their ability to diagnose and treat medical problems, are what distinguish them from other nursing personnel.

The concept of nurse practitioners originated in 1965 with a master's degree for pediatric NPs at the University of Colorado. Although some practicing NPs were educated through a certificate program, current NP programs are graduate-level programs that require students to obtain a bachelor's degree in nursing prior to acceptance. Many programs also require applicants to have at least 2 years of practice experience as a registered nurse.

In most states, NPs are required to carry dual licensure: licensure or certification as an NP in addition to their licensure as a registered nurse. The Nurse Practice Act of each state is the authorizing body that permits NPs to provide care in a variety of settings. The scope of NP practice varies depending on each state's regulations.

Although some NPs function in subspecialty roles and some work independently of a formal physician relationship, most NPs have a primary care focus and most work in collaboration with physicians. With a strong emphasis on primary care, NPs focus largely on issues of health maintenance, emphasizing prevention of illness and a state of complete physical, mental, and social well-being, not simply the absence of disease.

The collaborative relationship between physicians and NPs has been an effective approach to the delivery of health care for many years and has been well received by patients. This union has certainly helped in the *access* problem of health care by increasing the avenues by which patients can be seen without jeopardizing quality care. In fact, quality is maintained or even heightened, with the added benefit of cost-effectiveness.

The most successful physician-NP collaborations value the skills and expertise of each, and include strategies that promote "knowledge sharing." Making personal knowledge a group commodity benefits the providers, the practice, and most importantly, the patient.

How can alternative treatment modalities best be used in the physician-NP practice setting? First, practitioners should determine what aspects of alternative medicine will be employed. Next, they must commit to the concepts of the new therapy and work to increase provider knowledge in its appropriate use, potential side effects (if any), and possible interactions with traditional therapies. Then the physician and NP should agree about the appropriate times to initiate alternative therapy and the arrangements for appropriate patient follow-up care. As with any treatment modality, careful documentation of the patient's response to treatment is very important.

Case Study

Ms. H.W. is a 30-year-old African-American library assistant who lives on the Gulf Coast. Her job requires her to stand for many hours. She has been a patient of Dr. D. for about 3 years and has developed a rapport with Ms. E., the nurse practitioner, from previous visits. Her past medical-surgical history is relatively unremarkable except for childbirth via cesarean delivery 6 years ago. Although she does not engage in a routine exercise regimen, she consumes well-balanced meals and manages to maintain an ideal body weight of 115 lb. She is a nonsmoker and does not routinely take any prescription or over-the-counter medications. Her family history is significant for hypertension in her father and varicose veins in her mother and twin sister. She has seen multiple, small varicose veins in her legs for several years, but just recently began to experience symptoms from her varicosities, including occasional pain with a generalized "achy" and "tired" feeling in both legs. She has also observed mild to moderate swelling of both legs.

The physical examination was performed by Ms. E., the nurse practitioner. It confirmed the presence of several small- and moderate-sized varicose veins in both lower extremities, with evidence of bilateral trace ankle edema. The remainder of the physical exam was unremarkable. It was determined that Ms. H.W.'s current symptoms were secondary to her varicosities. All of the traditional medical treatment options were discussed, but surgery was not recommended, and Ms. H.W. was not interested in it. Neither was she completely satisfied with the idea of wearing support stockings during the day; she found them "very unattractive and too hot."

Ms. E. decided to consult with Dr. D., who is very knowledgeable in alternative therapies. Dr. D. suggested offering Ms. H.W. a trial of horse chestnut because aescin, its active ingredient, has been found to help patients with chronic venous insufficiency and varicose veins by promoting normal tone of vessel walls and aiding in venous return. Ms. H.W. was excited about having another treatment option and eagerly accepted the offer. Treatment was begun with an initial dosage of 100 mg once a day in conjunction with extremity elevation, exercise, and the use of support stockings primarily in the late evenings and at bedtime, the only times she would agree to wear them.

After 4 weeks, Ms. H.W. reported significant improvement. Although she was not sure if she noticed a decrease in the size of her varicose veins, her symptoms had definitely improved. It was decided that she should continue taking horse chestnut at a reduced maintenance dosage of 50 mg once a day and should return for follow-up evaluation in 4 to 6 weeks.

Practices teaming physicians and nurse practitioners have delivered traditional medicine for many years with excellent patient outcomes. The incorporation of alternative modalities into these practice settings will follow that same historical trend. Commitment, knowledge, skill, and dialogue are the elements required for success.

Chapter 7

Reimbursement, Liability, and Other Practice Issues

Seize opportunity by the beard, for it is bald behind.
—Bulgarian proverb

A practitioner of integrative care, however well intentioned and however competent in providing both conventional and alternative therapies, must understand the business aspects of health-care delivery systems to remain in practice (Berndtson 1998; Brown 1998; Dalzell 1999; Weber 1998). Programs of integrative care often bleed some red ink in their start-up phase, but to become sustainable they must develop a stable source of revenue to cover expenses.

In the model described through much of this book, integrative care doesn't require a separate facility or practice site. Skilled practitioners simply blend alternative practices into their existing practice. Even under these circumstances, however, key issues such as reimbursement, insurance coverage, liability, and the sale of products must be considered. In the case of a clinical practice dedicated entirely to an alternative practice, such as a hospital-supported program, there are challenges of center development, institutional and political support, marketing, and blending with the existing organization's mission (Kornblatt 1999).

■ REIMBURSEMENT ISSUES

Though the third party–payer climate is changing quickly in response to public demand, many alternative therapies such as acupuncture, homeopathy, therapeutic touch, massage, and over-the-counter herbs and supplements traditionally have not been covered by insurance. Patients paid out of pocket for these services or products, didn't get them, or engaged in bothersome debates with their insurance companies about getting these services covered—even when these services and products were cost-effective. I clearly recall resolving a back pain problem for one of my HMO patients using acupuncture. The series of treatments cost less than $300, but the HMO balked at paying it as a "noncovered service," even though a referral for an orthopedic evaluation plus the usual MRI scan would have cost the plan over $2000 before any treatment had even been initiated.

Fortunately, this situation is gradually changing as insurers respond to market demand for alternative therapies to be included in their product line and as they recognize the benefits of various alternative therapies in terms of safety and efficacy. Another driver of change has been legislation in certain states such as Alaska, California, Oregon, and Washington, which requires the coverage of alternative therapies in health care plans and authorizes the use of alternative practitioners as primary care providers. In some instances, chiropractors or naturopaths can be a patient's primary care provider.

Some therapies already have widespread insurance coverage. According to one survey, therapies commonly covered are chiropractic, biofeedback, hypnotherapy, preventive medicine, nutritional counseling, physical therapy, psychotherapy, massage, and acupuncture. Less frequently covered are herbal medicine, meditation, support groups, yoga, Ayurveda, homeopathy, naturopathy, and Reiki (Pelletier et al 1997). Other plans provide coverage for some additional therapies, such as acupuncture or massage, but stipulate certain terms such as licensure, clinical condition, or a limited number of treatments. Other insurers offer discounted fees for their members when they use alternative practitioners within their network. Several large plans offer discount cards that partially cover the costs of herbs and supplements. In capitated reimbursement plans, the addition of alternative practitioners in a carefully monitored case management program for difficult, expensive-to-treat diagnoses may result in overall cost savings to the plan.

Obstacles to incorporating complementary and alternative medicine (CAM) therapies into mainstream health care and health care reimbursement are "(1) lack of research on efficacy; (2) economics; (3) ignorance about CAM; (4) provider competition and divisions; and (5) lack of standards of practice" (Pelletier et al 1997). Nonetheless, state-mandated reimbursement for alternative providers is expanding, and insurance companies and HMOs are looking to this area as a method of market differentiation (to attract a younger and healthier group of patients interested in self-care) and potential cost reduction.

For the foreseeable future, many alternative practitioners will have to continue to require that patients pay out of pocket for services that insurance does not cover. Running a successful practice is a combination of many things. Proper staffing and control of overhead, supply costs, and other expenses are ever in the mind of the practitioner or organization trying to maintain a profit margin and a clinic's survival. Handling payment for self-pay patients is easier logistically and better financially than for insured patients. For insured patients, providers have to fill out and submit insurance forms for covered claims, negotiate insurance and managed care contracts, maintain their credentials with a third-party payer, and accept discounted fees as "usual and customary." These are not always familiar areas for alternative practitioners, especially non-physicians. Some do not welcome the involvement of third-party payment systems into their practice, seeing them as threats to autonomy and income that increase overhead and billing hassles— even though these systems hold out the promise of increased patient volume.

▬▬ LIABILITY ISSUES

As in every field of health care today, malpractice and professional liability issues are a continual challenge for both individuals and organizations. Although there is little case law in this area, so far it appears that the risk of providing alternative therapies is relatively low. Most of these therapies are gentler and safer than more aggressive medical therapies. Though chiropractors are sued for damages associated with using excess force, the rate of these claims and the payout on settlements is one-third of standard medical malpractice claims, or less. Massage therapists have also been subject to litigation, but the issue is less often physical injury than sexually inappropriate behavior.

One review of malpractice in this area concluded that primary care providers referring patients to autonomous alternative practitioners need not be excessively concerned about liability (Studdert et al 1998). If the referral is a reasonable one, particularly if the alternative practitioner is licensed and not known to be incompetent or unprofessional, negligence issues are minimal, even if an injury occurs. The alternative practitioner should be held to the standard of care of his or her own fellow practitioners.

Physicians, hospitals, or organizations that maintain a supervisory role over an alternative practitioner, however, are held to a higher standard. If there is a joint undertaking or a team practice, the liability of a member of a team who injures a patient through negligence may be assessed to other members or the sponsoring organization. This assignment of joint liability follows the customary legal practice of seeking the "deep pockets" in a case—the defendant who presents the most lucrative target because of having the greatest financial assets or the largest professional liability coverage. Organizations appear to be particularly liable in this scenario and therefore must be vigilant in verifying credentials, competence, and training. Establishing written protocols is often helpful in maintaining a high standard of care and in preventing a team member from straying errantly from what the rest of the group expects.

The issue of documentation of care is at least as important in the provision of alternative and integrative care as in conventional care (Kornblatt 1999). If a patient begins a course of unproved therapy instead of conventional care, he or she may experience a negative outcome or a delay in receiving conventional treatment. The practitioner must include in the documentation a discussion of the diagnosis and treatment options; what conventional therapies have been tried, refused, or have failed; and the patient's understanding of the risk and benefit of using an alternative therapy. Some legal experts even recommend a signed informed-consent document, particularly when the patient is being treated for a serious illness and has declined standard therapy. All conversations about risks, alternatives, deviations from conventional care or interruptions in it, care instructions, and follow-up must be documented clearly and legibly in a standard format such as the problem-oriented medical record and SOAP (Subjective, Objective, Assessment, Plan) format. As in conventional practice, good documentation is the best protection against liability problems. But it must be coupled with clear communication with the patient so that all parties are on the same level of understanding about the treatment plan and options. Regular communication, feedback, and clarification are the best ways to prevent misunderstanding, unrealistic expectations, and the creation of an angry, hostile patient who files a lawsuit. Even if an injury occurs, maintaining communication with the patient, avoiding defensiveness, and providing all possible assistance may alleviate the situation and prevent the need for legal recourse.

Finally, make sure that your professional liability carrier is aware of any type of alternative or integrative care that you practice. If you add a kind of treatment that you haven't offered previously, or if you sign on with a new insurance company, be sure to let the company know the scope of your practice. Adding a new treatment such as acupuncture may not cause the company to raise your premium, but if a claim arises from a therapy that the insurance company didn't know was being offered, the "blind-sided" company may decline coverage.

▰▰▰▰ SALE OF PRODUCTS TO PATIENTS

One source of income in many alternative and integrative practices is operating a natural pharmacy within the practice. Supplying patients with herbs and supplements, as well as health-related books, tapes, CDs, and other resources, can be a profitable sideline and conveys the message of whole-person health. You can select high-quality, standardized products with which you are familiar rather than having your patients purchase less predictable products at the local pharmacy or health food store. On the other hand, some critics have raised an ethical concern. Both prescribing and selling a product to a patient may seem to be a conflict of interest.

In my Colorado practice, I kept a supply of generic medications, vitamins, and supplements for my patients, because the nearest pharmacy was almost an hour's drive away. This was a convenience to them and supplied a small but steady percentage of my operating revenue. I also ordered cases of books that I found particularly helpful and provided them to my patients at cost. My prices for the drugs and supplements were comparable to those of local pharmacies and I was quite sure of what my patients were getting. I also was more confident that they would actually take what I prescribed when I handed it to them. Of course, you must maintain careful inventory, comply with state pharmacy laws, and make it clear to patients that they are free to obtain their products elsewhere.

Some clinics have set up a separate revenue pool for their pharmacies so that the provider's income incentive is not linked to the sale of products. This is more difficult to do in a small practice than in a practice owned by a hospital or organization. Another option is to put all pharmacy revenues into a charitable program supporting indigent care, research, or education.

▰▰▰▰ PRACTICES ASSOCIATED WITH A HOSPITAL OR OTHER ORGANIZATION

In my consulting and speaking engagements, I find increasing interest in the development of alternative and integrative practices associated with hospitals or other large-scale organizations such as HMOs, universities, or large group practices. These health care businesses have noted the increasing public interest in alternative therapies and want to move into what they see as a growth sector in the health care market. Many are simply trying to provide additional options for their patients, to improve outcomes, and to create better relationships with their communities. As businesses, however, they need to reduce costs and increase income. They believe that adding alternative or integrative practices or components will help them compete, get market differentiation, and be seen by potential patients as progressive, sensitive, and adaptive to patient demand.

This trend has both benefits and drawbacks for patients and for the field of alternative health care. On the positive side, these organizations bring to the table resources, public confidence, management expertise, and existing successful programs. On the negative side, the whole project can fall apart or never get off the ground unless there is an institutional commitment to change and innovation, a capable and dynamic staff of professionals trained in alternative care, and an overview of truly integrative care.

An organization wishing to develop an integrative care program has to overcome not only hurdles of adequate long-term reimbursement, but also initial resistance from some within the administration and staff who may not believe in the principles of integrative care. This resistance may be philosophical or may come from a real concern that resources invested in the new program will be diverted from other programs. Support for the program must come from the highest levels within the organization. In addition, any new program needs a solid business plan, including clear-cut goals and objectives. It must have a well-thought-out budget that projects the amount of time until the center is self-supporting. All revenue sources must be defined, whether from patients through self-pay or insurance, from foundation or other extramural support, from new-program development funds within the organization, or from some combination of these sources.

One of the easiest paths to success is to bring alternative and integrative therapies into existing programs to make them more humanistic and holistic. For example, imaging and relaxation therapy can be used to reduce anxiety before cardiovascular surgery, or practitioners of therapeutic touch or acupuncture and mind-body experts can be added to a pain management clinic. How about adding spirituality and mind-body programs to oncology and hospice–palliative care services? Another possibility is to bring massage and manipulative therapies into a center for chronic low back pain. Mind-body centers have been set up as part of symptom-reduction programs for patients with cardiovascular disease and other chronic illnesses. Bringing alternative practitioners into quality-improvement programs, research and experimental projects, and continuing education is another way to incorporate alternative and integrative practice concepts and providers into an organization that wants to move into this field, whether slowly or quickly.

Working in this way with an existing service allows the practitioners to get experience caring for patients within the large hospital or other organizational system. It also tells patients that the organization is seeking to care for them in innovative ways. It allows those who are resistant to see the new approaches in an incremental and nonthreatening fashion. And it gives time to educate the entire staff about this different approach and allows cultural change to occur gradually.

On the other hand, many organizations seek to set up an identifiable alternative or integrative clinic. To be successful, the new clinic will require a higher level of administrative, budgetary, and political support. A team must be built by a visionary leader, probably a physician skilled in both conventional and alternative therapies as well as administration and business (though this leader could equally well be a gifted holistic nurse). The choice of what therapies to include, the physical location and environment, the referral network, staffing, marketing, medical records development, and other practical matters must proceed in parallel with an overall philosophy of integrative practice. The center probably should be small to begin with, to avoid creating a large budgetary strain. It may consist of two or three physicians and nurses in a close working relationship. Alternative providers can be contracted to work on an incentive basis and come to the clinic as needed. Alternatively, a network of referrals can be developed and treatment given in satellite offices. This network model requires stringent attention to credentialing issues, team building, licensure, insurance, and the development of protocols to ensure quality of care.

Chapter 8

Continuing Education in Integrative Health Care

There is a time in every man's education when he ar-
rives at the conviction that envy is ignorance; that
imitation is suicide; that he must take himself for
better or worse as his portion; that though the wide
universe is full of good, no kernel of nourishing
corn can come to him but through his toil bestowed
on that plot of ground which is given to him to till.
— Ralph Waldo Emerson

Education is learning what you didn't even know you
didn't know.
— Daniel Boorstin

To offer integrative care requires the acquisition, cultivation, and development of knowledge, skills, and attitudes unique to alternative therapies. How do conventionally trained physicians, nurses, mid-level practitioners, and other team members acquire this additional information?

▬▬▬ READING

This book was written to introduce students in health care to the overall concepts, principles, and tools of integrative care. One expert in this area has estimated that about 30 hours of reading will give most health care providers an initial overview of the field (Gordon 1996). But this initial investment in time is unlikely to provide mastery of any of the major fields such as acupuncture, herbalism, or mind-body therapies. Such a short course of reading (this book, for instance) can provide the necessary foundation of terminology and concepts to enable the professional to speak intelligently with patients and apply some alternative therapies, and can serve as a catalyst for further learning. Many other excellent resources are listed in the Appendix.

A more focused approach is to do a short course of self-study and reading in the field of naturopathic medicine (Murray & Pizzorno 1998; Pizzorno & Murray 1999). This single effort will provide skills, knowledge, and attitudes regarding many helpful approaches such as supplements, herbs, lifestyle, and diet, and will provide a coherent framework for integrative care.

COURSES

Currently over two-thirds of U.S. medical schools and many nursing and mid-level programs offer either required or elective courses in the concepts of alternative therapy (Wetzel et al 1999, Gaudet 1998). These vary greatly in content, depending on their faculty, and are organized in various ways. They include 1-month electives, a series of special lectures, segments within required courses, journal clubs, seminars, reading electives, field visits to alternative practitioners, critical-thinking courses with alternative therapies as the topic, and student-interest groups who bring in guest lecturers on alternative therapies. Graduate programs in research methodologies in alternative therapies are offered at some nursing schools. Other options include electives or even required segments in many residency programs, and an innovative 2-year fellowship in integrative medicine. Many nursing programs include courses on principles of healing, the therapeutic relationship, therapeutic touch, energy medicine, spiritual dimensions of healing, and other alternative topics within their undergraduate and graduate programs.

CONFERENCES

One of the residents taking our elective in alternative and integrative care expressed an interest in going to a conference on the topic. I was surprised when she admitted that she didn't even know if there were such conferences or how she could find them. They just were not advertised in the standard medical journals she read. Of course, there are many annual conferences such as Columbia's course on botanical medicine, Harvard's alternative medicine clinical course, Dr. Larry Dossey's annual symposium, and the annual conferences of the Holistic Medicine and Holistic Nursing Associations, to name just a few. These conferences can help interested students or practitioners learn new skills; network with like-minded professionals; and be exposed to books, commercial products, and other resources in the field. Finding out about them is as easy as subscribing to one of the journals noted in the Appendix, such as Larry Dossey's *Alternative Therapies in Health and Medicine* or Andrew Weil's *Integrative Medicine.* Both of these provide a calendar of upcoming conferences and continuing education in the field. Once you get on the mailing lists of a few conferences, you will get information on many more.

More continuing education opportunities are offered every year by nationally known providers of traditional continuing education or are included as lectures or workshops within conventional programs. Hospital staffs, medical societies, and nurse practitioner or physician assistant groups have recognized that their members are interested in and need information on alternative and integrative therapy, so they often include relevant speakers and topics on their educational agendas.

ELECTRONIC RESOURCES

Internet sites related to alternative therapy abound. The greatest struggle is to sort out the sites providing quality information from those that are merely advocating products, services, and other commercial opportunities. In fact, one of our greatest challenges is to help our patients who use the Internet to become selective about the information they obtain. Most websites developed by professional, educational, and patient-support groups and by governmental entities are reliable sources of basic information, although they may not provide all the answers a provider or patient may seek. Our Alternative and Integrative Health Care Program website at the University of Texas Medical Branch (http://atc.utmb.edu/altmed) has reviews by our faculty to help rate the quality of websites. It also has information on curriculum, the Alternative and Integrative Therapies Journal Club, and other topics of interest in the field.

Some excellent databases, such as *HealthNotes Online*, are available in CD-ROM or Web-enabled format. This application is one I have found enormously useful in my own clinical practice, research, teaching, and speaking. It is written for the professional as well as the lay public, and I commonly print off a topic or two for patients to take home and read when they inquire about alternatives to conventional therapy or integrative approaches.

Excellent sites are listed in the Appendix and I am sure you will find some new ones. I like Dr. Andrew Weil's website (http://www.drweil.com), which includes an excellent searchable archive for answers to common questions and hot topics. I either bookmark it or keep it as my homepage. I find the information to be timely and relevant, although not always as research based as my professional colleagues would like. Online, for-credit curricula in such areas as herbal medicine are now available; for instance, the joint program designed by the Texas Medical Association and the American Botanical Council. I expect more of this kind of online learning in the future.

▰▰▰ SPECIAL SKILLS TRAINING

Beyond reading and participating in some general conferences, how can one learn the modalities of integrative health care in more depth? Certainly, including an alternative practitioner on your health care team or within your clinic is an opportunity for collaboration, and through the process of referral and co-management of patients you will learn the benefits, indications, and something about the techniques of a modality.

To learn a modality in-depth will require a longer commitment. Extended courses are available through classroom work, correspondence programs, or a combination. A physician colleague of mine recently enrolled in a naturopathic program conducted by mail. This program will allow him to learn many of the principles and practices of naturopathic medicine, including some aspects of homeopathy. He will be able to pace his learning to his own time availability and to spend less time away from his practice. Likewise, UCLA set up a course, "Medical Acupuncture for Physicians," designed to allow practicing physicians to learn acupuncture without taking a large block of time away from practice. An initial introductory weekend is offered, preceded by a set of readings. Then, more than 100 hours of videotaped lectures and demonstrations are shipped to the student, who can review them at home over a period of months. Finally, another hands-on session of about 2 weeks finishes up the training.

Similar programs are available in shorter or longer blocks in such fields as Ayurveda, energy medicine, herbalism, homeopathy, Reiki, nutritional therapy, mind-body therapy, yoga, meditation, movement therapy, and hypnosis. Some offer certifications or other diplomas of completion, although these may not be necessary or sufficient to practice in your state or under the existing practice acts. Investigate the rules and regulations of your state licensing board before taking training or adding a new modality to your practice. Certification tends to be less of a problem for physicians and nurses than for other types of practitioners, but everyone should consider it, because states vary in their requirements.

CHOOSING THE THERAPIES TO STUDY

How do you choose what to study in-depth from so many topics? Start by studying the modalities you are most interested in and the ones that you believe will best fit into your present or future practice. Every practice will benefit from enhancing skills in nutritional therapy, herbal medicine, and mind-body therapies. Practices are different, and the skills needed to treat an underserved urban population versus an upscale, highly educated, suburban community will vary enormously. Insurance coverage, cost of services or supplements, and the availability and affordability of group sessions all will affect the type of therapies you may choose to study and offer in your practice.

When choosing educational opportunities, look for known faculty in long-standing, well-developed programs; those that cover the best-evidenced modalities; and programs associated with well-respected professional or educational organizations. Further, in selecting the program, consider your budget, including both time and money (not only the actual expenses but also the loss of income while you are away from your practice).

Many courses have overlapping goals, which include personal growth and development along with learning a specific set of skills. For example, a program in journaling or music therapy can help you bring new skills to your practice and also will help in your own personal growth and transformation by encouraging attention to your inner realms. In fact, such learning is often the most effective because you will integrate the knowledge at a deeper, personal level. It is easier to recommend a therapeutic approach to a patient when you have used it effectively yourself. Experiential learning contributes to self-care as well as role modeling for your patients. Inner growth is an important aspect of continuing to provide quality integrative therapy over the years of practice.

A clinical practice that uses principles of integrative care must include ongoing staff training and education. As the integrative health care team develops and grows, patient needs and interests become more clear, and you find out what works and what doesn't work. Ongoing courses, offered either on-site, off-site, or on line, will help to expand services, improve skills in the services already offered, and refresh and re-energize the health care providers and staff.

Section
IV

Specific Therapies

Nothing is particularly hard if you divide it into small jobs.

—Henry Ford

The man who removes a mountain begins by carrying away small stones.

—Chinese proverb

This section is an introduction to the major categories of alternative therapies. It contains a wealth of background and specific information on when and how to integrate the various types of therapies into your clinical practice and your personal health care plan.

The chapters on *Herbals, Diet and Nutrition, Nutriceuticals,* and *Mind-Body Medicine* discuss these areas in some depth. The broad fields of *Alternative Systems of Care, Pharmacological and Biological Treatments, Bioelectromagnetic Therapies,* and *Hands-On Healing Techniques* are covered in more succinct summaries. Taken together these chapters provide the building blocks of a future integrative practice. Even if you know nothing about any of these therapies when you begin reading this section, you will walk away with an overview of most of the alternative therapies being practiced in this country today. And you will have in your hand tables, cases, references, and other types of information that tell you how to use these therapies to manage a wide variety of conditions.

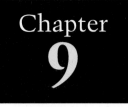

Chapter 9

Alternative Systems of Care

Study the past if you would divine the future.
> —Confucius

One must become humble as the dust before he can discover truth.
> —Mahatma Gandhi

If a man be gracious to strangers, it shows that he is a citizen of the world, and his heart is no island, cut off from other islands, but a continent that joins them.
> —Francis Bacon

Usually, when we talk about alternative systems of medical care, we are referring to culturally or scientifically defined systems different from our own. There are hundreds, perhaps thousands, of indigenous practices ranging from African and Caribbean folk healing to the practices of Amazonian rainforest shamans; many alternative systems in our own culture are based on unconventional scientific premises. I will cover here the most common examples, which in the United States are Ayurvedic medicine, originating in India; traditional Chinese medicine; Native American healing; *curanderismo*, or Hispanic folk medicine; homeopathy; and naturopathy.

▰▰▰ AYURVEDA

Based on traditional concepts of medicine as practiced in India, Ayurveda has been popularized in this country by Deepak Chopra, MD; Rudolph Ballentine, MD; Vasant Lad, MD; and Maharishi Mahesh Yogi. (See Chopra 1990 and 1993 and Ballentine 1999 to read further.) It is based on an 8000-year-old system from India that involves mind-body techniques such as yoga and meditative practices. It also stresses the use of proper nutrition, herbal medicine, massage, and a variety of beliefs and practices arising from Hinduism. In 1985, I spent a summer studying Ayurveda with the Maharishi's International University in Fairfield, Iowa. At that time, the Maharishi, who had made a big impact (and lots of money) teaching Transcendental Meditation (TM) around the world, was starting a series of clinics fostering Ayurvedic medicine. Dr. Deepak Chopra was one of our teachers and the medical director.

Like Chinese medicine, Ayurveda uses a system based on five elements. These exist throughout the universe, nature, and our bodies: fire, air, earth, water, and ether. These words sounded strangely out of place in today's world. Nonetheless, having paid dearly and having committed myself to being sequestered in a university filled with vegetarians and meditators for an extended period, I suspended my disbelief. I learned that these elements combined to form the three basic body types in Ayurvedic classification. These congruencies and forces are called the *three doshas—vata, pitta,* and *kapha.* They are a mixture of the elements: vata from ether and air, pitta from fire and water, and kapha from earth and water.

The three doshas, or tridosha, are used in diagnosing and treating patients in this system. Body type, pulse reading, and metabolism give the Ayurvedic practitioner a picture of the person, called a *prakriti.* This is the particular nature one has inherited. Harmonizing this nature with the doshas stimulates the process of improving one's health in the Ayurvedic program using various means such as herbalized massages, diet changes, herbs, meditative practices, breathing exercises, yoga, and detoxification treatments.

One particularly pleasurable aspect of my experience was the panchakarma treatment. After an Ayurvedic practitioner had determined that my dosha was pitta with a few imbalances, I was subjected to an exquisite massage of warm oil, specially formulated for my individualized diagnosis, prakriti, and dosha combination. Two masseurs poured warm, herbalized oil by the gallon over me for an hour and a half or more while I was lying on a special massage table that collected the oil into a pan for recycling. When I left the treatment, I felt as relaxed as Gumby after a sauna. My legs were like rubber, my mind in a heightened state of awareness, and I was in a blissful state of total physical and mental relaxation.

Individualization of Ayurvedic Therapy

A key aspect of this system is that each person's therapy is individualized based on his or her constitution and dosha configuration. The Ayurvedic practitioner asks, "Who is the patient?" rather than the Western diagnostic question of, "What disease does the patient have?"

Vata

The key feature of vata is *changeability.* Vata types are active, energetic, and thin. If we can use a metaphor from the canine world, the vata type is like a chihuahua. Problems that can occur include weight loss, anxiety, and emotional upset causing loss of appetite. Medical conditions that vata types are prone to include hypertension, insomnia, premenstrual syndrome, constipation, and restlessness.

Lighter exercise such as yoga, light dancing or cycling, easy paced tennis, and walking are all appropriate for these people, who tend to be overactive anyway. Certain foods that are warm and nourishing and grounding are helpful to this dosha. Relationships that are healthy for vata provide safety, reassurance, and stability to offset their proneness to anxiety.

Pitta

The key feature of pitta is *intensity.* Pitta types are of medium build, strong, and with good endurance. If this type were a dog, it would be a boxer. They tend to have a fair complexion, good digestion, and quick wit, and they are passionate, though sometimes prone to being argumentative, irritable, or angry. Skin and stomach problems, hemorrhoids, ulcers, and excess anger characterize medical conditions of this dosha.

Pittas tend to become overweight as they age, because they rely on youthful excellent digestion. They need to avoid spicy, sour, or salty foods, which overstimulate the appetite, and they also should avoid alcohol. Cooling foods are preferred. In good health, they have a lustrous complexion, a good intellect, excellent digestive abilities, and are in a state of contentment.

Exercise for these people needs to be active, such as skiing, mountain climbing, brisk walking or jogging, and swimming. Relational health should address their tendency toward resentment, self-criticism, and pride. It is important to avoid damaging the pride in relational disputes.

Kapha

The key feature of kapha is *relaxation.* The kapha type has a heavy, solid build, is strong, sleeps long and deeply, and tends to be slow to act and slow to anger. The canine counterpart of the kapha would be a large mastiff. Kapha types are prone to obesity, high cholesterol, sinus problems and allergies, asthma, and diabetes. Like the big, friendly dog, this type is affectionate, forgiving, and well-proportioned in a balanced state.

When unbalanced, however, they tend to eat compulsively without joy, procrastinate to excess, and become mentally dull and depressed. Active exercise, such as running, weight lifting, aerobics, dance, and rowing, is good for this type. They need to avoid sweets and rich foods and eat more salads, fruits, and vegetables. Because they tend to be shy, kapha types shine best in a relationship that praises their competence and is reassuring and supportive of their self-esteem. Kaphas often need to be brought out in conversation.

Integrative Use of Ayurveda

Ayurveda, or the "science of life," focuses on prevention and the treatment of the whole person as an individual. The diagnostic and therapeutic equation considers not only the physical but also the mental, spiritual, and psychological. Meditation, yoga, cleansing and detoxification treatments, and the evolution of consciousness are highly valued in this ancient healing art.

I consider a referral to an Ayurvedic practitioner based on patient preference and for many chronic diseases such as hypertension, addiction, and even cancer, where traditional Ayurvedic practices have been used for centuries. If I make such a referral, I want to be assured that the Ayurvedic practitioner will work with me to monitor the patient's progress, blood pressure, medications, and so forth.

Ayurvedic treatment often involves a number of major lifestyle changes, which may account for much of its success. The major studies that have been published about Ayurveda are mainly limited to an examination of the herbal remedies used and some of the meditative and yoga practices. These results are mostly encouraging and suggest we should look further into using this ancient healing art in our integrative approach.

▬▬▬ TRADITIONAL CHINESE MEDICINE

The way that can be told is not the eternal Way.
—Lao Tsu

As ancient as the Ayurvedic system, Chinese medicine has likewise existed for millennia. Using the metaphors of the five elements—fire, earth, metal, water, and wood—it is based on an apparently simple yet amazingly sophisticated system.

The first thing to realize when studying traditional Chinese medicine (TCM) is that you must be willing to enter a new paradigm of thinking, which includes new terminology. I remind my students of the old Chinese proverb that "a journey of a thousand miles begins with a single step." In fact, the journey to start the study of TCM starts with more than a step. It starts with a somersault! The worldview, language, and concepts more or less turn the world upside down from our usual way of thinking and conceptualizing. The concepts of paradox, polarity, something that both is and is not at the same time are quite foreign to ordinary Western thinking and require a major adjustment in our frame of reference. Let's take a spin.

Yin and Yang

Besides the five elements, the keys to the TCM are Yin and Yang and Qi (chee). No doubt, you have seen the symbol of the Yin and Yang, the two fishes, one white, one black, spinning in a perpetual circle (Figure 9–1). All of Chinese medicine centers on the balance between Yin and Yang. Health and disease result from an imbalance of these two elemental factors.

Yin refers to the feminine aspect of life. Yang is the counterbalancing male element. Beyond these general polarities are the differentiations of the passive and active elements of the universe. Yin literally means the shady side of the hill. Yang is the sunny side of the hill. Some of the characteristics of Yin and Yang are listed in the box.

In my undergraduate years I participated in a field experiment in which we mapped the plants and terrain of two sides of a small Arizona desert valley. To the untrained eye, the desert looked the same on the south- and north-facing slopes, which were less than 20 yards apart. Besides the rocks, sand, and so forth, there were about 20 different kinds of plants—sparse, hardy, spiny types ruggedly adapted to a climate with less than 10 inches of rain per year. Like the Chinese concepts of Yin and Yang, however, we found that even in the very tiny microclimate of this desert valley, the two sides of the hill were dramatically different. The north-facing (Yin) slope had a much higher density of plants than the south-facing slope. The south-facing (Yang) slope was subjected to the maximum intensity of the hot sun all year round. The little moisture that was available evaporated more quickly than on the Yin

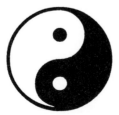

Figure 9–1   The symbol of Yin and Yang, which represents the balance between elemental factors in traditional Chinese medicine. The dark "fish" symbolizes Yin and the white "fish" symbolizes Yang.

SOME CHARACTERISTICS OF YIN AND YANG

YIN	YANG
Negative	**Positive**
Feminine	Masculine
Nourishing	Protective
Lower	Upper
Cool	Hot
Deficient	Excessive
Inside	Outside
Receptive	Creative

slope. Although they were only a few feet separated, the ecology of the two slopes was entirely different.

The ancients in China were keen observers of subtle differences in nature. In an agrarian culture, their livelihood depended on their awareness of small variations in natural patterns. They translated this essential life skill to their understanding of medicine. Each person was a composite of Yin and Yang, passive and active elements, and as in nature, summer and winter were needed to create spring and autumn. The cold and stillness of winter prepare to allow the burst of springtime. In turn, summer evolves with a flourishing of crops and growth, leading to the fall with its abundant harvest.

In the Chinese cosmology, human life is not separated from nature, as it often is in our Western worldview. Instead, life and health are seen as inextricably and intimately tied up with nature in all of its aspects.

Qi

In addition to the Yin and Yang polarities, another important notion in TCM is that of *Qi*. What is Qi? This term is best translated as "vital energy" or "life force." An ancient Chinese philosopher tried to describe Qi by telling the story of a recently deceased sow pig. Her eight piglets continued to suckle hungrily. Suddenly, they looked up en masse, realized that her life force or Qi was gone, and ran off.

Despite our highly refined science and measurements of physiological function, we have no measurement of this vital energy or life force.

But anyone who cares for others is clearly aware of the difference between its presence or absence. The "will to live" is clearly a thin line between survival and death in our patients. We cannot measure it, find it, or even describe it, but the Chinese have defined it for centuries as Qi.

According to Chinese medical theory, this energy flows in patterns or channels referred to as *meridians*. These are like underground rivers, carrying the ceaseless flow of the Qi throughout the body. Like irrigation channels, they flow into all parts of the body to nourish, support, protect, and bring health and healing.

Diagnostic Methods

In TCM, a balance in Qi results in health, longevity, and well-being. An imbalance results in pain, disability, degeneration, and ill health. Diagnosis is made by the four examinations: asking, looking, feeling, and smelling. An interesting dimension of the history of TCM is that male physicians (and all Chinese physicians were males in the obscure mists of historical times) were not permitted to examine female patients directly. Instead of relying on a physical exam, a female attendant would show the doctor pins stuck into a doll at the sites of her mistress's pain and discomfort. The fair lady would sit behind a screen and pass her delicate hand through an opening in a curtain, laying it on a silk pillow. The doctor would carefully palpate the pulse, observe the face and tongue, listen to the history, and make a diagnosis. Even today, examination of the pulse, tongue, and facial appearance is essential to the diagnostic process in Chinese medicine.

The sound of the voice and preferences for tastes, colors, and seasons are all essential to the diagnosis. The system of five elements, also referred to as five phases or five correspondences, is shown in Table 9–1 to demonstrate the various dimensions considered in a TCM exam. The ancient Chinese were by nature very conservative, probably a habit resulting from their sometimes harsh and grueling agricultural life. Nothing was discarded, including any data or observation about the human body or the human experience. As a result, many things that we discard as irrelevant to medical history taking are considered valuable in TCM. As Table 9–1 shows, preferences for color, flavor, and time of day or year are all parts of the diagnostic system.

Treatment

Imbalances in the Qi or Yin and Yang are treated through a variety of methods. One of the best known is acupuncture, in which small needles are inserted into a variety of points along the body's meridians. An

Table 9–1 THE FIVE ELEMENTS OF TRADITIONAL CHINESE MEDICINE

Correspondence Systems	Five Phases				
CARDINAL DIRECTION	**East**	**South**	**Center**	**West**	**North**
ELEMENT	**Wood**	**Fire**	**Earth**	**Metal**	**Water**
Season	Spring	Summer	Harvest	Autumn	Winter
Yin organ (Zang)	Liver	Heart	Spleen	Lung	Kidney
Yang organ (Fu)	Gall bladder	Small intestine	Stomach	Large intestine	Bladder
Color affinity	Liver: blue; Gall bladder: green	Red	Yellow, earth tones	White	Black, dark blue
Flavor preference	Sour, citrus, acid	Bitter, roasted	Sweet	Flavorful, spicy, piquant	Salty
Voice timbre	Shouting	Laughing	Singing	Weeping, sobbing	Moaning, groaning
Psychological characteristic	Anxiety, irritability (Hun)	Joy, creative thinking (Shen)	Thought, introspection (Yi)	Sadness, grief (Po)	Will, ambition, fright (Zhi)
Sensory function	Vision	Taste	Touch	Olfaction	Audition, balance

Source: Helms, J: Acupuncture Energetics. Berkeley, CA: Medical Acupuncture Publishers, 1995:217 (with permission).

imbalance in Qi can be restored by the needles, which are thought to somehow release, unblock, or rebalance the disturbed energy patterns.

The mechanism by which acupuncture needles work is still poorly understood by Western scientists. Release of endorphins, hormones, and various cytokines have been linked to acupuncture's effects. These kinds of explanations are more acceptable to the Western mind than notions of Qi and vital energy.

Nonetheless, the National Institutes of Health (NIH) has released a consensus statement recognizing the beneficial effect of acupuncture on many conditions, based on evidence of efficacy from clinical trials. The NIH panel found particularly strong evidence for the efficacy of acupuncture for nausea induced by anesthesia, pregnancy, or chemotherapy, and for dental pain. A number of other conditions were listed for which acupuncture is "probably effective": stroke rehabilitation, addiction, headache, menstrual cramps, carpal tunnel syndrome, epicondylitis, asthma, and pain. Its usefulness for these conditions is undisputed by acupuncturists, but the quality of the scientific studies was not adequate for the NIH to make a conclusive statement. Of course, studying acupuncture in randomized, controlled, double-blind studies is methodologically difficult, as you might imagine.

Herbal therapeutics is particularly well developed and sophisticated among practitioners of TCM. A blend of 3 to 15 herbs is used to cool, heat, stimulate, sedate, and otherwise balance the system. A form of massage known as *Tui Na* or *An-Mo* is used to release energy and to effect relaxation. Dietary modifications are important in this system, as are exercises such as the martial arts of *Tai Chi* and *Qi Gong*. These exercises stimulate energy flow, heal imbalances, and reduce stress. Coupled with synchronous deep breathing, postural movements, and meditations, they are thought to be a complete system of fitness.

Prevention First

The Chinese medical practitioner of old was paid only when his patient was well. As soon as the patient became ill, payments were stopped. This was perhaps the earliest form of prepaid health insurance! Because of this interesting economic arrangement, the physician was prompted to keep the patient well, and preventive medicine was stressed.

Consequently, the physician would see the patient regularly, usually when the seasons changed. The physician would take a history and use the other traditional diagnostic methods I've described, including looking, feeling, and smelling, especially looking at the tongue and feeling the pulse, to make a diagnosis. Then, using the system of the five elements (see Table 9–1), the physician would determine what adjustments might be necessary to maintain health. It was said that the superior physician would treat a disease *before* it occurred, whereas the inferior physician, like a man who started to dig a well when he became thirsty, would treat a disease *after* it occurred. Acupuncture, herbs, exercise, massage, or diet would be prescribed to the patient as dictated by the examination, even if the patient had not yet developed a complaint.

Indications for Referral and Treatment Using TCM

TCM is particularly useful for chronic problems such as back pain and other musculoskeletal pain, arthritis, ulcers and other gastrointestinal problems, headaches, nausea (including the nausea of pregnancy and that due to chemotherapy or anesthetics), dental pain, chronic fatigue, and other conditions often not responsive to standard Western medical therapy.

In most modern medical practices, acupuncture is most often used or recommended for pain. Having studied and practiced acupuncture for over 15 years, however, I find it useful for a wide array of conditions. My daily practice includes administering acupuncture to treat back and neck pain; arthritis; headache; neuritis, sciatica, carpal tunnel syndrome, and other kinds of neuropathy; musculoskeletal indications such as tennis elbow, plantar fasciitis, tendinitis, and knee pain; fibromyalgia; nausea; irritable bowel syndrome; and chronic fatigue syndrome. These are the most common and helpful applications of acupuncture I have found, but many skilled acupuncturists and TCM practitioners can do much, much more.

TCM practitioners more typically use herbal therapy plus acupuncture rather than acupuncture alone. Most states regulate and license these practitioners, who may study for up to 4 years. It is important that the TCM practitioner to whom you refer patients be able to communicate with them in a way that is understandable regardless of the patient's ancestry. Acceptance and open-mindedness on both sides are necessary to allow the therapeutic relationship to evolve and bridge the cultural gap between the practice of TCM and the patient who is used to a Western medical approach.

As a system of healing that has existed for thousands of years, TCM deserves our deepest respect and admiration. The approach to the patient is truly holistic and involves humility in the face of the challenge of deeply knowing another person and his or her problem. It is also spiritual in the sense that TCM encourages us to see the other person through the mind's eye or the spirit (*shen*) rather than just through the physical eye. And it emphasizes the prevention of disease as a superior form of medicine. Many conditions that either do not respond to conventional Western medicine or are not well characterized by our standard diagnostic terminology and methods may be successfully approached by this ancient system of healing. (See Eisenberg 1987, Filshie 1998, Helms 1995, Kaptchuck 1983, and Micozzi 1996 to read further.)

▬▬▬ NATIVE AMERICAN HEALING

The Native Americans traditionally lived in close intimacy with nature. They held—and many still believe to this day—that there is a close connection between man and his environment, that all living things are sacred, and that life forces or deities inhabit every plant, animal, stone, and so forth. The indigenous peoples of both North and South America were master herbalists and had medicine men or shamans who served as healers in their cultures. These healers were very comfortable in both the physical world and the spiritual world. They saw illness as an imbalance in the relationship between the two worlds and often entered into trances and other altered states as part of the healing ritual.

Besides smoking sage and a mild species of tobacco, the shamanistic healers often used hallucinogenic substances such as ayahuasca, peyote, mescaline, and ebena snuff, which induced trance states that the healers used to increase their contact with the spirit world, not for mere personal pleasure. In these states, they would attempt to diagnose, treat, and transform their patients. The healing might involve "recovering the soul," which was thought to be somehow lost through illness.

Their support for these healing rituals involved not just the individual patient but also the community. The beliefs, expectations, and prayers of one's neighbors were often part of the healing process. The rituals of dancing, drumming, singing, chanting, and so on were all a part of the shared experience of the community, which contributed to healing encounters.

Native healers still exist in many parts of the Americas, from reservation to rainforest. They are excellent pharmacologists and toxicologists, knowing the benefits of many local plants. The accelerating loss of cultures and environments has put this knowledge in danger of being lost, however. The study of their work by ethnobotanists, anthropologists, and others is essential because it not only provides rich opportunities for cultural awareness but also hints about plants that are potentially useful for pharmacological purposes.

In some indigenous American societies, the medicine man or woman is still an important part of the healing culture and often deals with primary care problems. Recently I met a nurse who told me about her experiences as a paramedic on an ambulance crew near Albuquerque, New Mexico. Around that modern city are several Native

American reservations. When an ambulance was called out, the native healer was also notified. Before the ambulance crew was permitted to begin work, the healer performed a purification or other healing ritual on the afflicted person. She didn't tell me of a specific incident in which the native ritual had critically delayed conventional care, but clearly it was a major concern to the ambulance crew. On the other hand, someone with the high stress level, elevated circulating catecholamines, and pulse and blood pressure changes that accompany a myocardial infarction, for instance, might well be calmed and relieved by the presence of a comforting and trusted local healer and the gentle rituals of smoke and chant. Contrast that with being rushed into a brightly lit ambulance with radios, sirens, and flashing lights, the kind of climate you would expect to *raise* stress levels rather than lower them. The ritual allowed the person to make a transition between the traditional, known world and the foreign, unknown one. My hypothesis, which seems to me to be worthy of study, is that the few minutes of calming ritual might do much to preserve that patient's myocardium and improve the benefit of the usual oxygen, aspirin, nitroglycerin, and morphine.

Of course, one can rely too much on these rituals. I recall a man who needed hospitalization after his pneumonia was ministered to for several days with burning sage, drumming, and prayer chants. Another man I cared for was found unconscious and incontinent of feces after too long a session in the sweat lodge. Both of these men were non-Native Americans, however, who had poor understanding of the context and the power and spirit of these ancient rituals.

Patients often self-refer for therapy by this kind of healer. If you are familiar with a skilled medicine man or shaman in your community, building a collaborative relationship may help you care for your mutual patients.

Little formal research into these therapies has been done; much is needed. I can think of many fascinating questions that can be asked and studied in the context of traditional Navajo healing or other practices. The rituals of sand-painting, the sweat lodge, and the sacred journey all speak to a healing that goes beyond the physical and into the deeper, spiritual layers of being. Mehl-Madrona (1999) presents a nice review of this topic.

▬▬▬ *CURANDERISMO*

Practiced in the Hispanic culture by folk healers, this widely popular system incorporates herbalism, spiritualism, mysticism, energy medicine, and a mix of Native American and Spanish cultural beliefs. The primary aspect of this system is its association with faith healing. An encounter with a *curandera* or *curandero* (female or male folk healer) is likely to involve candles, pictures of Jesus and the saints, and other religious trappings.

If you practice in the U.S. Southwest or in an urban community with a large Hispanic population, you should be aware of the power of this parallel health system. The curandera (most are female) may be giving advice that supports, interacts with, or contradicts your standard therapies. On the other hand, employing the power of the curandera in the community is a way to improve communication, compliance, and follow-up. For instance, one recent Hispanic graduate of our family medicine program told me about the relationship of her father, a cardiologist who works mainly among Hispanics, and his mother, a curandera. They often collaborate. When a case seems to require it (often it involves some psychological, emotional, or spiritual issue), he refers the patient to the curandera, who frequently obtains an effect beyond the ability of modern medicine. On the other hand, the curandera can sense when a purely physical problem, such as unstable angina, is out of her realm and sends the patient to her son, the cardiologist. It's all in the family but is a beautiful example of integrative medicine addressing the special needs and cultural issues of a population.

Beliefs common to curanderismo include *empacho*, a blocked bowel; *mal de ojo*, the evil eye; the *caida mollera*, or sunken fontanelle; and the *susto*, a frightening event that causes an illness. Treatments include placing an egg under the bed, casting out spirits, and sucking on the fontanelle. In addition, curanderas often administer herbs that have been used in this culture for many generations, do brushings with their hands to eliminate energy blockages, offer prayers and incantations, and light candles.

Sometimes the curandera may recommend treatments that contradict conventional advice. Herbs or mixtures of herbs may interact with medications. If the curandera does not trust the health care system, the patient may come to your office but entirely ignore the treatments you recommend. For this reason, a collaborative model is best.

One Hispanic professor of medicine gave the following perspective on the role of curanderismo: "A poor Hispanic will go to the curandera when sick and to the doctor when desperate. A rich Hispanic will go to the doctor when sick and to the curandera when desperate!" This tongue-in-cheek description is not entirely accurate, but it does highlight the sacred and central role that the system plays in the life of the Hispanic community, in their consciousness, and in their health care. Combining the use of herbs and other traditional Hispanic treatments with conventional medical care is quite common, especially among the elderly. (See Micozzi 1996, pp. 259–277, for more detail.)

■■■■■ HOMEOPATHY

A common disparaging remark about a dose of medication is that it is a "homeopathic dose." This comment usually means that the dose of the active medication was too low to have any real effect. In fact, homeopathy is an entire system of medicine. The term *homeo* means "like," and the central concept of homeopathy is that "like cures like."

This system of healing was developed by Samuel Hahnemann, a German physician in the 19th century. He believed that low doses of a substance would effect a cure. His theory of "like treats like" says that if the administration of a substance causes a certain effect (such as ipecac syrup causing vomiting), the same substance can be employed in extremely minute doses to treat the same condition. This bimodal effect is contrary to contemporary theories in physics and chemistry but falls under the concept of energy medicine, which will be discussed later in this book.

For example, to treat vomiting, some ipecac is placed in a 1:10 dilution of water (on the decimal scale, written "1X"). It is then shaken, or "succussed," rediluted to 1:100 (on a centesimal scale, this is written "1C"), succussed again, and diluted again and again (2X, 3X, 4X, or 2C, 3C, 4C) and on up as desired. Depending on the potency wanted, it can be diluted to below Avogadro's number of molecules. For you chemistry buffs, this essentially means there is no ipecac left in the homeopathic dilution after about 12C (see the following) dilution. Nonetheless, the homeopath administers this remedy for the successful treatment of nausea and vomiting.

Paradoxically, in fact, the more dilute a substance is, the more potent it is thought to be, again contrary to intuition. The thought is that if a high dose of a substance is poisonous, a moderate dose can cause side effects or illness symptoms, but an extremely dilute dose can relieve the exact symptoms that it causes at higher doses. In clinical practice, any dilution may be used, but the most popular for self-care are the 6th, 12th, and 30th (X or C) (Jacobs 1999, Micozzi 1996). The "M" scale is 1:1000 and is used primarily in professional settings with even higher dilutions commonly prescribed. These are logarithmic notations: For example, 6X dilution is 10^{-6}, 200C dilution is 10^{-400}, and 1M is 10^{-2000}.

An example may be in order. A woman came to the homeopath asking him to see her husband. Their marriage was falling apart because of the husband's extreme jealousy and fits of rage. He would hardly let his wife out of his sight for fear that she was developing another relationship. At the least provocation, he had extreme bouts of anger accompanied by redness and flushing of the face, head, and neck. The homeopath interviewed him and found that he had had a rather dramatic change in his personality after an auto accident a few years before, in which his liver was injured. None of this behavior was present before the accident.

He also had developed an extreme craving for sour citrus fruit, eating up to six lemons or limes a day. After interviewing him at length, the homeopathic physician decided that the proper remedy was belladonna. In pharmacological doses, belladonna causes flushing, redness, and mental agitation. After taking the belladonna homeopathic extract for less than a week, the husband's rage and jealousy had abated, and his wife reported that he was back to his old self.

An anecdote like this by no means proves the effectiveness of homeopathy, but it does illustrate the power of a system of medicine that is outside our usual concepts of how things work. Some have said that a placebo response is the only way homeopathy could work. The homeopathic practitioner, who may be an MD, conducts an extremely long and detailed interview with new patients, often of 1-1/2 hours or longer. In addition to noting the usual complaints leading to a diagnosis, the unusual aspects of a personalized complaint are given great credence. The prolonged patient encounter may in some way be curative by itself, but trials of the remedies without the homeopathic interview have also shown effectiveness (Reilly et al 1986, Reilly 1997, Jacobs 1994). Meta-analyses of placebo-controlled trials (Linde et al 1997, Kleijnen et al 1991) found that homeopathic remedies, administered in a small lactose tablet about the size of a nitroglycerin tablet, were more effective than placebo for a number of conditions, including hay fever and asthma. More methodologically rigorous studies are clearly needed.

Homeopathy is widely accepted in England, in other parts of Europe, and in India, and is increasingly accepted in the United States despite its implausible mode of action. Even though highly diluted homeopathic substances have little or no active chemical content, it is thought that an energy "imprint" is left. One untested explanation is that homeopathic remedies leave a signal in the water and create unique patterns called "clathrates," which are like the patterns we see in snowflakes. I personally favor this idea of a retained energy pattern or memory of water left behind in the homeopathic formula when the original substance has been diluted out.

Mixtures of homeopathic compounds are commonly available at pharmacies and health food stores. Their safety is remarkable and the potential for benefit, as shown by tradition, history, and science, indicates that they have a rightful place in modern medicine. A colleague of mine, an MD classically trained in homeopathy, declared that *Arnica montana*, a homeopathic remedy for strains, sprains, and bruises, should be available in every emergency room. Such an approach seems safe enough to consider in acute injury.

The most common applications of homeopathy are in conditions such as allergies, asthma, colds, flu, headaches, digestive complaints, sprains, vertigo, skin problems, emotional disorders, and arthritis. Though off-the-shelf homeopathic remedies may have some value, the maximum benefit is obtained by a consultation with a well-trained, sensitive, and skilled homeopathic practitioner. Toxicity considerations are nonexistent because of the extremely low dosages of the active substance. Like many alternative systems, homeopathy stretches our concepts of science and healing, but it may offer substantial and safe benefit to our patients.

▬▬▬ NATUROPATHY

While in medical school, I had a quotation taped to my wall. It was spoken by my childhood hero, Thomas A. Edison, inventor of the light bulb. He said, "The doctor of the future will prescribe no medicine but will interest his patients in diet and exercise and the care of the human condition." Henry David Thoreau likewise captured the spirit and essence of naturopathy when he said, "Nature is doing her best each moment to make us well. She exists for no other end. Do not resist. With the least inclination to be well, we should not be sick."

Michael Murray and Joseph Pizzorno (Murray & Pizzorno 1998) have written extensively about naturopathy. To quote them:

Naturopathy is a system of medicine that focuses on prevention and the use of non-toxic, natural therapies.

Naturopathic medicine is based on seven principles:

1. First, do no harm (*primum no nocere*).
2. Nature has healing powers (*vis medicatrix naturae*).
3. Identify and treat the cause (*tolle causam*).
4. Treat the whole person.
5. The physician is a teacher.
6. Prevention is the best cure.
7. Establish health and wellness.

Having read this far, you will recognize that all of these principles are core to the integrative medicine of the whole person that we have been discussing.

Naturopathy draws from deep roots of healing wisdom based in several of the systems we have already discussed, such as Ayurveda and TCM, as well as the European tradition from the Greek Hippocrates. In general, naturopathic practitioners do not prescribe medication. Instead, therapies include clinical nutrition and nutritional supplements, botanical medicine, homeopathy, traditional Chinese medicines and acupuncture, hydrotherapy, physical medicine, counseling, and lifestyle modification.

Naturopathy is clearly eclectic, with a diversity of approaches and methods. Its unifying concept, however, is that it approaches the whole person with goals of wellness and prevention using gentle, natural therapies. This seems to make sense when you consider that a recent study showed that over 100,000 people died in U.S. hospitals in 1 year as a result of medication toxicity (Lazarou & Pomeranz 1998).

What I like best about naturopathy is its commonsense approach to problems. It builds on the "four cornerstones" of good health (Murray and Pizzorno 1998):

1. A positive mental attitude
2. A healthy lifestyle: exercise, sleep, and good health habits
3. A health-promoting diet
4. Supplementary measures such as nutritional supplements, vitamins, and minerals, and such physical modifications as breathing, posture, and bodywork, in addition to exercise

The naturopath integrates multiple therapies in supporting the natural tendency of the body to heal itself. Many of the therapies we discuss in this book, from herbs to supplements, are consistent with the naturopathic model of care. The in-depth studies done by naturopathic scholars into the biochemistry, physiology, and effects of natural substances such as vitamins, antioxidants, and botanicals sometimes leap from the lab into the clinic with less than full scientific support, yet by and large, they are safe and rational approaches.

Only a few states, about seven at last count, grant licensure to naturopathic doctors (NDs), and these practitioners have limited or no prescriptive authority in most states in which they are licensed. Because they do not have the option to give a drug in cases where conventionally trained physicians do, they keep the focus on lifestyle issues longer.

An example of a patient who might benefit from a naturopathic approach is Bill W., a 57-year-old man with known coronary artery disease. Bill is obese, with high cholesterol, a history of a myocardial infarction at age 55, and hypertension. Yet this 260-lb patient apparently had been doing some reading, and began asking a series of well-thought-out questions. Already receiving maximal medical therapy from the cardiologist for his vascular problems, he asked about the possibilities of taking antioxidants for his vascular health, along with ginkgo biloba for memory and circulation, and niacin to further lower his cholesterol. He also asked about a referral to a stress-management class. If we could have reached Bill about 20 years ago, a visit with a naturopathic practitioner would have included recommendations for a positive mental attitude; active exercise; a low-fat diet; supplements including antioxidants, vitamins, and flaxseed oil; and increased fresh fruit and vegetables. These changes would have been encouraged gradually and progressively. With proper coaching and support, Bill might have avoided having a myocardial infarction at age 55. Though both conventional and naturopathic methods will be helpful and necessary at this stage, Bill's treatment is now definitely not proactive or primary prevention but a reaction to already advanced disease.

Naturopathic physicians are not necessarily better at preventive education and motivation. But it is sometimes tempting to tell a patient like Bill to lose 20 lb, exercise 4 times/week, cut out the high-fat foods, quit smoking, reduce the sodium in his diet, and come back and see us in a few months when all those changes have taken place. This is a tremendous burden to place on a patient.

The naturopathic approach is often gentler, firmer, and more realistic. The naturopath would have suggested many of the same things, but the naturopath would have kept on working with the patient to achieve these simple, preventive changes. In conventional health care, we often pay lip service to the kinds of changes patients need to make to prevent later problems, but we give up in frustration when they don't make them. Then we give an antihypertensive or a lipid-lowering drug that patients must take for the rest of their lives.

Perhaps patients who choose to see naturopathic practitioners are self-selected. Maybe they are people who are highly motivated to make the kinds of lifestyle choices that will keep them healthy (our dream patient!). However, in a general primary care setting we take all comers regardless of motivation. But we often may find that encouraging the patient interested in a natural approach can be a helpful point of departure to making the major lifestyle changes needed to regain or maintain excellent health and wellness. Knowing some of the principles, techniques, and treatments of naturopathy can be helpful in this phase of the journey. It gives us one more set of options to pull out of our pocket besides the prescription pad. If conventionally trained health practitioners study naturopathy, it will provide a strong foundation for integrative care. Even a few dozen hours of reading will give you tools that last a lifetime.

Several excellent schools such as Bastyr University in Seattle train naturopathic physicians in a 4-year curriculum as rigorous and demanding as medical school. Some correspondence programs teaching naturopathy may not offer the high quality and clinical exposure needed to manage patients optimally, but some are of high caliber.

OTHER ALTERNATIVE SYSTEMS OF CARE

We might discuss literally hundreds of other systems of care. With so many cultures worldwide, native and local practices abound.

In the National Center for Complementary and Alternative Medicine (NCCAM) categorization, Alcoholics Anonymous is mentioned as a healing system for people whose lives are damaged by the consumption of alcohol. Many other 12-step programs exist for treatment of conditions from substance abuse and addictions to dysfunctional family problems and unhealthy personal practices such as overeating.

Environmental medicine focuses on toxic substances and allergens in food, air, water, and the environment as a cause of illness. The multiple chemical sensitivity syndrome and the sick building syndrome are two chronic conditions that cannot be explained by other theoretical systems and are addressed by this system.

Fields such as functional medicine, Cayce-based systems, and orthomolecular medicine are also included in the NCCAM listing as Unconventional Western Systems. Each of these has its own rich literature, practitioners, and adherents.

CONCLUSION

As you can see, there are many ways of looking at healing in the world. They originated in different times, in different cultures, and in response to different levels of medical need. Besides being culturally sensitive to various ethnic belief systems, the excellent integrative practitioner of the future will provide patient-centered care and will learn to work collaboratively with practitioners of alternative systems. Knowing the underlying beliefs, vocabulary, and methods of these systems gives you a diverse palette of methods to use with patients who, for various reasons, prefer to try another system of care. By cooperating with them, you retain their goodwill and improve the continuity and quality of care.

Finally, by the study and practice of some of these alternative systems, you broaden the options your professional practice can offer to patients. If you become competent in some aspect of an alternative system such as acupuncture, homeopathy, or naturopathy, you can adapt this type of care, integratively, into almost any conventional health-care practice.

Chapter 10 *Herbals*

The use of herbal or botanical medicinals for common ailments is one of the fastest growing areas in alternative therapies. In most countries, herbs are considered mainstream to their healing systems rather than alternative. Single herbs (monotherapy) or preparations of mixtures of herbs have been used for centuries and continue to be used to this day. Acknowledging the popularity of herbs and their central position in many cultural healing practices, the World Health Organization (WHO) has taken the following balanced position: *the traditional, historical use of herbal preparations is evidence of safety and efficacy in the absence of scientific evidence to the contrary* (Blumenthal 1998, p 16). This means that herbal therapies need not be subjected to double-blind, randomized, controlled studies to be acknowledged as valid medicines.

Until the last century, *phytomedicines,* or plants and plant products used for healing, were the primary means of administering medicinally active compounds. As manufacturing of drugs began with the first purified plant extracts of morphine from the opium poppy in 1805 and proceeded to the highly sophisticated chemical laboratories of today, herbal use declined. The pharmaceutical industry flourished because of the ease of administration and standardization of the purified, pharmacologically active ingredients in its products, as well as the potency of newer drugs such as antibiotics.

The rational use of herbs in medicinal applications follows the same rules as for manufactured drugs:

■ *Dose-response relationship.* Varying doses of an herb may create different effects, not just more or less of the same effect. Just as intravenous dopamine can be given in either renal

GLOSSARY OF HERBAL EFFECTS

Adaptogen—balances body systems and improves resistance to stress
Alteratives—purify blood and balance a particular body function
Anticatarrhals—eliminate or counteract formation of mucus
Astringents—constrict or bind tissues and reduce secretions
Carminatives—relieve gas
Cholagogues—promote flow of bile
Demulcents—sooth and protect injured or inflamed tissues
Diaphoretics—induce sweating
Emmenagogues—promote menstruation
Galactogogues—increase milk secretion
Hemostatics—arrest hemorrhage
Lithotriptics—help dissolve stones
Nervines—calm nervous tension
Rubifacients—increase blood at skin surface
Tonics—promote functions of the organs and whole body system
Vulneraries—encourage wound healing

or cardiac doses, an herb like goldenrod has no diuretic effect at low doses, a positive diuretic effect at medium dose, and an antidiuretic effect at high doses.

■ *Efficacy-constituent relationship.* A plant preparation may have several chemically active constituents that contribute to its effectiveness, rather than one component only. For example, the most commonly identified active ingredient of St. John's wort (SJW) is hypericin, which works synergistically with other substances such as flavonoids and hyperforin.

■ *Combination of ingredients vs. isolated constituents.* A total plant extract contains a combination of ingredients that may act together as coeffectors and will work better than an individual, isolated ingredient.

■ *Pharmaceutical quality.* A high level of pharmacological quality and standardization are necessary for phytomedicines to be effective. This requires proper plant identification, use of the correct part of the plant, careful attention to time of harvesting, and exacting manufacturing and handling processes. In Europe, where botanicals are very commonly used in mainstream practice, manufacturing standards are high, but preparations in the United States often are of unpredictable quality and potency. This single factor, more than any other, restricts the value and credibility of the use of many herbs in this country.

In this country, herbs are most often administered for a single indication. Much as we use an antibiotic to treat a specific type of infection, we tend to match one herb with one disease, such as saw palmetto for prostatism. Though this is useful, it reflects our relative lack of sophistication in the use of herbs, especially compared to Ayurvedic or Chinese practitioners who subtly balance the effects of multiple herbs in their prescriptions.

Given that herbal therapy is not widely taught in professional schools, how is the health-care practitioner to learn to recognize and use herbs effectively? How do they work? Can they be recommended for patients? In what forms are they used? (See "Herbal Preparations.") What are the appropriate dosages? What are their side effects? How about drug-herb interactions? The herbal literature is vast, has its own particular vocabulary, and is difficult to apply clinically. Much of the information about herbals has been developed in Europe and has not been published in mainstream American medical journals. One of the best works is the recently translated German Commission E Monographs (Blumenthal 1998), which report on the efficacy, safety, and indications of herbal products—but they analyze nearly 400 herbs and mixtures. The sheer volume of herbs makes most clinicians shudder at the prospect of learning to use herbs at all.

Fear not. I have in this chapter and Table 10–1 carefully summarized the most commonly used herbs for a primary care setting. For simplicity of association, key **indications** for each herb in the text are in **bold type.** If you learn these couple dozen herbs, you will be well on your way to integrating safe, effective herbal therapies into your practice. Be aware of the toxic herbs such as coltsfoot, comfrey, and chaparral, which ought to be avoided. Know that some of the indications take their validity from traditional use, as supported by WHO, rather than from scientific study. Recognize the challenge of finding standardized, reliable products from companies that provide the best, most active ingredients. Finally, remember that *herbs are drugs.* As you delve into the herbal literature, you will find that the active chemical constituents in herbs are well-characterized amines, glycans, alkaloids, phenolics, lignins, terpenoids, flavonoids, tannins, saponins, and other compounds that you may recall from your study of biochemistry or organic chemistry.

Because our patients interested in self-care often self-prescribe herbs, we must become knowledgeable so we can advise them about safety, efficacy, and interactions with conventional therapy. Having said all that, "A journey of a thousand plants must begin . . . with something useful!"

HERBAL PREPARATIONS

Bath—A form of hydrotherapy. Immerse the full body in a bath with 500 mL or 1 pt of infusion or decoction. The full-strength herbal infusion or decoction is used for foot or hand baths.

Capsule or pill—Powdered herbs may be enclosed in gelatin capsules or pressed into a hard pill. The powder can also be rolled into a pill with bread or cream cheese. This is one of the most common ways herbs are supplied and used.

Compress—Also called a *fomentation*. A clean cloth is soaked in an herbal infusion or decoction and applied over injured or inflamed areas.

Crude herb—The fresh or dried herb in an unprocessed form. Measurements are expressed by weight.

Decoction—An aqueous preparation of hard and woody herbs, which are made soluble by simmering in almost boiling water for 30 min or more. If the active ingredients are volatile oils, it is important to cover the pan to prevent vaporization. The decoction is then strained while hot and either stored or consumed as needed.

Essential oils—Volatile oils, usually mixtures of a variety of odoriferous organic compounds of plants.

Extract—Concentrated form of natural products obtained by treating crude herb with solvent and then discarding the solvent to result in a fluid extract, solid extract, powdered extract, or tincture. Strength is expressed as the ratio of the concentration of the crude herb to the extract; e.g., 5:1 means 5 parts crude herb is concentrated in 1 part extract, and 1:2 means 1 part of extract is comparable to 0.5 parts herb.

Fluid extract—Concentrated tinctures with a strength of 1 part solvent to 1 part herb.

Fomentation—See *Compress.*

Infusion—The preferred method used for soft plant parts such as leaves, flowers, or green stems, an infusion is prepared just like making a *Tea.* In the case of volatile oils or heat-sensitive ingredients, soaking in water or milk for 6 to 12 hours in a sealed earthenware pot makes a cold infusion.

Liniment—Usually a mixture of herbs and alcohol or vinegar to be applied topically over muscles and ligaments.

Lozenge—Dissolvable tablet often used for upper respiratory and throat problems. They are made by combining a powdered herb with sugar and viscous jelly obtained from either an edible gum or mucilaginous plant.

Ointment—An herb or mixture of herbs in a semi-solid mixture such as petroleum jelly. This is applied externally for injuries or inflammation. If made with volatile oils, it can even be used as a respiratory anti-catarrhal. Also known as a *Salve.*

(Continued)

HERBAL PREPARATIONS *(Continued)*

Powdered extract—A solid extract that has been dried to a powder.
Poultice—A raw or mashed herb applied directly to the body or wrapped in cheesecloth or other clean cloth. It is used either hot or cold for bruises, inflammation, spasm, and pain.
Salve—See *Ointment.*
Tincture—An alcohol-based preparation. Alcohol is a better solvent for many plant ingredients than water, so mixing herbs in alcohol such as vodka or wine with a specific water/alcohol ratio is a common method of extraction. The mixture is soaked for about 2 weeks. Then the herbs are strained out and the liquid is saved in a dark, well-stoppered bottle. These preparations are much stronger volume-for-volume than infusions or decoctions. Strengths are typically 1:5 to 1:10.
Tea—Made by steeping herbs in hot water (the same as an *Infusion*). Place 1 tsp dried herb or 2 to 3 tsp fresh herb into 1 cup (250 mL) hot or boiling water. Steep for 5 to 15 minutes. For larger quantities, use 1 oz (30 g) of herb in 1 pt (500 mL) of hot water. Bruise or powder seeds before making an infusion or tea. The shelf life of these bioactive fluids is short, even in the refrigerator. Discard them after 8 to 12 hours.

- **ALOE**

Aloe vera is a common succulent houseplant. Long kept in the kitchen for soothing **burns**, it is now available in commercial preparations for such indications as sunburn and the treatment of **stomach ulcers**. The solidified gel from the leaves, which extrudes when they are broken, can be used directly on the affected areas of the skin and is useful in many **skin conditions** as a *vulnerary* (promotes wound healing). For internal use, it comes in a diluted liquid form. The *Aloe barbadensis,* from which the latex-containing anthroquinone glycosides are derived, is a cathartic laxative used for **constipation** and is not to be confused with the gel form.

Aloe can be a powerful *cathartic* and an *emmenagogue* (increases menstrual flow). It also has *purgative* effects and so should be avoided during pregnancy and lactation. Hypokalemia from the purgative effects of the aloe latex leaf preparation results in drug interactions with cardiac glycosides, antiarrhythmics, thiazide diuretics, corticosteroids, and licorice root. These effects are not found in use of the pulp juice (in the absence of diarrhea) or gel topical extract.

For external use, simply put some of the juice or gel from the plant on the affected area. The internal dosage is 0.1 to 0.3 g of juice or 10 to 30

Text continued on page 127

Table 10–1   HERBS COMMONLY USED IN PRIMARY CARE

Herb	Common Usage*	Activity	Adverse Effects and Contraindications	Dosages	Drug Interactions
Aloe Aloe vera	**Burns and wound healing** Gastritis Ulcers Psoriasis	Anti-inflammatory Antiseptic	Dermatitis GI upset (PO) Diarrhea Avoid in children and pregnancy	30 mL/dose Juice: <1 qt/d Topical	None known for gel extract
Bilberry Vaccinium myrtillus	**Eye disorder** **Antidiarrheic** **Circulatory disorders**	Antioxidant Collagen stabilizer Vasoprotectant Astringent	None reported	20–40 mg t.i.d. antho- cyanosides 25% extract 80–160 mg t.i.d.	None known
Black Cohosh Cimicifuga racemosa	**Menopause symptoms** **Menstrual problems**	Estrogen-receptor blocker Luteinizing-hormone suppressant	GI upset ↑ BP Avoid in pregnancy/lactation	4 mg t.i.d. or as per label Decoction from 1 tsp root t.i.d. 1 mL tincture t.i.d. (40 mg/d of drug) 2 mg b.i.d. of standardized extract (Remifemin)	None known
Cat's Claw Uncaria tomentosa	**Arthritis** Cancer HIV	Immune stimulant Anti-inflammatory	Avoid in pregnancy/lactation, autoimmune illness, multiple sclerosis, TB	1 g/250 mL tea, drink q cup t.i.d. 1–2 mL tincture t.i.d. 20–60 mg standardized dry extract daily	Avoid combining with hormone drugs, insulin, vaccines, iron, NSAIDs, salicylates

*The most frequent indications are shown in boldface type.

(Continued)

Table 10–1 HERBS COMMONLY USED IN PRIMARY CARE (Continued)

Herb	Common Usage	Activity	Adverse Effects and Contraindications	Dosages	Drug Interactions
Cayenne Capsicum annum	**Arthritis Muscle pain Neuralgia** Post-mastectomy pain Psoriasis	Substance P (pain peptide) blocker ↓ Lipids ↓ Platelet aggregation	Eye irritation Burning, local and mucous membrane Gastritis Diarrhea (with internal use)	Extract of 0.025–0.075% as tolerated t.i.d.–q.i.d. 4–5 times daily topically	Warfarin: ↓ platelet aggregation with internal use
Chamomile Matricaria recutita Matricaria chamomilla	**Gastrointestinal complaints Skin and mucous membrane problems Stress and anxiety**	Antispasmodic effect Sedative effect	Avoid if allergy to a member of daisy family (Asteraceae) such as ragweed, asters, chrysanthemums.	3–4 c of the tea a day as needed 300–500 mg t.i.d–q.i.d. capsules 4–6 mL t.i.d. tincture between meals Topical	Caution if using with tranquilizers or CNS depressants
Cranberry Vaccinium macrocarpon	**Urinary tract infections**	↓ Bacterial adherence to bladder endothelium	Diarrhea	90 mL /day (prophylaxis) 360–960 mL/day (treatment) (Power capsules also available)	None known
Dong Quai Angelica sinensis	**Dysmenorrhea Other menstrual disorders Menopause symptoms** Allergies	Phytoestrogen Antimicrobial effects Smooth muscle relaxant IgE inhibition	Photodermatitis Uterine stimulant	1–2 g dried root in tea b.i.d.–t.i.d. 3–5 mL tincture t.i.d.	Coumarin

Herb	Uses	Actions	Precautions/Contraindications	Dosage	Interactions
Echinacea *Echinacea spp*	**Colds and flu** **Upper respiratory infections** **Urinary tract infections** Wound healing (topical) Recurrent candida vaginitis	Immunostimulant ↑ Macrophage phagocytosis Lymphocyte activity stimulant Anti-inflammatory Antimicrobial properties	Avoid in: HIV/AIDS, autoimmune disease, collagen vascular disease, multiple sclerosis, tuberculosis Avoid if allergy to sunflower seeds or to a member of daisy family (Asteraceae) such as ragweed	300 mg t.i.d. (do not exceed 6–8 wk) of freeze-dried extract 0.5–1 g/t.i.d. of dried root or as tea Juice 2–3 mL t.i.d. 2–3 mL tincture t.i.d. Topical	None known
Ephedra *Ephedrae herba* *Ma huang*	**Asthma** **Bronchitis** **Cough** **Decongestant** **Energy** **Weight loss** Diuretic	Sympathomimetic activating alpha and beta 1 & 2 receptors CNS stimulant Uterine contraction stimulant	↑ B/P, root ↓ B/P, above the ground Anxiety/restlessness Headaches Irritability Nausea, vomiting Urinary obstruction with BPH Addictive potential Dysrhythmias Alters DM control Kidney stones Caution in heart disease, hypertension, diabetes, or thyroid disease	15–30 mg t.i.d. adults 1–4 g/t.i.d. tea Tincture (1:4) 6–8 mL t.i.d.	Cardiac glycosides Halothane Guanethidine MAOIs Oxytocin Antihypertensive medication (↑ blood pressure) Must be protected from the light.

(Continued)

Table 10-1 HERBS COMMONLY USED IN PRIMARY CARE (Continued)

Herb	Common Usage	Activity	Adverse Effects and Contraindications	Dosages	Drug Interactions
Evening Primrose Oil *Oenothera biennis*	**Fibrocystic breast Eczema** Diabetic neuropathy PMS	Source of gamma linoleic acid (GLA)	Headache GI symptoms	500–2000 mg t.i.d./q.i.d.	Phenothiazines
Feverfew *Tanacetum parthenium*	**Migraine prophylaxis and treatment**	↓ Platelet aggregation Smooth muscle relaxant ↓ Prostaglandin synthesis and serotonin release from platelets and WBCs	Stop 2 weeks before major surgery Oral ulcers Rash Rebound migraine Avoid in pregnancy/lactation, and if allergy to sunflower seeds or to a member of daisy family (Asteraceae) such as ragweed	25–50 mg 0.2% cap b.i.d. 125 mg/d of dried leaves (or 2 fresh leaves/d)	Warfarin: ↓ platelet aggregation.
Garlic *Allium sativum*	**Hyperlipemia Hypertension** Cancer prevention Antimicrobial	Platelet aggregation inhibitor ↑ Fibrinolysis Antioxidant	Heartburn GI upset Flatulence Body/breath odor ↓ Blood glucose Stop 2 weeks before major surgery	At least 4 mg/day of allicin 1–2 fresh cloves/d Up to 3 g powder/d	May potentiate anti-thrombotic effect of anti-inflammatories, warfarin

| **Ginger**
Zingiber officinale | **Antiemetic**
Nausea
Motion sickness
Arthritis | Intestinal tone and peristalsis stimulant
Cholagogue
Anti-inflammatory
Antioxidant
Positive inotrope
Platelet aggregation inhibitor | GI upset
Caution if patient has gallstones
Stop 2 weeks before major surgery | 250 mg to 1 g q.i.d.
1–2 g is antiemetic dose
Can also take as candied or crystallized ginger
100–250 mg t.i.d. of 20% extract | Warfarin: ↓ platelet aggregation |
| **Ginkgo**
Ginkgo biloba | **Cerebrovascular insufficiency**
Peripheral vascular disease
Vascular dementia
Alzheimer's disease
Memory
Vertigo
Tinnitus
Macular degeneration
Depression
PMS
Diabetic neuropathy
Impotence | Membrane stabilizer
Anti-platelet activating (PAF)
Free-radical scavenger
Antioxidant | GI upset
Allergies (whole plant)
Spontaneous bleeding problems
Headaches
Avoid in pregnancy
Stop 2 weeks before major surgery | Dose standardized to 24% flavone glycosides
6% terpene lactones
40–80 mg b.i.d./t.i.d.
Higher dose for CNS effects and for established problems; lower for peripheral effects and prophylaxis | Warfarin
Aspirin (↓ platelet aggregation)
MAOI (↑ effect) |

(Continued)

Table 10–1 HERBS COMMONLY USED IN PRIMARY CARE (Continued)

Herb	Common Usage	Activity	Adverse Effects and Contraindications	Dosages	Drug Interactions
Ginseng *Panax ginseng* *Ginseng radix* *Eleutherococcus senticosus*	**Fatigue** **Weakness** **Energy** **Immunity** Libido Stress-induced GI ulcers Postoperative stress	Immune enhancer Platelet aggregation prevention Tonic effect	Agitation Insomnia (PM doses) BP Edema Hypertonia Stop 2 weeks before major surgery	1–2 g of dried root/d standardized as 3–8% ginsenoides *Caution*: standardization and dosing is quite inconsistent with ginseng products.	Warfarin: ↓ platelet aggregation Corticosteroids (↑ side effects) Digoxin (↑ serum levels) Opioids, diuretics (↓ effect) MAOIs, hypoglycemics (↑ effect)
Goldenseal *Hidrastis canadensis*	**Cold** **Immunity** Diarrhea	Antimicrobial	Avoid in pregnancy, diabetes (may lower glucose) Mouth irritation	250–500 mg t.i.d. Do not exceed: 2 mo (Endangered species, should probably not use)	Often combined with echinacea
Grape Seed Extract *Vitis vinifera*	**Atherosclerosis** **Retinopathy** **Venous insufficiency** Hepatic protective Dental caries	Proanthocyanidins: powerful anti-oxidants Vascular renewal and stability Collagen support	None reported	25–250 mg b.i.d.	None known

Herb	Uses	Actions	Side Effects/Cautions	Dose	Interactions
Hawthorn *Crataegus laevigata*	**Congestive heart failure** **Hypertension** **Angina**	Cardioactive glycosides Positive inotropic ACE inhibition Mild diuretic Collagen stabilizer Coronary vessel dilator ↓ Peripheral resistance	Hypotension Arrhythmia	100–250 mg t.i.d. of standardized extract (1.8% vitexin-4'-rhamnoside) Fluid extract (1:1) 1–2 mL t.i.d., Freeze dried berries 1–1.5 g t.i.d.	None known Can be used safely with digoxin and other cardiac drugs
Horse Chestnut *Aesculus hippocastanum*	**Venous insufficiency** **Varicose veins** **Nocturnal leg cramps** **Pruritus and swelling of legs** Topical treatment for hemorrhoids, skin ulcers, varicose veins, sport injuries, trauma	Aescin component reduces lysosomal activity, improves venous tone, inhibits capillary protein permeability Diuretic	GI irritation Pruritus Nausea Standardized seed extracts safe, though whole herb may be fatal Avoid in pregnancy/lactation, liver, renal disease	Initial dose of 90–150 mg aescin/d with maintenance dose 35–70 mg aescin/d	None known
Kava *Piper methysticum*	**Anxiety** **Restlessness** **Insomnia** Anticonvulsant Oral anesthetic	GABA receptor-like actions Limbic system modulation Inhibits voltage-dependent sodium channels in brain	Dermatitis Sedation May impair reflexes and judgment for driving in high dose Avoid in pregnancy/lactation, depression, Parkinson's disease	45–70 mg t.i.d. for anxiety 180–210 mg h.s. for sleep	Alcohol Benzodiazepines Barbiturates Anti-Parkinson drugs Other psychopharmacological agents General anesthetics (Note: Kava is nonaddictive)

(Continued)

Table 10–1 HERBS COMMONLY USED IN PRIMARY CARE *(Continued)*

Herb	Common Usage	Activity	Adverse Effects and Contraindications	Dosages	Drug Interactions
Milk Thistle *Silybum marianum*	**Cirrhosis** **Alcoholic and viral hepatitis** **Mushroom poisoning (Amanita)** **Other hepatotoxins**	Cell membrane stabilizer Ribosomal protein synthesis stimulator Free-radical scavenger Antioxidant	GI upset	70–210 mg t.i.d. of silymarin (calculated as silibinin) Phosphatidylcholine bound form of silybin dose 120–240 mg b.i.d. Used IV (20 mg/kg) in Europe for Amanita poisoning	None known
Peppermint *Mentha piperita*	**Dyspepsia** **IBS** **Biliary dyskinesia** **Digestive aid** Myalgia Neuralgia Nasal decongestant Headache (topically)	Antispasmodic Cholagogue Menthol is active ingredient Antibacterial Antiviral Gastric secretion stimulant Coolant	Non-enteric dosage may worsen heartburn in esophageal reflux/hiatal hernia Caution in small children (choking from menthol) Allergic reactions Bradycardia Muscle tremor Dermatitis, skin rash	1–2 tsp. leaves in 1 c of water as tea up to t.i.d. 1–2 enteric-coated capsules t.i.d. between meals (0.2 mL/capsule) Topically t.i.d./q.i.d.	None known

	Indications	Side Effects	Dosage	Interactions
Saw Palmetto *Serenoa repens*	**BPH (stages I and II)** **Prostatitis** Antiandrogenic (5 alpha-reductase) Bladder muscle spasmolytic Anti-inflammatory	GI side effects Diarrhea Avoid in pregnancy Potential risk of aggravation of estrogen-sensitive tumors	1–2 g of seeds/d 10 g b.i.d. crude berries 320 mg lipophilic ingredients daily (160 mg b.i.d.) Water-soluble components and tea not active pharmacologically.	None known
St. John's Wort *Hypericum perforatum*	**Depression** **Anxiety** **Insomnia** Contusions First-degree burns Wound healing Anti-inflammatory (topically) Affects neurotransmitters serotonin, dopamine, catecholamine, and possibly MAOIs, reduction of interleukin-6 Antiviral Antibacterial	Avoid in pregnancy (possibly uterotonic) GI side effects Photodermatitis Allergy Fatigue Restlessness	300 mg t.i.d. standardized solid extract (0.3% hypericin) Tincture (1:5) 3–6 mL t.i.d. Fluid extract (1:1) 1–2 mL t.i.d. Standardized fluid extract (0.14% hypericin: 1.0 mg hypericin/3 mL) 0.5–0.9 mL t.i.d.	Potential interaction with SSRIs general anesthetics, benzodiazepines: lowers levels of indinavir and other retrovirals used in AIDS, digoxin, oral contraceptives No longer contraindicated: use with MAOIs, tyramine-containing compounds, L-dopa, 5-hydroxytryptophan Lowers serum levels of cyclosporine

(Continued)

Table 10–1 HERBS COMMONLY USED IN PRIMARY CARE *(Continued)*

Herb	Common Usage	Activity	Adverse Effects and Contraindications	Dosages	Drug Interactions
Tea Tree Oil *Melaleuca alternifolia*	**Skin infections** Mucosal and vaginal lesions Fungal infections (skin/nails) Acne		Contact dermatitis	Topical: Few drops of oil	None known
Valerian *Valeriana officinalis*	**Insomnia** **Anxiety**	GABA domain effects Improves latency and quality of sleep Improves slow-wave sleep	Overdose with temporary GI, chest, CNS symptoms ? use in pregnancy	150–300 mg dried extract (1.0%–1.5% valtrate or 0.5% valerenic acid) Solid extract (4:1) 250–500 mg, tea from dried root 2–3 g Tincture (1:5) 4–6 mL Use doses t.i.d. for anxiety take 30–45 min before sleep	Avoid with benzodiazepines, barbiturates, general anesthetics (Note: Valerian is not habit-forming)

mL of gel t.i.d. Commercial preparations of the juice also are available for internal use and up to 1 qt/day may be taken. For constipation, 50 to 200 mg/day of aloe latex in capsule form may be taken.

- **BILBERRY**

Vaccinium myrtillus is the European blueberry or huckleberry. It contains anthocyanosides that benefit **vision problems**, **glaucoma**, **cataracts**, **macular degeneration**, **diarrhea**, and **circulatory disorders.** During the Second World War, Royal Air Force pilots used this herb before nocturnal bombing runs to improve their night vision, a beneficial effect thought to result from "recharging" the visual purple in the retina. Its traditional use has been for diarrhea, but it is more commonly used these days for its circulatory and eye benefits. Bilberry anthocyanosides act as powerful antioxidants in protecting against atherosclerotic damage, strengthening connective tissue in blood vessels, preventing platelet aggregation, and fostering smooth muscle relaxation. As a result, it has uses in venous insufficiency, varicose veins, and protecting against vascular damage in diabetes. Studies suggest benefit in inflammatory conditions such as rheumatoid arthritis and in improving uric acid excretion in gout. It has no reported side effects and is even considered safe in pregnancy and lactation. Likewise, no drug interactions have been reported.

Dosages for bilberry are based on the anthocyanoside content and are 20 to 40 mg t.i.d., 80 to 160 mg t.i.d. of 25% extract, or 50 to 120 g (about ½ to 1 cup) t.i.d. of the fresh berries. (Note that these are not the same as the usual American blueberries found in supermarkets. Their purple or blue pulp reflects their higher anthocyanidin content.)

- **BLACK COHOSH**

Cimicifuga racemosa is best thought of as a female herb. Its traditional uses include the relief of **menstrual cramps** and **PMS**. It has been studied and found to be useful in treating **symptoms associated with menopause** such as hot flashes, mood and sleep disturbance, and vaginal atrophy. The American Indians used it for these indications and for dysmenorrhea. Its active ingredients are triterpenes and flavonoids, some of which act on the pituitary to suppress luteinizing hormone. It does not alter the production of follicle-stimulating hormone and prolactin. Stomach upset and occasional lowered blood pressure are the only reported side effects, and no other contraindications or drug interactions are reported. Some experts recommend limiting treatment to 6 months because long-term safety has not been evaluated.

A contemporary preparation of black cohosh is *Remifemin*, which is provided in a convenient tablet form for both dysmenorrhea (q.d. or b.i.d.) and menopause (2 tabs b.i.d.). A therapeutic dosage is 40 mg daily. Black cohosh can also be taken as a tea made of ½ to 1 tsp of the dried root drunk 3 times daily or 2 to 4 mL of tincture 3 times daily.

- ## CAT'S CLAW

Uncaria tomentosa is a popular South American herb and was listed among the top 10 herbs sold in natural food stores in the United States in a recent year. Why all this interest in Cat's Claw? Traditionally, it has been used by peoples in the Andes for a very wide range of indications including inflammation, gastric ulcers, tumors, dysentery, arthritis, and as a contraceptive. A renewed interest in this country has occurred in its use for support in cancer and HIV disease, though convincing studies are not yet available. It is used most commonly as an agent for **arthritis** because of its anti-inflammatory action.

Because of its imputed action as an immune stimulant, it should be avoided in autoimmune disease, multiple sclerosis, and tuberculosis. It has not been proven to be safe in pregnancy and breast-feeding; with its traditional use as a contraceptive, I would recommend avoiding it in these conditions.

This popular herb is taken as a tea, which is prepared with 3 c of water and 1 g of the root bark. After steeping for 15 minutes, the liquid is strained and a cup is then drunk 3 times/day. It is also available in a tincture (1–2 mL b.i.d.) or as a standardized dry extract, of which 20 to 60 mg can be taken daily in divided doses.

- ## CAYENNE

Capsicum annum is the hot fruit of the pepper plant and contains the active ingredient capsaicin. The irritant effect of the cream applied topically is thought to deplete substance P, a pain-transmitting neuropeptide, from peripheral C-type nerve fibers. Thus, painful stimuli are not perceived at a central level. It has found its most popular use topically for **arthritis**, **muscle pain**, **neuralgia**, and **neuropathy**, and also is helpful in some cases of postmastectomy pain and psoriasis. As an ingredient in food, it is used as a digestive aid in relieving dyspepsia, gas, and cramps. It has been found beneficial in cardiovascular disease, reducing the rate of atherosclerosis in rats fed a high-capsaicin diet. It is thought to reduce cholesterol, triglycerides, and platelet aggregation while increasing fibrinolytic activity.

Topical applications can cause local burning and irritation, which cause some patients to stop using it before substance P depletion can occur. It can also irritate mucous membranes, so patients should be reminded to wash their hands after application and prior to touching eyes, genitalia, or other sensitive areas. Gastritis and diarrhea can result if too much is taken internally. Because of its effects on platelet aggregation, high internal doses may require the adjustment of warfarin dosage.

The cream is available in 0.025% to 0.075% strength and is applied to the skin 4 or 5 times daily. Dietary intake is as tolerated.

- **CHAMOMILE**

Matricaria recutita, also known as *Matricaria chamomilla* or chamomile, is a safe and useful classic herb so popular that it was voted "Medicinal Plant of the Year" in Germany in 1987. It is widely used for **gastrointestinal complaints**, **skin and mucous membrane problems**, **stress**, and **anxiety.** The active ingredients are the volatile oil bisalbol compounds and the flavonoids apigenin, quercetin, and luteolin. The distilled oil is a beautiful blue color and is only applied topically.

Taken internally, chamomile is used most widely for its antispasmodic effects, for such gastrointestinal problems as colic, irritable bowel syndrome (IBS), cramps, flatulence, and stress-related GI complaints. It is safely used for colic even in children and infants and is a good substitute for a bedtime bottle of juice or milk. It also can help to calm the teething infant. Chamomile is a mild sedative and can be relaxing as a soothing tea in cases of stress and anxiety.

Topically, it has been applied for a wide variety of skin complaints such as eczema, psoriasis, and dry skin, and seems to promote skin healing. It can also be used as a wash or gargle for canker sores and gum disease, or in a bath, poultice, or wash for anogenital irritation.

Chamomile has no known drug interactions and is reported to have no contraindications in pregnancy or lactation. There is a risk of allergic reaction by those with a sensitivity to members of the daisy family (*Asteraceae)* such as ragweed, asters, and chrysanthemums. Tyler believes this precaution has been overemphasized and reports a reaction rate of only 1.7% in a large skin-testing study (Robbers & Tyler 1999, p. 70). Because of its sedative effect, perhaps some caution is advisable with tranquilizers or CNS depressants.

The dosage of chamomile is 3 to 4 cups of the tea per day as needed. This is prepared with a heaping tablespoon (about 3 g) of the flower tops in a cup of hot water. It also comes in capsules, taken as 350 to 500 mg t.i.d.–q.i.d. A tincture form is taken 4 to 6 mL t.i.d. between meals. Topically, it is applied as a poultice of the flower tops, mixed in a bath as 50 g per 2½ gallons of water, or used as a 3% to 10% infusion as a rinse or wash.

- **CRANBERRY**

Vaccinium macrocarpon is the common cranberry, which is most widely known for its effects on **urinary tract infections (UTIs).** Although initially the mechanism of action was thought to be acidification of the urine, this is no longer thought to be the case. To acidify the urine adequately to suppress bacterial growth would require the intake of at least a quart of the juice (which contains hippuric acid) at a sitting. The effectiveness of lower doses in treating bladder infections appears to result primarily from decreasing the adherence to the bladder and urethral epithelium of *Escherichia coli,* the organism most commonly causing cystitis.

Cranberry cannot be recommended for upper urinary tract infections such as pyelonephritis, which require antibiotics. Patients with urinary complaints accompanied by high fever, flank pain, or abdominal pain (especially children and the elderly) should seek attention for possible antibiotic prescription. Drinking large amounts of commercial, sweetened cranberry juice can load the body with sugar, so it is better to use fresh juice sweetened with other juices such as apple or grape. Blueberry juice is also useful for the treatment of cystitis.

The usual dose of cranberry juice is several glasses (360 to 960 mL) per day for treatment of UTI; 90 mL/day has been recommended as prophylaxis for those with recurrent UTIs. Concentrate in capsule form is also available and should be taken 2 to 4 times daily.

- **DONG QUAI**

Angelica sinensis is an Asian herb widely respected as a "women's remedy." It has been widely used for **dysmenorrhea**, **irregular or prolonged uterine bleeding**, and **symptoms related to menopause**. Dong quai (pronounced *dong kwhy*) is useful in stabilizing estrogenic activity and relieving hot flashes. Its imputed mechanism of action is via phytoestrogens and it also contains ferulic acid, ligustilide, vitamin B_{12}, and vitamin E. It has been shown to have both a relaxing and stimulating effect on the uterus.

Some patients may have hypersensitivity that can cause excess bleeding and fever. Dong quai also can be photosensitizing. It should not be used during pregnancy and lactation, though various sources disagree on this point. Overall, the evidence is better for the use of black cohosh than dong quai for menstrual disorders and menopause. I suspect this is because dong quai's traditional use in Chinese medicine was a part of a formula including several other herbs and a high-soy diet. There is a potential drug interaction with coumarin.

For PMS, dong quai should be taken 3 times/day starting on day 14 of the menstrual cycle, as either 1 to 2 g of powdered root or tea, 1 tsp of tincture, or 1/4 tsp of fluid extract.

- **ECHINACEA**

Echinacea angustifolia is best known as an **immune stimulant**. Long favored by the American Indians, echinacea (ek-ih-NAY-sha) is considered as an antibiotic, useful against both bacterial and viral infections. It is one of the best-selling herbs in health food stores in the United States.

Its imputed actions are encouraging the swarming of white blood cells to the site of an infection, stimulating phagocytosis, improving lymphocyte production, and increasing interferon production. Some sources recommend against its use in autoimmune disease or tuberculosis. It is not recommended during pregnancy. Side effects are not reported. Cross allergy with the daisy and ragweed families is possible.

Dosage is 3 to 4 cups of tea/day, or 300 mg of freeze-dried extract, 1 to 4 mL of tincture, or 2 to 3 mL of fresh juice 3 times/day during an infectious episode such as a **common cold** or **chronic respiratory tract infection**. Though sources vary, a cycle of 5 days on and 2 days off during an infection is widely recommended. Taking it all the time is not considered as useful, and in any case, it should not be taken for longer than 8 weeks.

- **EPHEDRA**

Ephedra sinica or *ma huang* contains alkaloids, ephedrine, and pseudoephedrine. It is widely used in **asthma**, **allergy**, **low blood pressure**, **cerebral insufficiency**, as a **stimulant**, and for **weight loss**. It has marked sympathomimetic effects and can be overused or even abused. Its CNS effects have been characterized as stronger than those of caffeine but weaker than those of amphetamines.

It is best avoided by hypertensive or anxious patients and those with cardiac arrhythmia, glaucoma, benign prostatic hypertrophy (BPH), or diabetes. Ephedra may be habit forming. It can interact with cardiac glycosides, halothane, guanethidine, monoamine oxidase (MAO) inhibitors, and oxytocin.

Dosage is 1 to 2 tsp (1 to 4 g) of dried herb steeped as a tea for 10 to 15 minutes and taken 3 times/day. The adult dose is 6 to 8 mL of the tincture (1:4) or 15 to 30 mg total alkaloid, calculated as ephedrine, given 3 times/day. Ephedra is also found mixed in many other over-the-counter preparations.

- **EVENING PRIMROSE OIL**

Oenothera biennis produces seeds that are a source of omega-6 essential fatty acids. This oil, also known as EPO, has a fairly long list of indications but it is most commonly used for **atopic eczema**, **cyclical and noncyclical mastalgia**, and **fibrocystic breasts**. Psoriasis and diabetic neuropathy are sometimes improved with EPO. Some trials have used it without benefit in multiple sclerosis and PMS. Its actions are thought to be related to antioxidant effects and to the correction of deficiencies of the essential fatty acids linoleic acid and gamma-linolenic acid (GLA). It should not be used with phenothiazines, because it may precipitate seizures. Side effects are mild gastrointestinal distress and headache.

Doses for atopic eczema (based on a standardized GLA content of 8%) are 2 to 4 g/day for children and 6 to 8 g/day for adults. For mastalgia, the usual dosage is 3 to 4 g/day.

- **FEVERFEW**

  Tanacetum parthenium is a primary remedy in the treatment of **migraine headaches** as well as associated nausea and vomiting. It may also be useful in dizziness and tinnitus as well as dysmenorrhea. It should not be used during pregnancy (it stimulates the uterus) or lactation. It may cause mouth ulcers in some people, particularly those chewing the leaves. It treats and prevents migraine by inhibiting the release from platelets of blood vessel–dilating substances, inhibiting inflammatory mediators, and regulating vascular tone. The active ingredient is parthenolide, which should be present in at least a 0.2% concentration in preparations. Rebound migraine can occur when use is discontinued abruptly.

  The dosage is 1 fresh or frozen leaf 1 to 3 times/day. The leaf is chewed because parthenolide is not water-soluble and so cannot be made into a tea. The drug equivalent is 0.2 to 0.6 mg of parthenolide, which is equivalent to 50 to 200 mg of dried aerial parts (not the root) in tablets or capsules. It also is available in a tincture of 1:5 in 25% ethanol; the usual dose is 5 to 20 drops. Continuous use for at least 4 to 6 weeks is recommended for prophylaxis at a dose of not less than 125 mg/day of dried feverfew containing a minimum of 0.2% of the parthenolide active ingredient.

- **GARLIC**

  Allium sativum is a favorite kitchen herb in many cultures but it also has many health effects, including antiplatelet activity (at about 1 clove/day) and antibiotic and immunity-enhancing effects. The volatile oil is largely excreted via the lungs and is useful in respiratory infections. Studies have shown its benefit in reducing **high blood pressure** and **cholesterol** levels. The active ingredient is allicin. Fresh garlic has compounds such as S-allylcysteines and gamma-glutamylpeptides, which also exert beneficial effects. Possible gastrointestinal side effects include nausea, diarrhea, vomiting, or a burning sensation. It may potentiate the antithrombotic effects of anti-inflammatory drugs or warfarin.

  Dosages of up to 3 cloves/day are recommended, or garlic oil capsules may be used. These should deliver at least 2 to 5 mg of allicin. The German Commission E, which reviewed herbal products, recommended that commercial preparations contain not less than the equivalent of fresh garlic. Preparations of garlic oil (2 to 5 mg/day) or tincture 1:5 in 45% alcohol (2 to 4 mL t.i.d.) are also available. To be sure of receiving an adequate dose of the active ingredients, take fresh garlic or standardized preparations. Cooking removes some of the benefits of garlic. Many people prefer the garlic capsules to reduce the odor of garlic on the breath.

- **GINGER**

  Zingiber officinale is another favorite among Asians and other cooks everywhere. It has many uses, including as an **anti-inflammatory**, a **digestive aid**, a gargle for sore throats, and a compress for abdominal and gynecological problems. A recently marketed preparation claims effectiveness for **rheumatologic problems** via inhibition of leukotrienes and prostaglandins. It has been widely used against **nausea**, particularly in pregnancy, when a tea made from fresh-grated ginger root, ginger ale, lemon, and a bit of honey or sugar is sipped in the morning. Ginger stimulates intestinal tone; this is thought to be the way in which it reduces nausea. Its anti-inflammatory and antiplatelet functions may account for its imputed effectiveness in some kinds of migraine.

  Because it stimulates bile flow, it may create problems in those with gallstones. Excessive doses of ginger can also cause gastrointestinal upset.

  The antiemetic dose is 1 to 2 g. The dosage for other indications is a standardized capsule, 250 mg to 1g, taken 3 to 4 times/day. An infusion is prepared by pouring boiling water over the sliced root or a decoction can be made using 1½ tsp of dried root powder or finely chopped ginger root. The tea or decoction can be drunk as needed. Ginger also is available in a tincture (1.5 to 3 mL 3 times/day) and a 20% extract, of which 100 to 150 mg can be taken 3 times/day. Candied or crystallized ginger, available in Asian markets, is a pleasant form to use, especially for children. A compress made from fresh grated root in cheesecloth soaked in hot water and applied to the abdomen has long been favored as a stimulant for digestive and gynecological functions.

- **GINKGO**

  Ginkgo biloba is the most widely sold herb in Europe, where it is used for **cerebrovascular insufficiency**, **peripheral vascular disease**, **vascular dementia**, **Alzheimer's disease**, and **memory problems**. Other indications are vertigo, tinnitus, macular degeneration, depression, PMS, diabetic neuropathy, and impotence. Studies have recently indicated its effectiveness in slowing the progression of Alzheimer's disease and multi-infarct dementia. Its mechanism of action is thought to be from its function as an antioxidant, a free-radical scavenger, a membrane stabilizer, and an inhibitor of platelet-activating factor. This effect makes its use in conjunction with warfarin or aspirin potentially a problem. Clotting studies need to be followed carefully if ginkgo is to be used with either of these drugs. Rarely stomach or intestinal upsets, headaches, or skin rashes can occur. Avoid its use in pregnancy.

Standardized extracts contain 24% mixed flavonoid glycosides and 6% terpene lactones. For memory problems and dementia, the dosage is 120 to 240 mg daily, taken in 2 to 3 doses. A lower dosage, not more than 160 mg/day in 2 or 3 doses, is used for vertigo, tinnitus, and peripheral vascular disease. An initial period of 6 to 8 weeks is recommended to assess the effectiveness of ginkgo.

• GINSENG

Panax ginseng, Panax quinquifolius, Eleutherococcus senticosus (Asian, American, and Siberian species) is widely reputed as a **tonic for stress, fatigue, or weakness**, and a **booster for energy and immunity.** A favorite among Asians for centuries, it is considered an *adaptogen*—that is, a substance that helps restore homeostasis during periods of physiological or psychological stress. Probably the simplest statement about ginseng is that the claims about its effectiveness are contradictory and difficult to verify. Nonetheless, it remains one of the top three best-selling herbs.

Siberian ginseng, *Eleutherococcus*, was introduced as a cheaper substitute for the expensive and difficult-to-cultivate *Panax* species. Its active components are not ginsenosides typical of the *Panax* varieties, but it has at least some of the adaptogenic qualities of standard ginseng. In experimental studies it has been found to be radioprotective, to inhibit carcinogenesis, to be endocrinologically active and immunosupportive, and to affect glucose control and hypertension. Despite its common name, however, aficionados of ginseng do not consider eleuthero to be a true ginseng.

Ginseng has been claimed to improve athletic performance, sexual potency, memory, immune function, circulation, and longevity, and to treat cancer. The origin of the word *panacea* comes from the name *Panax*, derived from the Greek word meaning "all-healing." Evidence of its effects on the endocrine system has been shown with increases in pituitary and adrenal hormones. Direct effects on potency have not been proven. It may reduce cholesterol levels. Many of the studies have been in animal models. Problems of source, standardization of dosing, and opposing effects of the active ginsenosides account for the difficulty in studying this herb and proving its wide range of imputed effects.

The ginsenosides belong to a chemical group called saponins, which are similar in composition and structure to steroids such as testosterone, estrogen, and adrenocorticotropic hormone (ACTH). Korean ginseng may raise blood pressure. The use of ginseng requires caution for patients with cardiac problems, diabetes, psychosis, or agitation, or if they are receiving steroid therapy or MAO inhibitors, and possibly during pregnancy. Excessive doses may cause edema and hypertonia.

A standardized preparation includes 4% ginsenosides. Daily dosages vary from 0.5 to 2 g of root or equivalent preparations for healthy young persons over a short term. Older and unhealthy people should take about half that amount. It can be taken continuously in chronic states. My conclusion on ginseng is that it is a mild stimulant tonic and probably best for older people rather than for the young and healthy, though it is generally quite safe in both groups. Because of the high cost of ginseng, some preparations have little or no active ingredient. Buy from reputable suppliers only.

- **GOLDENSEAL**

Hydrastis canadensis is a widely used **immune stimulant** and **natural antibiotic**. It has an astringent effect and its most common use is for **sore throats** and **colds**. It is sometimes sold together with echinacea for these indications. The berberine alkaloid of goldenseal exerts antibiotic effects and has been shown to inhibit the attachment of group-A streptococci to the endothelial lining of the throat. It has effects against other microorganisms such as *Staphylococcus, Candida, Giardia, E. coli, Trichomonas vaginalis, Entamoeba histolytica*, and others. The alkaloid, berberine, also has been shown to activate phagocytosis. As an external agent, goldenseal is used for eczema, ringworm, pruritis, earache, and conjunctivitis. It may be used internally for infectious diarrhea, gastritis, infection and inflammation of mucous membranes, and digestive disorders. Because of its stimulant effect on the uterus, it should not be used during pregnancy and also should be avoided in lactation. It may reduce glucose levels in diabetics.

Goldenseal is usually taken 3 times daily, as either 0.5 to 1 g of the dried root and rhizome, 2 to 4 mL of a tincture (1:10, 60% ethanol), 0.3 to 1 mL of liquid extract (1:1, 60% ethanol), or 250 to 500 mg of the extract standardized to contain 5% hydrastine. Goldenseal is an endangered species, so it should probably not be used. In any case, do not use it for more than 2 months.

- **GRAPE SEED EXTRACT**

Vitis vinifera is a source of procyanidolic oligomers, which are powerful antioxidants. These substances are also found in other plant sources such as grape skins, red wine, pine bark, lemon tree bark, citrus peels, peanuts, and cranberries. Collectively, the term *pycnogenols* has been used to describe this group of proanthocyanidin complexes. Because of powerful antioxidant effects, grape seed extract and the other pycnogenols are useful in **atherosclerosis**, **retinopathy**, and **venous insufficiency**. They help maintain collagen, act as free-radical scavengers, and have approximately 50 times the antioxidant effects of vitamin

C and vitamin E. Other uses are for dental caries, macular degeneration, capillary fragility and other microvascular disorders, disorders of visual function, and hepatic protection.

These agents are considered safe, with no described drug interactions. Grape seed extract is used in dosages of 75 to 150 mg twice daily. Grape seed extract is equivalent in effects to pycnogenol *Pinus pinaster*, another form of procyanidin that comes from the pine tree.

- **HAWTHORN**

Crataegus laevigata is best known as a **cardiac tonic.** Hawthorn berries have been used for centuries in Asia and Europe for their beneficial effects on the cardiovascular system. Hawthorn is a traditional heart tonic, often used in conjunction with digoxin. Testing has shown that hawthorn increases myocardial contractility and coronary blood flow while decreasing heart rate and oxygen consumption. Its active constituents are proanthocyanidins and cardiotonic amines. It also contains antioxidant flavonoids, which are produced in highest quantity from the young floral buds and leaves. It also inhibits angiotensin-converting enzyme (ACE) and acts as a vasodilator and mild diuretic. It is used clinically in angina, congestive heart failure, and hypertension, though it is best used as an adjunctive therapy in severe cases. The extracts are well tolerated, show no drug interactions, and have a wide therapeutic index.

The dosage is 2 tsp of berries and leaves infused for 20 minutes and drunk 3 times/ day for several months. Hawthorn can also be taken 3 times/day as a tincture (2 to 4 mL) or a capsule (150 to 250 mg). Capsules of the extract should contain 1.8% vitexin-4'-rhamnoside or 10% procyanidins.

- **HORSE CHESTNUT**

Aesculus hippocastanum is suggested by the German Commission E for **venous insufficiency, nocturnal leg cramps, pruritus,** and **swelling of the legs.** The extract of the seed is taken internally for these indications, and it also is used topically for hemorrhoids, skin ulcers, varicose veins, sports injuries, and trauma. It is often combined with witch hazel in the topical form. The active ingredient is aescin, which reduces lysosomal enzyme activity involved in chronic venous pathology, reduces transcapillary filtration of fluid and low-molecular-weight proteins, increases venous tone, and acts as a mild diuretic. Horse chestnut offers a useful herbal alternative for patients who might be candidates for venous ligation surgery, sclerotherapy injections, and compression stockings. Butcher's broom, *Ruscus aculeatus*, is also used for varicose veins and affects venous tone, but it is less well studied than horse chestnut.

Side effects are mild and may include gastrointestinal complaints and nausea as well as pruritus from the oral form. Rare renal and hepatic reactions and anaphylaxis have been reported with the intravenous form. Pregnancy and nursing are contraindications. The topical form may cause allergic dermatitis.

The standardized extract of the horse chestnut seed can be given at an initial dosage of 90 to 150 mg of aescin per day, which can be reduced to a maintenance dose of 35 to 70 mg of aescin once the clinical effect has been obtained. *Whole herb preparations of horse chestnut are toxic and potentially fatal.*

- **KAVA**

Piper methysticum is a Polynesian euphoriant that is used primarily to treat **anxiety**, **restlessness**, and **insomnia.** The active ingredients are kavalactones. In the crude form, these have a greater gamma-aminobutyric acid (GABA) receptor domain effect than does the pure extract. It is a member of the pepper family. Small doses of kava (also known as kava kava) improve mental function; before serious negotiations, chiefs of Polynesian tribes often drank it, prepared by chewing on the root and then spitting the extract into a large pot of coconut milk for brewing. Kava may push limbic system impressions forward, according to some sources, and may have anticonvulsant properties. It also has some benefit as a skeletal muscle relaxant for patients with nervous tension and stress headaches. Studies with kava showed no depression of mental function, no impairment in driving or operating heavy equipment, and increased memory in standard doses.

Traditionally, the cups of kava are drunk quickly because it numbs the mouth. Kava should not be used in Parkinson's disease or with benzodiazepines; the combination may cause disorientation. At high doses, kava may impair judgment while driving. It should be avoided in pregnancy, nursing, and possibly in severe depression. Doses of 400 mg/day or more over long periods may cause a scaly rash that resolves with discontinuance of the herb. Very large doses (several hundred grams per week) lead to not only dermatitis but also stupefaction, weakness, hematuria, hematologic effects, and pulmonary hypertension. Clinical studies, mainly from Germany, have shown kava to be nonaddictive and safe at normal dosages.

For anxiety or depression, the dosage is 60 to 70 mg 3 times daily. For insomnia, 180 to 210 mg is taken 45 to 60 minutes before retiring. Dosage is based on the kavalactone content in the standardized preparation. The dosage of the dried rhizome is 1.5 to 3 g/day; the alcoholic 1:2 extract is taken in a dosage of 3 to 6 mL/day. Kava's effects are potentiated by alcohol. In its traditional social context, the bowl drunk by a group will have about 250 mg of kavalactones and one person may consume several bowls at a sitting.

- **MILK THISTLE**

  Silybum marianum contains the active constituent silymarin. This herb acts as an antioxidant, inhibits leukotriene formation, stabilizes membranes, and is a choleretic and lipotropic. It has a decongesting effect on the liver and is best known for preventing **liver damage**, including fibrosis and **toxic or chemical-induced cirrhosis**, as well as damage from **viral hepatitis.** No toxicity has been found in animals or humans. Patients with hepatitis C have shown a 30% reduction in abnormal liver enzymes with 2 to 3 months of use. Milk thistle is also useful in psoriasis. It promotes milk secretion and is safe during lactation. It also can stimulate bile production and thus may have a cathartic effect.

  The standard dosage based on silymarin content is 70 to 210 mg 3 times/day. A form bound to phosphatidylcholine is available, to be taken at a dosage of 120 to 240 mg twice daily. A tea prepared from 1 tsp of the dried herb and leaves infused for 10 to 15 minutes in a cup of boiling water may be drunk 3 times/day. A tincture also is available; 1 to 2 mL can be taken 3 times daily, but the tincture is not advised in liver disease owing to its alcohol content.

- **PEPPERMINT OIL**

  Mentha piperita, peppermint is considered a candy and breath mint, yet it has significant medicinal value. Its presence at the checkout counter of most restaurants has to do with not only its breath-enhancing benefits but also its effects on the lower esophageal sphincter. Peppermint reduces the lower esophageal sphincter tone, allowing for comfortable belching and the improved comfort of restaurant-goers. Herbalists refer to it as a *carminative,* a digestive aid that stimulates peristalsis, relaxes the stomach, and prevents gas. Its volatile oils, mainly menthol, have been found useful in **irritable bowel syndrome (IBS)** when administered in the form of enteric-coated peppermint oil (ECPO), which reaches the small and large intestines. ECPO acts as a smooth muscle relaxant via its calcium channel–blocking effects, is an antispasmodic, and reduces bile output. A study published in *Gastoenterology* showed that it has significant effects in reducing abdominal pain, distension, stool frequency, borborygmi (loud bowel sounds), and flatulence in patients with IBS (Liu 1997). Other common uses of peppermint are for **nonulcer dyspepsia**, **biliary dyskinesia**, and as a **digestive aid**. Topically, its cooling effects are soothing for myalgia, neuralgia, and tension headache. It can treat nasal congestion when used topically or as an inhalant.

  Because it relaxes smooth muscle, however, peppermint may worsen heartburn and esophageal reflux, especially with hiatal hernia. Small children and infants may choke from the vapors, and allergic reactions, muscle tremors, and bradycardia have been described with its use. Although some practitioners of naturopathy use it to dissolve gallstones, it should be used with caution for this indication. Topical preparations can cause a rash.

The dosage for IBS is 0.2 to 0.4 mL of ECPO or a tincture of 1 to 2 mL 3 times daily, half an hour before each meal. The preferred method of taking peppermint for **dyspepsia** is 1 tsp of the herb infused as a tea and taken as often as desired.

- **SAW PALMETTO**

Serenoa repens, the saw palmetto plant, yields berries that contain fatty acids, sterols, and carotenes. These chemical compounds inhibit steroids essential to prostate metabolism, such as 5-alpha-reductase, and have a mild alpha-1–receptor antagonism. As a result, saw palmetto is clinically beneficial for **benign prostatic hypertrophy (BPH)**. Saw palmetto (along with zinc, echinacea, and bearberry) also can be used for **prostatitis**. It has been shown to be more effective than placebo in BPH. Some sources claim that it does not reduce prostate-specific antigen levels, but others disagree. In any case, it is a safe product that has few side effects such as the hypotension experienced by some patients who take prescription alpha-1–receptor antagonists.

Saw palmetto is also considered a tonic for the male reproductive system that boosts male sex drive. Quality-of-life indicators show marked improvement with saw palmetto, perhaps in large part because it reduces nocturia, thus improving the quality of sleep.

Before relying on saw palmetto, patients should be examined to rule out more serious problems of the prostate, especially prostate cancer in men older than 50. Side effects are mild and are limited to occasional gastrointestinal complaints and diarrhea. Saw palmetto was used by the Native Americans in Florida as a food source, so it is clearly a safe herb. Some believe that because of its hormonal effects it should not be used by patients who are pregnant or who have estrogen-sensitive tumors. No drug interactions are known.

The extract, containing 85% to 95% fatty acids and sterols, should be given in a dosage of 160 mg twice daily. Teas contain primarily water-soluble components of saw palmetto and have no benefit in prostate conditions. Most patients taking saw palmetto receive relief within a month of beginning treatment.

- **ST. JOHN'S WORT**

Hypericum perforatum is a well-researched herbal product used primarily for mild to moderate **depression, anxiety**, and **insomnia**. It has active ingredients in the anthraquinone class, such as hypericin and hyperforin, as well as flavonoids. In Germany, SJW is the most-prescribed agent for **depression**; its sales exceed those of fluoxetine by a large multiple. The treatment of depression is its largest use in this country as well. It has been tested against tricyclic antidepressants and found to have improved depression scales with a significantly reduced side effect profile. It acts primarily as a selective serotonin reuptake inhibitor (SSRI). It has additional effects on the monoamine oxidase inhibition (MAOI) pathway as well as on catecholamine methyl transferase (COMT). An interesting discovery is that SJW affects interleukin-6 and, through that immunomodulator, affects the hypothalamic-pituitary-adrenal axis. This psychoneuroimmunological effect demonstrates the interplay of the immune system with the nervous system. It also has been found to have antimicrobial activity; more long-term studies are needed to confirm preliminary reports of a benefit in AIDS and other viral infections such as chronic fatigue syndrome. The topical preparation, a red oil, is useful in wound healing. It has both anti-inflammatory and antibiotic effects.

Though much has made of a potential interaction of SJW with MAOIs, no clinical evidence of a problem has been found. There also seems to be no reason to prohibit patients taking SJW from consuming tyramine-containing foods such as aged cheeses, wine, and beer. Its use with SSRIs is of some concern, however. The potential of a serotonin syndrome if SJW is used together with such common antidepressants as paroxetine, fluoxetine, and sertraline requires caution. Experts in this area recommend tapering the SSRI while starting SJW. Several other drug interactions have been reported recently (see Table 10–1).

Photosensitivity is a potential concern, especially in fair-skinned individuals, although the sunburn reported with SJW primarily has been in range animals eating large amounts of the raw herb. Other side effects are mild and infrequent; they include gastrointestinal irritation, hypersensitivity, fatigue, and restlessness. Perhaps the greatest advantage of SJW is patient compliance because of its lack of side effects. It is also much less expensive than leading SSRI antidepressants. SJW is not recommended during pregnancy or lactation because of a lack of toxicity data.

Dosage is based on the standardized hypericin content of 0.3%. The usual daily dosage in capsules is 300 mg 3 times/day. For insomnia, the dose is 900 mg an hour before retiring. Tea is prepared by pouring boiling water over 2 to 4 g of the herb and steeping for 5 to 10 minutes; this is drunk 3 times daily. There is a standardized fluid extract (0.14% hypericin—1.0 mg hypericin/3 mL), of which 0.5 to 0.9 mL is taken 3 times/day, and a fluid extract (1:1) that is taken at a dosage of 1 to 2 mL t.i.d. The tincture (1:5) is taken in a dosage of 3 to 6 mL t.i.d.

- **TEA TREE OIL**

Melaleuca alternifolia is an Australian plant from which an essential oil is extracted. Tea tree oil is considered a useful **dermatolog-**

ical with **antibacterial, antiviral, and antifungal properties.** It is used topically in full strength on boils, wound infections, and acne. At least one study showed improved healing of boils and reduced scar formation, presumably from its effect on *Staphylococcus aureus.* Another study showed it to be as effective as clotrimazole for tinea pedis. It has also been used in vaginitis, by inserting a tampon soaked in 40% tea tree oil for a 24-hour period or douching daily with a 0.4% concentration of the oil in a quart of water.

Tea tree oil has a minimal tendency to irritate skin despite its penetrating qualities. Occasionally, it can cause contact dermatitis and irritation and will need to be diluted or even discontinued for a while.

- VALERIAN

Valeriana officinalis yields valerenic acids, flavonoids, and valepotriates from its root. Valerian is used for **nervousness, anxiety,** and **insomnia.** It has been shown to improve the quality of sleep by improving slow waves in those with low baseline values. It is nonaddictive, unlike many other sleep aids and anxiolytics, particularly benzodiazepines. It stimulates release of GABA and inhibits its reuptake. Its components bind directly to GABA receptors. Several studies have shown that valerian does not cause daytime drowsiness, reduced concentration, or reduction in physical performance.

Because of its mechanism of action, it theoretically may potentiate the action of sedative medications that depress the CNS. It does not have a synergy with alcohol. Although no evidence has shown it to be harmful in pregnancy or lactation, it probably should be avoided during these times, like most herbs. There are no known side effects except occasional mild stomach upset, and there are no known interactions with other drugs.

The dosage for insomnia is 150 to 300 mg of 0.8% valerenic extract before sleep. For anxiety, give 150 to 300 mg 3 times/day. A solid extract (4:1) is dosed at 250 to 500 mg t.i.d. or h.s. The tea can be drunk as needed t.i.d. or at h.s. and is made from steeping 1 to 2 g of the root in boiling water for 10 to 15 minutes. A tincture (1:5) is available and 4 to 6 mL is recommended t.i.d. Unfortunately the odor of valerian has been likened to dirty socks.

▬▬ CONCLUSION

This chapter provides a fundamental background in botanical medicine, emphasizing commonly used herbs. The references on pages 362–363 include a more in-depth review of the subject and should eventually find their way to your bookshelf.

Chapter
11

Diet and Nutrition

The doctor of the future will give no medicine, but will interest his patients in the care of the human frame, in diet, and in the cause and prevention of disease.
—Thomas Edison

The only way for a rich man to be healthy is by exercise and abstinence, to live as if he were poor.
—Sir William Temple

Our diet is a key to the prevention of illness and the maintenance of good health. It is somewhat bizarre that nutrition and diet can be considered "alternative" therapy. We live in a culture in which cracking open the chest to sew leg veins onto the heart is considered mainstream medical practice. Yet the low-fat (10%) Dean Ornish diet, which includes yoga, relaxation, exercise, and relational healing, is considered alternative. What's wrong with this picture?

People in our society take many different attitudes toward food. My colleague Don Ardell (1999) has cleverly described the healthy and not-so-healthy eaters that you'll encounter in your practice in a piece called "The Health Enhancer (and Other) Diets" (see Box).

Many diets claim to reduce the risk of heart disease, cancer, arthritis, and other conditions. The value of many of them is yet to be determined. The Gerson diet, Hoxsey treatment, Livingston-Wheeler diet, wheatgrass diet, and others have not been proven to cure or reverse cancer. No diet has. Most of these diets stress increasing the use of fresh fruits and vegetables (not a bad idea) and also promote more dramatic changes in how you shop, cook, and eat.

Clearly, the intake of certain foods is associated with risk reduction for various diseases. For example, increased fruits and vegetables reduce the risk of cancer and cardiovascular disease, as assessed across a number of studies. Whether this is because of protective carotenoids, lignans, and flavonoids in the plant-based foods, their higher fiber content, or simply the fact that they replace many of the higher-fat foods in the diet is unknown.

A problem is that many diets, fad weight-loss programs, and dietary supplements have become very popular through sales of books,

142

THE HEALTH ENHANCER (AND OTHER) DIETS

Survivors eat to stay alive. They would not eat at all if they did not have to. Food is not a high priority with this nothing-for-lunch bunch. These people are simply uninterested in spending time thinking about food or eating. They eat just about whatever finds its way to their plates, while thinking about something (anything) else. Food bores them; nutrition is of little interest. There are not a lot of survivor eaters.

Vaudevillers are the overwhelming majority of eaters. In this case, food is seen and experienced as entertainment. The emphasis is on how it tastes—period. Nutritional considerations, body-shape implications, the mood of the diner, the source, and the methods of delivery—forget it. All that matters is how it looks, smells, tastes, and feels going down the gullet. Vaudevillers account for the popularity of junk food. For these folks, mealtimes are the high spots of the day. They get up early for breakfast, then start thinking about lunch and supper. The evening meal is the major event of the night, followed in importance only by the midnight snack.

Disease avoiders are the products of health educators, cardiologists, diet authors, and nutritionists. They worry a lot about food. They are obsessed with "scare" research linking one more disease with yet another food they love but henceforth must avoid. They comprise the vast number of persons who try to eat only those foods that have not been identified as possible carcinogens. Thus, their food choices are rather limited. They constantly wonder what kind of edible goody will be their eventual undoing.

Fat fighters are the unhappiest of eaters. They, like the vaudevillers, love to be entertained by food. However, though they may eat more of it, they enjoy it a lot less. Everything they eat turns to hideous adipose (fatty) tissue, or so they believe. Food is associated with guilt, shame, and pounds. Fat fighters spend a lot of money on diet books, spas, doctors, and, naturally, restaurants and supermarkets. For them, food is a four-letter word.

Food faddists are the hardest to take. They want you to worry, feel guilty, or get angry about food. If it's not organic, homegrown, or purchased in a "health" food store, they regard it as poison. There are lots of food faddists in my area. A woman friend takes megadoses of Geritol. She mixes the stuff in a blender with wheat germ, Valium, and bone meal. Her blood's so iron-rich she attaches her earrings with magnets.

Health enhancers are the small but growing band of individuals who eat for health, enjoyment, and performance. They are as concerned about, and interested in, the quality and atmospheres (internal and external) of the nutritional experience as they are with the taste. These are the wellness eaters.

Source: Ardell D: *14 Days to Wellness—The Easy, Effective, and Fun Way to Optimum Health.* Novato, CA: New World Library, 1999: 104–105 (with permission).

testimonials, and other promotional measures. Separating the wheat-grass from the tofu seems a Herculean effort, yet here goes. . . .

▬▬▬ WE AREN'T EXACTLY STARVING DOWN HERE

The major nutritional problem in the United States is that we consume **too many calories**. Any dietary plan to lose weight may wind up being an instant best-seller, even without scientific validation. Many of the currently popular diets, such as the Zone or Sugar Busters or Atkins diet, manipulate the distribution of calories among fats, carbohydrates, and proteins (Stein 1999). Immediate weight loss is often seen, owing to water loss. On close examination, though, it turns out that these diets often recommend an intake of about 1200 calories or so per day, which is a weight-loss diet for almost anyone.

Americans are dying to lose weight (literally), but generally they want an easy way to do it, forgetting that the lard that has accumulated over many years is unlikely to leave in a fortnight. For example, consider the case of John Carlos.

John Carlos is a 43-year-old musician (jazz and blues) and parking lot attendant. He is 238 lbs and has a BP of 150/100 and a total cholesterol of 242. He prefers to take a lipid-lowering statin drug for cholesterol instead of changing his diet to include more fruits, vegetables, and grains and less fat. John Carlos also would rather pop a medication to lower his blood pressure than lose weight or exercise. His idea of stress management is a couple of martinis at lunch and an occasional benzodiazepine when things get really rough, rather than some simple mind-body relaxation therapies. So you can see that dietary modification is really outside the way of life that John Carlos has come to accept as normal. How can we help him?

Perhaps he would consider one of the approaches to diet described below. Let's take a closer look at several common alternative diets so you will at least have a clue about them when patients ask.

The Atkins Diet

The Atkins diet, around since the 1970s, is enjoying a resurgence. The book, *Dr. Atkins' New Diet Revolution,* is a recent best-seller (1999). This diet drastically lowers the intake of carbohydrates, ordinarily our main source of nutritional energy. (Most diets get about 50% or 60% of their calories from carbos.) On this diet you can reportedly eat all the fat and protein you want, and you will still lose weight. For example, when the pizza comes, scrape all the cheese, pepperoni, and sauce onto your plate and eat that, but don't touch the crust! Strange as it sounds, people are able to lose weight and lower lipid levels on this diet, primarily because it pushes the body to burn fat into ketones by not providing much carbohydrate. It also causes your breath to smell like the south end of a northbound mule due to chronic ketosis, but don't worry. Some low-calorie breath mints—the kind that curl your lip—could help, but they contain sugar, *verboten* on this diet (oops!).

Much to my surprise, however, I have had several patients over the years who have used this diet quite successfully. Though this is anecdotal, I have had physician colleagues tell me how they got patients off of taking over 140 units of insulin daily by using the Atkins diet. I haven't had the courage to try this tactic yet, but in view of the biochemistry, the lowered carbohydrate load certainly would be expected to lower insulin requirements.

The Atkins diet has been around for almost 30 years, so it seems to be safe enough. The weight loss must be maintained with reduced calories and regular exercise after stopping it, or those unwanted pounds will just return. Nutritionally oriented practitioners like me are concerned that the absence of fiber, fruits, and vegetables in this diet may have some adverse long-term health consequences. Clearly, fruit and vegetables can reduce the risk of heart disease and cancer, so replacing them with high-protein and high-fat foods is a concern. But many patients do well on this diet and one could argue that the loss of double-digit amounts of fat may offset the risk of missing phytochemicals, fiber, antioxidants, and other goodies in a diet that is more plant based. The new version of the diet does have a gradual phase-in of fiber, fruits, and vegetables.

Hypertension, heart disease, diabetes, hypercholesterolemia, and osteoarthritis can all be improved by a major weight loss. Patients starting this diet should be monitored medically with regular lab work and checkups, particularly if they have liver, kidney, or gastrointestinal disease or diabetes. Maybe staying on this diet for a month or two and then going off would be a safe approach. Keep an open mind about the Atkins diet, especially since some of your patients will be on it whether you believe in it or not (Merrell 1999).

The Ornish Diet

Dr. Dean Ornish has devised a diet for cardiovascular risk reduction that really seems to work. Even the Medicare program is studying it in comparison to cardiac bypass surgery and angioplasty. Its acceptance could have major implications in terms of health care costs in this country (Kostreski 1999). As mentioned before, it includes an extremely low amount of fat (10% of calories). It also employs mind-body techniques, relaxation, yoga, exercise, and dealing with emotional and relational dysfunction as a program to heart health. In his recent book, *Love & Survival: The Scientific Basis for the Healing Power of Intimacy* (1998), Dr. Ornish reviews his earlier studies (1990, 1983), showing a reversal of angiographically proven stenosis in coronary artery disease with this approach, also introducing fascinating data about the value of positive, caring relationships and social support to our cardiac health.

The major problem with this effective approach is that few in our society care to make the radical lifestyle changes involved. The diet alone requires a lot of motivation and discipline. To reduce fat content from the usual American diet, which consists of over 40% fat, to less than 10% requires an essentially meatless or vegetarian diet. This is a huge change for most of us. In the guise of tasty, entertaining foods, our omnipresent fast-food outlets offer us things that are higher in fat than a sow's belly.

Several other diets in this vein (or artery) are noteworthy. The Pritikin diet, like Ornish, focuses on cardiovascular risk reduction. Again, it moves people from the typical high-fat American diet to more plant-based food sources. Without going to the extent of the Ornish program, many sensible vegetarian or even semi-vegetarian (occasional fish or fowl) diets offer us the lower-fat, higher-fiber balance recommended in the recently released food pyramid (Fig. 11–1).

Vegetarian Diet

As you can see from the food pyramid, it is possible to get most of our nutrition from plant sources. "Vegetarians" follow a variety of regimens. The vegan diet has no animal products at all, whereas the lacto-ovo vegetarian diet includes milk and eggs. It is clear that vegetarians live longer and are afflicted with fewer of the modern diseases such as heart disease, diabetes, hypertension, and cancer (Key 1999, Janelle 1995, Fraser 1993, National Research Council 1989, Sacks 1974). Although I have seen obese vegetarians, they are rare and they usually didn't get obese on a pure vegetarian diet (and I don't mean french fries or potato chips with orange soda!). The data are good that these are healthy diets and people do well on them.

There are some potentials for deficiencies in some of the strict vegan diets and vegetarian diets in children. Vitamin B_{12}, calcium, zinc, iron, and some essential amino acids may be missing in these diets. These deficiencies can be anticipated and managed with supplements or proper food mixing. Overall, vegetarian diets not only are safe, but because of their high fiber, phytochemical, and antioxidant levels, they are quite healthy. Because they are much lower in fat than the standard American

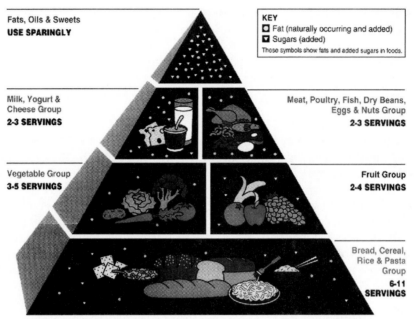

Source: U. S. Department of Agriculture, Human Nutrition Information Services

Figure 11–1   Source: U.S. Department of Agriculture, Human Nutrition Information Service.

meat-based diet, they also are wonderful for weight loss, protection against lipid and cardiac problems, and diabetes.

Though I try to resist despair, my heart often sinks when someone who is 40 or 50 lbs or more overweight comes to me wanting to lose weight. I realize that weight loss is essential to their health, but many of them are just not willing to commit to the slow and consistent lifestyle change required. What I have begun recommending to these struggling folks is a vegetarian diet. When they grimace, I back off and say, "OK, how about a semi-vegetarian or pesco-vegetarian diet, one with occasional fish or even fowl?" That seems to work better in our society, or at least among my patients.

DASH Diet (Dietary Approaches to Stopping Hypertension)

The DASH diet (Appel 1997) was found to improve blood pressure by using whole foods such as vegetables, fruits, and low-fat dairy products, with reduced saturated and total fat. This diet reduced fat to 27% and was high in fruits and vegetables. This was not a vegetarian diet, yet those following it showed a significant blood pressure reduction in just 11 weeks compared to the control group. Best of all, it had enough dairy and meat products to make it palatable to those who might not accept a full vegetarian diet.

Mediterranean Diet

The Mediterranean diet (Jossa 1996; DeLorgeril 1994, 1998) emphasizes the kinds of food eaten in that part of the world. Lots of fresh vegetables, pasta, olive oil, and fish and poultry are staples. This diet is lower in sodium than the traditional U.S. diet, and the olive oil tends to lower LDL without lowering HDL cholesterol levels. Grapes, wine, artichokes, and other yummies are part of this diet, and they offer their own health benefits as antioxidants, protecting from heart disease and liver disease, among others. This diet may not be the best for losing weight, but it certainly has many health benefits and is delicious and readily available.

Macrobiotics

The macrobiotic diet is derived from the Japanese diet and is essentially a vegetarian diet with small amounts of fish (pesco-vegetarian). This diet features soy, rice, seaweed, pickled vegetables, and other staples of the Japanese diet. It has been advocated as a cancer prevention and treatment (Kushi 1983, Lerner 1994, pp. 285–318). The diet became quite popular in the early 1980s when a physician with metastatic prostate cancer clearly visible on a bone scan was interviewed by a popular magazine. After 6 months of eating miso soup, seaweed, rice balls, and other healthful but radically non-American foods, a follow-up bone scan showed complete remission of his lesions (Sattilaro 1982). Proof, coincidence, or association? I worked for a time with Keith Block, MD, a physician in the Chicago area who used this strict diet with cancer patients. His clients came from far and wide to learn how to cook and eat macrobiotically. As much as I enjoyed the flavor and novelty of the macrobiotic diet, I found it too difficult to shop, cook, and eat in this way regularly. Though I enjoy a meal at a Zen-style or macrobiotic restaurant whenever I can, this kind of program is too radical for most patients. In any case, it may be too little, too late. If food is primarily a preventive for disease rather than a treatment, then those with advanced cancer may have benefited from the diet earlier, though their motivation to try it would not have been as high. In any case, Block and his colleagues propose the macrobiotic diet as a sensible part of an overall program of cancer therapy, which includes chemotherapy, surgery, and radiation as necessary. They also emphasize compassionate caring, stress management, and a holistic fitness program including body, mind, and spirit (Lerner 1994, pp. 335–351).

Zoned, Busting Sugar, and Your Blood Type?

Three popular diets deserve mention here because they are so widespread. They resemble each other in their pseudoscientific terminology, wide claims for efficacy, and lack of scientific studies supporting them. The "Zone Diet" advocates a complex set of rules to maintain a strict intake of 40% carbohydrate, 30% protein, and 30% fat (Sears 1995). By reducing insulin secretion, which is stimulated by carbohydrates, this diet claims to help with weight loss. The "Sugar Busters" diet is similar in terminology and tone (Steward et al. 1998). It uses the term "glycemic index" to rate foods by their tendency to produce insulin release. It forbids a huge range of foods including potatoes, white bread, white pasta, corn, beets, and even carrots. It fails to notice that we eat these foods not individually but with other foods. Both the Sugar Busters diet and the Zone diet need more emphasis on exercise and reduction of total calorie intake.

Eat Right for Your Type takes a medical anthropology approach, claiming that people with certain blood groups evolved from different populations (D'Adamo 1996). For example, blood type B evolved from nomads, and therefore people with this blood type should consume dairy products, little meat, and no chicken. People with type A blood (agrarians) cannot digest meat and should all be vegetarians, and blood types AB should eat no wheat, but can eat soy, dairy, seafood, and a little meat. Many people (type O blood) should go on a meat-based, low–plant-food diet because they evolved from hunters. This seems risky in view of what we know of the benefits of plant-based diets and the dangers of high fat consumption. The author bases his concern on the fear that if one eats the wrong type of food, the proteins (lectins) in that food will produce antibodies, which will cause all kinds of health problems.

Using Soy Products

Another current hot controversy in dietary manipulation is the use of soy products. There are several lines of reasoning about the increased use of soy in our diet. I trained in the Midwest, where we were surrounded by miles of soybeans and corn. This was profitable agriculture, but most of this plant material was used not for human food but for fodder, to feed livestock. The hogs and cattle turn these highly nutritious vegetables into tasty but high-fat foods. Maybe this is not as good a tradeoff as it seems.

Women in Asia have a much lower risk of breast cancer than those in the United States. Perhaps this difference is because of less fat in the diet, more breast-feeding, or other lifestyle factors. However, one hypothesis is that the use of more soy in their diets provides some protection from these cancers, perhaps because of its phytoestrogen content. Phytoestrogens are compounds in soy and other plants that have weak estrogenic properties and actually block estrogen receptors that are associated with the more aggressive forms of cancer.

Recent research at MD Anderson Cancer Center in Houston, Texas, has suggested that the use of soy products *after* the diagnosis of breast cancer may not be safe because even the weak estrogenic properties may stimulate tumor growth. The data are still not in for a final risk assessment. For now, I am advising my patients to avoid significantly increasing their soy intake if they have had known estrogen-receptor–positive cancer of the breast.

Overall, however, as a preventive measure and also as a means of lowering fat intake, the addition of tofu, soybeans, soy milk, and artificial meat products made from soy may offer some measure of protection from cancer.

■■■■ GENERAL RECOMMENDATIONS ABOUT DIETS

I learned about several of these diets from my patients and then had to read about them on the Internet, in books and magazines, and finally in some peer-reviewed literature. My approach to this continual procession of diets (several more will have hit the bookracks by the time you read this) is somewhat pragmatic. First, I figure that at least my patients are taking an interest in weight loss, however far-out the diet may seem. That is good because it shows motivation. Rather than condemning the diet out of hand, I am challenged to learn about it. As in the case of the Atkins diet, some people do remarkably well. In the end, if I realize my patients are being duped or at least misinformed, I'll let them know and recommend a diet I consider more sensible, such as the vegetarian or Mediterranean diet or the pyramid plan.

I think the best we can say is that shifting our diet to more carbohydrates in the form of fruits, grains, and vegetables will be beneficial in reducing the major scourges of our society, such as obesity, heart disease, hypertension, diabetes, and some forms of cancer. These benefits mostly seem to accrue as a result of increased fiber, reduced fat, and protective flavonoids, carotenoids, lignans, and antioxidants in the plant-based foods.

And What about Losing Weight?

Reducing weight, a veritable preoccupation in our society, is a challenging issue in every medical setting. Very-low-calorie diets, fat reduction, and vegetarian diets all can play a role. The key issue, however, is weight maintenance, not just weight reduction. Maintaining weight loss requires changing one's lifestyle. Dietary changes that helped folks lose weight need to be continued in the post-diet phase. Also key to the success of any diet plan is the maintenance of an active exercise program. Those who are able not only to lose weight but also to keep it off as measured a couple of years down the road have maintained exercise as a regular part of their lifestyle, at least to the tune of a half-hour a day or so.

Self-Image Issues

A minister friend of mine talked about how to handle the self-image issues associated with being overweight. As long as you "need to lose weight" and keep telling yourself that, you always will. This phrase sets up a self-defeating inner affirmation that you "need to. . ." rather than being in the "process of . . . ." Think of fat as "out of control, underexercised muscle!" and you have created a more useful paradigm that encourages better choices.

Another aspect of the weight-loss problem is the stress generated by societally induced negative self-images. I read of an ethnic German community in Pennsylvania where all the adult members were, to put it gently, portly. They weighed 250 to 300 lbs yet curiously did not die of obesity-related problems like heart disease at a higher rate than the general population of the state. They more or less accepted their body habitus as normal and not unsightly or unhealthy. In other words, they had a high degree of self-acceptance. When they moved out of their community to live in mainstream American society, however, where the emaciated supermodel is considered the ideal, they started to have heart disease, hypertension, diabetes, and so forth at the same rate as the general population. No doubt there is an obesity-related bias in this country. Jobs, marriage, and other healthy pursuits are often denied the portly because of their weight, even when they are qualified, lovable, and otherwise suitable. This is a tremendous blow to self-esteem and would be expected to be hard on one's health.

Lesson: Some degree of healthy self-acceptance, self-esteem, and self-love protects against even the well-known risks of being overweight. At a bookstore yesterday, I saw on the health topic table several fat-rights books addressing this issue, with titles like *Fat. . .So?* One had an obese lady (rather cute I thought) in a bathing suit beauty contest on the cover. Even the 1999 *Sports Illustrated Swimsuit Edition* (I read it for the articles) had an ad featuring a pizza and beer bubba–type of guy happily lying on his side in a swimsuit on the beach. The quote was something like, "Pizza. Pork rinds. Beer. Put him on the cover. . .Because he's never looked better. . .What you live is what you get." These are all attempts—healthy ones, I think—to consider the healthy pleasures of eating, to accept our imperfections, and to accept ourselves as worthwhile human beings even though we are carrying around too much of that unexercised, out-of-control muscle (Ornstein & Sobel 1989).

Helping Obese Patients

Don't give up hope for patients who have a sincere interest in weight loss and are ready to try anything that promises to help them, including fad diets. Encourage self-care, nutritional awareness, regular exercise, self-esteem, and a gradual process of health improvement and weight normalization. It is helpful to ask about their target weights. Usually they mention a goal weight they last were at when they finished high school or college. They may see this as ideal and realistic even though that was 100 lbs and 25 years ago. I encourage a more realistic goal, perhaps segmenting the weight loss into 10- to 20-lb mini-goals rather than trying to climb off that discouraging mountain of weight loss at one jump. This builds confidence and success. Slow, steady weight loss of ½ to 1 lb weekly, accompanied by regular exercise, is the proven formula for sustained weight loss. It is all about lifestyle change and not just shedding the pounds. Eat well to be well.

Chapter 12

Nutriceuticals

The wise man does at once what the fool does finally.
—Baltasar Gracian

Health is so necessary to all the duties, as well as pleasures, of life, that the crime of squandering it is equal to the folly.
—Samuel Johnson

DEFINITION

Let us now turn from diets to the topic of "nutriceuticals." These are agents such as vitamins, minerals, and other dietary supplements, which, though not truly considered foods, can be useful in improving health, making up for dietary deficiencies, and even treating certain conditions (Goodwin et al 1998). Where does the word "nutriceutical" come from? It is made up from the words "nutrition" and "pharmaceutical" and implies the use of nutritional agents in the treatment of health conditions. You'll also see it spelled "nutraceutical." For our purposes, the two are interchangeable. Spelling it with "a" emphasizes the pharmaceutical aspect, whereas spelling it with "i" emphasizes the nutrition aspect (or so I've heard). The term most often refers to amino acids, enzymes, essential fatty acids, minerals, and vitamins. In the newest classification from the National Center for Complementary and Alternative Medicine (NCCAM), some of the pharmacological and biological agents that I cover in the next chapter could be discussed here.

Why would we need to supplement our diets in an admittedly overfed society? Though we take in plenty of calories, we may not always choose our food wisely. Beta carotene, for instance, a highly available nutrient in fresh fruits and vegetables, may not be taken in adequate quantities if our daily diet is low in these natural foods. In addition, picking vegetables and fruits before they are ripe may reduce their nutritional content. Also, certain pesticides used in agriculture contain hydrazine and other chemicals that reduce the availability of such essentials as vitamin B_6 (pyridoxine).

Plants do not require the same elements for growth that humans do.

For instance, selenium, chromium, and iodine are unnecessary for plants but are essential to humans and may need to be added to the diet.

Finally, some people require more or less of a given vitamin, mineral, or other nutrient because of biological individuality. The general Recommended Daily Allowance (RDA), though helpful, may not meet every person's daily needs.

Speaking of vitamins and minerals, just what do they do? Although their functions vary, they serve as essential cofactors in the wide range of enzymatic and energy transfer processes in the body. Without their actions as catalysts and cofactors in chemical reactions, we would not exist. They also serve as antioxidants, protecting the body from the damaging effect of free radicals, protecting us from toxins and the body's own waste products, and combining to activate the enzyme systems on which we rely. Some, such as vitamin C and calcium, provide supportive elements to connective tissue and organs.

▬▬▬ AMINO ACIDS

Amino Acids
● ●

ESSENTIAL
Isoleucine
Leucine
Lysine
Methionine
Phenylalanine
Threonine
Tryptophan
Valine

SEMIESSENTIAL
Histidine

NONESSENTIAL
Alanine
Arginine
Asparagine
Aspartic acid
Glycine
Proline
Serine
Tyrosine

The amino acids are the building blocks of proteins. Those considered essential to complete nutrition are listed in the box. There are also several compounds of amino acids, such as carnitine, made from the combination of other amino acids. Naturopathic physicians and many other nutritionally oriented practitioners and physicians such as Alan Gaby and Jonathan Wright, who teach extensively about nutritional therapy (Gaby & Wright 1998), use amino acids therapeutically.

There is literature supporting most of these uses as primary therapies, but I prefer to use them as adjunctive, integrated with conventional therapies. Because amino acids are foods, these therapies are largely safe. We do need to be vigilant in the clinical setting, however, and watch these and other natural products for side effects and reactions, perhaps from contaminated products or from use at supraphysiological levels. For instance, L-tryptophan was used

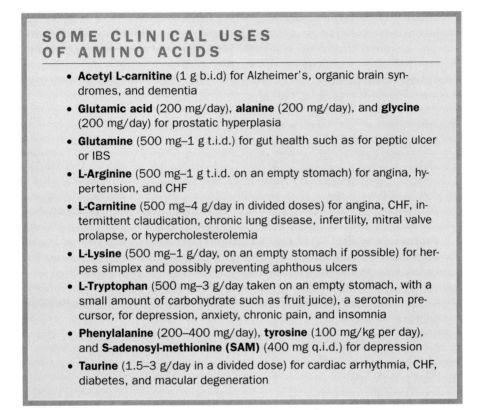

SOME CLINICAL USES
OF AMINO ACIDS

- **Acetyl L-carnitine** (1 g b.i.d) for Alzheimer's, organic brain syndromes, and dementia
- **Glutamic acid** (200 mg/day), **alanine** (200 mg/day), and **glycine** (200 mg/day) for prostatic hyperplasia
- **Glutamine** (500 mg–1 g t.i.d.) for gut health such as for peptic ulcer or IBS
- **L-Arginine** (500 mg–1 g t.i.d. on an empty stomach) for angina, hypertension, and CHF
- **L-Carnitine** (500 mg–4 g/day in divided doses) for angina, CHF, intermittent claudication, chronic lung disease, infertility, mitral valve prolapse, or hypercholesterolemia
- **L-Lysine** (500 mg–1 g/day, on an empty stomach if possible) for herpes simplex and possibly preventing aphthous ulcers
- **L-Tryptophan** (500 mg–3 g/day taken on an empty stomach, with a small amount of carbohydrate such as fruit juice), a serotonin precursor, for depression, anxiety, chronic pain, and insomnia
- **Phenylalanine** (200–400 mg/day), **tyrosine** (100 mg/kg per day), and **S-adenosyl-methionine (SAM)** (400 mg q.i.d.) for depression
- **Taurine** (1.5–3 g/day in a divided dose) for cardiac arrhythmia, CHF, diabetes, and macular degeneration

widely as a natural sleep aid and antidepressant. As a serotonin precursor, there was good therapeutic rationale for its use and many of my patients benefited from it. It was taken off the market in the early 1990s when a contaminated batch caused several deaths from eosinophilia myalgia syndrome (EMS). It is now available again. Interactions with drugs also may be a concern. For example, it may be best to avoid using L-tryptophan with selective serotonin reuptake inhibitors (SSRIs) because of the potential of a serotonin syndrome.

ENZYMES

An enzyme you will hear a lot about these days is **CoQ10**, or Coenzyme Q10, which is an important coenzyme in the electron transport chain. Because it is required for all energy-dependent reactions in the body, tissue-level deficiencies are likely in metabolically active tissues.

CoQ10 has been widely studied for use in such conditions as

congestive heart failure (CHF) (Baggio et al 1994, Morisco et al 1993), hypertension, and diabetes. HIV support, mitral valve prolapse, chemotherapy support, gingivitis, and male infertility are other applications of this useful and ubiquitous substance. (Its other name is *ubiquinone*, emphasizing its presence in every part of the body.) It may be deficient in certain people with CHF and also in those who are taking an HMG-CoA reductase inhibitor such as Mevacor for lowering cholesterol.

I tend to use CoQ10 in my patients with CHF who are at the maximal dosage of their conventional therapy of an angiotensin-converting enzyme (ACE) inhibitor, diuretic, or other medication. Several studies indicate that it improves ejection fraction and reduces symptoms. Its natural sources include broccoli, spinach, nuts, meat, and fish.

Bromelain is another agent that is an enzyme, this one derived from the pineapple. It is useful as a digestive aid; an anti-inflammatory for minor injuries, muscle bruises, aches, and sprains; and a treatment for angina, asthma, and urinary tract infections.

Several digestive enzymes are available, including **pancrease, lipase,** and **lactase**. A mixture called **pancreatin**, composed of protease, lipase, and amylase, is useful in those with pancreatic insufficiency and to help digest proteins, fats, and carbohydrates. Conditions such as cystic fibrosis, chronic pancreatic insufficiency, and even some types of heartburn and indigestion may benefit from this mixture. Those with lactose intolerance, the inability to digest the simple mild sugar lactose, may benefit from adding lactase to the diet. Such conditions as irritable bowel syndrome (IBS), migraine, some kinds of diarrhea, and indigestion and heartburn may be helped by this enzyme.

▬▬ ESSENTIAL FATTY ACIDS

Despite our society's general overconsumption of fat, certain kinds of fat are healthy. The omega-3 and omega-6 fatty acids and alpha-linolenic and linoleic acid are protective against heart disease, stroke, autoimmune and inflammatory conditions such as rheumatoid arthritis, skin diseases such as eczema and psoriasis, and possibly multiple sclerosis (Murray & Pizzorno 1998). These essential fatty acids are components of the synthesis pathways of prostaglandins, which are involved in a wide variety of inflammatory processes in the body. The omega-6 pathway produces arachidonic acid, primarily from animal products in the diet. The omega-3 series is predominantly from plant sources and produces particularly beneficial prostaglandins. Seeds, nuts, and oily fish such as halibut are sources of essential fatty acids. Many nutritionally oriented practitioners encourage the addition of a daily tablespoon of flaxseed oil, a rich source of omega-3 fatty acids. Omega-3 fatty acids are from fish oils such as cod liver and halibut; flaxseed, which contains about 53% alpha-linolenic acid; black currant seed oil; and walnut and soybean oil. Sources of omega-6 fatty acids are safflower, sunflower, and soybean oil, which yield linoleic acid. Evening primrose oil, borage oil, and black currant seed oil also yield gamma-linolenic acid, the dehydrogenated form of linoleic acid.

Increasing the dosage of these essential fatty acids may also increase the need for vitamin E in the diet. Adding a vitamin E capsule to a bottle of the essential fatty acid or oil will prevent oxidation into less active forms. Keep the oil in a sealed bottle in a refrigerator. Keep in mind that taking large doses of these oils may mean consuming excess calories and fat.

Clinical indications are dry skin, heel fissures, eczema, and dandruff. Other indications are hypertension and hyperlipidemia. Omega-6 fatty acids can reduce serum cholesterol but the tradeoff may be the increased amount of fat in the diet. For rheumatoid arthritis and other autoimmune disorders, the appropriate supplements are borage oil, which provides 1.4 g/day of gamma-linolenic acid; black currant seed oil, 10.5 g/day; and fish-oil concentrate, 10 to 12 g/day. According to Gaby and Wright (1998), there are a series of other indications for the variety of essential fatty acids:

- Fish-oil concentrate, 3 to 12 g/day
- Cod liver oil, 5 to 15 mL/day
- Flaxseed, sunflower, or safflower oil, 5 to 30 mL/day
- Evening primrose oil, 2 to 6 g/day
- Borage oil, 1 to 6 g/day
- Black currant seed oil, 2 to 20 g/day.

They suggest that flaxseed oil or flaxseed oil alternated with sunflower oil on alternate days may be helpful for benign prostatic hypertrophy. Flaxseed oil is also indicated for constipation and may reduce cancer risk. (The new cyclo-oxygenase-2 inhibitors, which are involved in the same pathways as the essential fatty acids, are now thought to reduce the risk of colon and possibly other cancers.) Gaby and Wright also suggest that diabetic neuropathy may benefit from using evening primrose oil for a year, and familial tremor may suggest the use of sunflower/safflower oil or flaxseed oil. Another intriguing set of studies suggests a benefit of sunflower oil, evening primrose oil, or cod liver oil combined with a low-fat diet for multiple sclerosis.

MINERALS

Minerals are essential to complete health. The use of supplemental minerals is useful in a number of therapeutic situations. Table 12–1 summarizes the minerals most commonly used in a primary care setting. By and large, minerals either are cofactors in important biochemical reactions in the body or contribute to structural aspects of the body.

Calcium does both. It is the major element sustaining our skeleton, which keeps us from slithering along the ground like your ordinary ameba. It is also essential in many important physiological reactions, especially the contraction of muscles. Nutritionally oriented physicians and others recommend it in high doses, such as 1000 to 1500 mg/day for the prevention of osteoporosis, building strong bones in children, muscle cramps, dysmenorrhea and premenstrual syndrome (PMS), migraines, some kinds of depression, and as an adjunctive agent for hypertension and hypercholesterolemia. Natural sources are green leafy vegetables, canned fish with bones, tofu, and dairy products. To absorb calcium, the body requires vitamin D either in supplement form or as converted within the body from sunshine.

Chromium is another essential mineral, particularly in energy transfer. It is most widely known for its use in diabetes. A number of studies have shown it to be useful in the dosage of 200 µg/day of chromium picolinate to improve blood sugar control in some people. It is also marketed as a weight-loss aid (another sure-fire claim for commercial success), but I have yet to see any scientific studies to document this assertion. The daily dosage is between 50 and 200 µg, most of which can be obtained from such natural sources as corn, beef, apples, sweet potatoes, mushrooms, nuts, tomatoes, broccoli, and eggs.

Copper is not only a nice coating for cookware, but has widely reputed effects on certain types of arthritis. Many of my patients have claimed that wearing copper bracelets improved their rheumatoid arthritis or osteoarthritis. I saw one study (Walker et al 1976) that reported that the weight of a copper bracelet decreased significantly over a 2-week period when worn by arthritis sufferers but remained the same in healthy controls. I don't know that this means anything conclusive, but copper bracelets continue to be advertised and sold for this indication. Those taking large doses of zinc also need to supplement with copper, because copper can become less available in the presence of zinc. Copper performs a number of functions in the body, mainly as a cofactor or catalyst for chemical reactions. The requirement is 2 to 3 mg daily for adults. Food sources of copper include potatoes, avocados, beef liver (yecch!), oysters (yum!), and lobsters (yum-yum!). If your home has copper pipes, you may get all you need that way.

Table 12–1   MINERALS MOST COMMONLY USED IN PRIMARY CARE*

Nutrient	Benefits and Therapeutic Uses	Therapeutic Range	Risks	Sources	RDA
Calcium	**Bone and teeth formation** **Osteoporosis** **Rickets** **Dysmenorrhea** **PMS** Migraines Depression Hypertension Hypercholesterolemia Muscle cramps Pre-eclampsia	1000–1500 mg/d	Excess may interfere with absorption of other minerals Kidney stones	Green leafy vegetables Sardines, canned salmon Tofu Dairy products	1000 mg/d
Chromium	**High cholesterol** **Hypoglycemia** **Glucose metabolism** **Diabetes** Athletic performance Weight loss Obesity Energy transfer	200 µg/d	Diabetic patients require medical supervision	Corn, sweet potatoes, mushrooms, tomatoes, broccoli Beef, eggs, oysters Apples, rhubarb Nuts, barley	50–200 µg

*Most important benefits and indications shown in boldface type.
PMS = premenstrual syndrome, RBC = red blood cells, BPH = benign prostatic hypertrophy, URI = upper respiratory infection

(Continued)

Table 12-1   MINERALS MOST COMMONLY USED IN PRIMARY CARE* (Continued)

Nutrient	Benefits and Therapeutic Uses	Therapeutic Range	Risks	Sources	RDA
Copper	**Wound healing** Collagen and RBC formation Iron absorption Benign prostatic hyperplasia Hypoglycemia Rheumatoid arthritis Catalyst for chemical reactions Bone strength	2–3 mg/d	Neurological and gastrointestinal (GI) symptoms	Potatoes Avocados Beef liver, oysters, lobsters	1.5–3 mg/d
Iron	**Hemoglobin synthesis**	50–300 mg/d	GI symptoms (stomach upset, constipation) Hemochromatosis Heart problems	Peanut butter, almonds Broccoli, beans, spinach Wheat cereals, barley Chicken, meats, liver, oysters Raisins, molasses	6 mg/d (infants) 30 mg/d (pregnant women) 10–15 mg/d (adults)
Magnesium	**Cardiac arrhythmias** **CHF** **Hypertension** **Migraine** Asthma Chronic fatigue syndrome Diabetes Osteoporosis PMS	500 mg t.i.d.	Excess may increase prostate cancer Neurotoxicity	Peanuts, nuts, oatmeal Bananas, avocados Milk Broccoli, dark-green leafy vegetables, collard, okra Potatoes, whole wheat bread	30 mg/d (newborns) 300–400 mg/d (adults)

Mineral	Indications	Dose	Toxicity	Food Sources	Recommended Intake
Manganese	**Antioxidant** **Hypoglycemia** **Bone and connective tissue growth** Heavy menstrual flow Arthritis	5–15 mg	Unknown	Tea Blueberries, pineapple, oranges Nuts, whole grains, beans Spinach, carrots, broccoli Raisins	1 mg/d (children) 5 mg/d (adults)
Molybdenum	**Cofactor in various metabolic pathways** **Antioxidant** Asthma		Joint pains	Whole grains, beans Green leafy vegetables Lean meats, organ meats Milk	15–150 mg/d (children) 75–250 mg/d (adults)
Potassium	**Hypertension** **CHF** Muscle and nerve function Muscle cramps Stroke prevention		Fatal heart dysrhythmias	Watermelon, bananas, citrus fruits Beans Potatoes Milk	2000 mg/d
Selenium	**Antioxidant** **Detoxifying agent** **Immunity** **Cancer risk reduction** Asthma Coronary artery disease Eye disease (macular degeneration)	200 µg/d	GI symptoms Neurotoxicity Death	Seafood Lean beef, organ meats Chicken Nuts	10–30 µg/d (children) 40–75 µg/d (adults)

Continued

Table 12–1   MINERALS MOST COMMONLY USED IN PRIMARY CARE* *(Continued)*

Nutrient	Benefits and Therapeutic Uses	Therapeutic Range	Risks	Sources	RDA
Zinc	**Metabolism of over 200 different enzymes and hormones**	30–100 mg/d		Oysters, lean meats Turkey (dark meat) Beans Almonds	5–10 mg/d (children) 15 mg/d (adults)
	Antioxidant				
	Male fertility and potency				
	BPH				
	Wound healing				
	URIs				
	Skin and nail problems in diabetics				
	Memory loss				
	Olfaction and tasting problems				

Iron is essential to the function of the protein hemoglobin, which carries oxygen in the blood. Most people absorb enough iron from their diet, but they may need supplements if they are highly athletic, pregnant, or suffering from any chronic blood loss, including menstruation. Small children and toddlers need plenty of iron to avoid anemia, which can seriously affect growth. However, iron supplements can be toxic to small children. Too much iron is also a hazard to those with a rare iron-storage disease called *hemochromatosis*. An excess of iron also has been found to increase the risk of heart disease in men. There really are not many alternative treatments using iron. Daily requirements range from 6 mg in infants to 30 mg in pregnant women. Usually about 10 to 15 mg is enough for adults. It is available from such food sources as wheat cereals, meats (including chicken), molasses, raisins, beans, and spinach. Cooking in an iron skillet also adds iron to your diet.

Magnesium is a valuable adjunctive treatment for many conditions. As a kid I used to stand delighted when I threw magnesium shavings from my dad's shop into a fire and watched them sparkle. Besides its use in pyrotechnics (that's fireworks) and airplanes, it can be helpful in CHF, hypertension, cardiac arrhythmia, migraine, asthma, bone health, kidney stones, chronic fatigue syndrome, PMS, and diabetes. The daily requirement varies by age from 30 mg in the newborn to around 300 to 400 mg in adults. Higher doses are commonly prescribed for such problems as hypertension or arrrhythmias (500 mg). Food sources include peanuts, bananas, milk, dark-green leafy vegetables, oatmeal, potatoes, and whole wheat bread.

Manganese is found in most antioxidant formulas and is useful primarily for that effect. It is a cofactor in many biochemical reactions and is useful for bone and connective tissue growth, may help reduce heavy menstrual flow, and assists the action of glucosamine for arthritis. The requirement for this element is low and deficiency is rare; children need about 1 mg/day and adults up to 5 mg/day. It is present in tea, some fruits and vegetables, nuts, whole grains, raisins, and some other foods.

Molybdenum, like manganese, is found in many antioxidant products and functions as an important cofactor in the production of several enzymes. Deficiency is rare and most adults get their daily requirement of 75 to 250 µg from food. Children require as little as 15 to 150 µg/day, depending on their ages. The amount of molybdenum in foods depends on its presence in the soil in which they are grown. Sources include whole grains, green leafy vegetables, lean meats, organ meats, and milk.

Potassium is an essential salt and may be useful in hypertension. Those taking diuretics often require supplemental potassium in the prescription strength. You'd have to take 15 or 20 over-the-counter potassium supplements to make up for the prescription strength. I have found potassium to be helpful for muscle cramps, particularly of the nocturnal variety. (Calcium can also help with this troubling problem.) Potassium is also helpful for hypertension, mainly because those eating a lot of high-potassium foods are eating less sodium-rich food. It may be useful to prevent strokes. There is no minimum requirement. It is certainly highly available in lots of fruits and vegetables; in fact, you can get all of your daily potassium from these sources. Particularly rich in potassium are watermelons, bananas, and citrus, with lesser amounts in potatoes, milk, and beans. A nephrologist recently told me, however, that although bananas have a reputation of being a rich source, with an average of 1 mEq of potassium per inch of banana, you'd have to eat about 5 *feet* of bananas a day to get your total daily requirement!

Selenium is another antioxidant mineral. Whether it is present in foods depends on whether it occurs in the soil in which the food has been grown. Selenium is essential to the function of glutathione peroxidase, an essential detoxifying agent and antioxidant. Also, those whose diet is deficient in selenium are prone to cancer, which isn't the same as saying that selenium prevents cancer. It may be useful in coronary artery disease and in boosting immunity. It facilitates the function of vitamin E. It is included in formulas for treating macular degeneration, an eye disease. Supplements should be taken with food for adequate absorption. Usual supplemental doses are 200 µg but the RDA is lower, about 10 to 30 µg in children and 40 to 75 µg in adults. Selenium occurs in seafood, lean beef, chicken, some nuts, and organ meats.

Zinc is one of my personal favorite minerals. It is a key element in making over 200 different enzymes and many hormones. I learned about its usefulness from a patient who took it to stave off flare-ups of his chronic prostatitis. Whenever he felt an attack starting, he would boost his daily dose of zinc from 30 to 100 mg and was convinced that this often kept him from needing antibiotics. Zinc also has been touted as a boost to male fertility and potency, because it seems to concentrate in the prostate. Some studies show it to be useful in benign prostate hyperplasia. It also acts as an antioxidant and has been included in formulas for eye health to prevent or treat macular degeneration. Zinc lozenges are available to treat sore throats and upper respiratory infections, but it doesn't seem to offer dramatic benefit. It also is helpful in wound healing, skin and nail problems, some cases of diabetes, and memory loss. I also recommend it to patients who are having troubles with tasting and olfaction. The RDA is 5 to 10 mg in children and 15 mg in adults. Food sources are oysters, the dark meat of the turkey, lean meats, beans, and almonds.

This has been a whirlwind tour of common applications of minerals in alternative and integrative care. There are a number of other minerals such as boron, cobalt, fluoride, iodine, nickel, silicon, sodium, sulfur, tin, and vanadium. In my experience, these are less important therapeutically. There are also toxic minerals like aluminum, arsenic, cadmium, lead, and mercury. You certainly should be aware that heavy toxic metals like lead and cadmium can be present in certain herbs, particularly patent Chinese formulas.

▅▅▅▅ VITAMINS

Vitamins have long been popular as safe and effective agents in the health food scene. We have many, many opportunities to use them clinically. (See the sidebar for a typical regimen that I would recommend.) The literature on vitamins is broad, covering both laboratory and clinical experiments. I will not attempt here to review the entire area of vitamins and vitamin therapy, but I hope to cover a goodly sample of the use of vitamins in nutritionally oriented therapy. Table 12–2 summarizes the vitamins most commonly used in a primary care setting. Keep in mind that vitamins are water-soluble (vitamins B, C) or fat-soluble (vitamins A, D, E, K), which affects how they are absorbed, transported, and used in the body.

> **Dr. Victor Sierpina's Nutritional Supplement and Diet Program**
> •
> - Vitamin C, 500 mg morning and evening
> - Vitamin E (d-alpha tocopherol), 400 IU morning and evening
> - High-potency vitamin B complex with trace minerals and antioxidants, daily
> - High-fiber, low-fat (25% or less) diet with 5-7 servings of fruit and vegetables daily
> - Garlic, olive oil, red wine, green tea as tolerated
> - Thankfulness for your food. . . .

Vitamin A

Vitamin A promotes the integrity and healing of epithelial tissues and enhances immune function. Of all the vitamins in this list, it is the most toxic in excessive doses. Anything over 10,000 units/day in a pregnant woman is considered potentially teratogenic and over 25,000 units/day in others may be toxic. Vitamin A can also cause liver damage, a condition of the brain called pseudotumor cerebri, and such side effects as fatigue, headache, joint and muscle pain, diarrhea, irritability, and dry skin.

Nonetheless, vitamin A can be useful therapeutically. Think of using it to support healthy epithelial tissues such as skin, gastroin-

Text continued on page 171

Table 12-2   VITAMINS MOST COMMONLY USED IN PRIMARY CARE*

Nutrient	Benefits and Therapeutic Uses	Therapeutic Range	Risks	Sources	RDA
Vitamin A	**Integrity and healing of epithelial tissues** **Immune function** **Eyes** Skin Peptic ulcer Prevents some kinds of cancer Recurrent infection Wound healing	5000–25,000 IU/d 50,000 IU for 1–2 days	Headache Fatigue Teratogenic (>10,000 IU/d) Liver damage Pseudotumor cerebri Joint and muscle pain Diarrhea Irritability Dry skin	Beef and chicken liver Fatty fish Milk, cheese Some vegetables Egg yolk	5000 IU (males) 2500 IU (females)
Beta Carotene	**Immune enhancer** **Antioxidant** **Eye function** Strokes Heart attacks	25,000–50,000 IU/d	Avoid in smokers	Squash, pumpkin, yams Cantaloupe, pink grapefruit, mangoes, apricots Tomatoes Carrots, potatoes Watermelons Green leafy vegetables	25,000 IU
Vitamin B₁ (Thiamine)	**Nerve function** **Energy metabolism (memory)** **Beriberi** **Alcoholic psychosis** Fibromyalgia Canker sores Diabetes	10–100 mg/d	Unknown	Pork, liver, fish Oranges Peas, beans Peanut butter Wheat germ, seeds, nuts Brown rice, whole grains	0.3 mg (infants) 1.2–1.5 mg (males) 1.0–1.3 mg (females) 1.6 mg (nursing)

	Benefits/Indications*	Dosage	Side Effects	Food Sources	RDA
Vitamin B$_2$ (Riboflavin)	**Metabolism of carbohydrates** **Health of mucous membranes** **Migraine headache prophylaxis** Regulation of cell growth Improved immune function Improves the health of eyes, nerves, skin, nails, and hair May improve memory Cataracts and macular degeneration Athletic performance	5–100 mg/d 400 mg/d (for 3–4 mos)	Interferes with other B vitamins	Dairy products Liver, fish Broccoli, spinach, collard greens, asparagus Mushrooms Avocados Enriched flour	1.1 mg (children) 1.4–1.7 mg (males) 1.2–1.3 (females)
Vitamin B$_3$ (Niacin)	**Cholesterol/triglycerides** Depression Anxiety, schizophrenia Alzheimer's disease Osteoarthritis Diabetes Cerebrovascular insufficiency Dysmenorrhea Dermatologic conditions	1000–3000 mg/d 500–1000 mg bid 1000 mg tid 500–1000 mg tid 100 mg/d 200–500 mg/d 100 mg every 2–3 hrs	Hot flushes Itching Liver damage Rhabdomyolysis if used with HMG-CoA reductase drugs	Chicken, turkey Peanut butter, nuts Potatoes, rice, whole grains Salmon, tuna Beef, liver, pork	5–13 mg (children) 15–20 mg (males) 15 mg (females)

*Most important benefits and indications shown in boldface type.
RBC = red blood cell

(Continued)

Table 12-2 VITAMINS MOST COMMONLY USED IN PRIMARY CARE* *(Continued)*

Nutrient	Benefits and Therapeutic Uses	Therapeutic Range	Risks	Sources	RDA
Vitamin B$_5$ (Pantothenic acid, Panthetine)	**Cholesterol/triglycerides** **Obtaining energy from food** Hypoadrenalism Wound healing Postoperative ileus Allergic rhinitis	300 mg tid (pantethine) 100–1000 mg bid/tid	Diarrhea	Most food: Whole grains, beans Mushrooms Avocados Eggs, dairy products Liver	4–10 mg
Vitamin B$_6$ (Pyridoxine)	**Metabolism of amino acids** **Carpal tunnel syndrome** **Antibody formation** **RBC and nerve function** **Neuropathy** **Kidney stones** **Cardiac risk** **Atherosclerosis** **PMS** **Depression**	50–100 mg/d 10–50 mg/d	Nerve damage (doses ≥500 mg) Anemia	Beef, liver, chicken, fish, pork Milk Bananas, avocados, mangoes Potatoes Whole grains	1.7–2.0 mg (males) 1.4–1.6 mg (females)
Vitamin B$_9$ (Folic acid)	**Formation of new cells** **Neural tube development in fetus; pregnancy support** **Immune function** **Prevention of atherosclerosis, stroke, myocardial infarction** **Depression** Ulcerative colitis	0.4 mg/d 1–2 mg/d	Excess may mask B$_{12}$ deficiency and interferes with other nutrients and some drugs.	Beans Spinach, beets, asparagus Beef and chicken liver	150–200 µg (males) 150–180 µg (females)

Nutriceutical	Uses/Functions	Dosage	Side Effects/Cautions	Sources	RDA/Amount
Vitamin B$_{12}$ (Cobalamin)	**RBC formation** **Production of myelin** **Megaloblastic anemia** **Cardiovascular health** **Neurologic problems** Dementia Childhood asthma Chronic fatigue syndrome	1000–5000 µg (injection) 100–500 µg (oral) 1000–3000 µg/d	None	All animal products	0.5 µg (infants) 2 µg (adults) 2.6 µg (pregnancy)
Vitamin C (Ascorbic acid)	**Antioxidant** **Integrity of collagen** **Wound healing** **Immune system** **Lowering of blood lipids** **Antibiotic properties** **Cold/flu**	500–3000 mg/d 500 mg tid	Diarrhea Kidney stones Worsening of gout May precipitate sickle cell crisis	Citrus fruits, berries Green vegetables Brussels sprouts, broccoli, cauliflower Melons	50–60 mg
Vitamin D	**Metabolism and absorption of calcium** **Bone and tooth development** **Osteoporosis** **Rickets** Osteomalacia Psoriasis Scleroderma Some eye conditions Migraine	200–400 IU	Diarrhea Headache	Sun exposure Milk Cod liver oil, oily fish: herring, mackerel, sardines, salmon, tuna Cereals Egg yolk Butter Liver	5–10 µg (10 µg = 400 IU)

(Continued)

Table 12–2 VITAMINS MOST COMMONLY USED IN PRIMARY CARE* *(Continued)*

Nutrient	Benefits and Therapeutic Uses	Therapeutic Range	Risks	Sources	RDA
Vitamin E (Tocopherol)	**Antioxidant** **Inhibition of platelet aggregation** **Enhanced immune system** **Stability of cell membranes** **Reduced cardiovascular risk** **Intermittent claudication** Autoimmune diseases Diabetes Fibrocystic breasts Prevention of some cancers	100–800 IU	Bleeding problems	Almonds, sunflower seeds, peanuts Safflower, sunflower, or olive oil Sweet potatoes Wheat germ Avocados, mangoes Asparagus	10 mg (males) 8 mg (females) (1 mg d-alpha tocopherol = 1 IU alpha tocopherol)
Vitamin K	**Improved blood clotting** **Osteoporosis** **Calcium regulation** Pain	45–80 mg/d 20–30 mg/d (injections)	Bleeding Jaundice	Green leafy vegetables Broccoli, cabbage, cauliflower Liver Green tea Eggs	45–80 mg (males) 45–65 mg (females)
Biotin	**Dermatitis (for infants)** **Brittle nails** ↓ **Blood glucose in diabetics** Pain Muscle weakness	10–15 µg/d 8–16 mg/d	None	Beef liver Brewer's yeast Egg yolks Whole grains, nuts	Unknown; estimated to be 30 µg/d

testinal tract, respiratory tract, and conjunctiva, and for its benefit for vision. It can also be used to support immune function, to promote healing of peptic ulcer and inflammatory bowel disease, and possibly to prevent some kinds of cancer. It can be used to reduce recurrent infections.

The usual dosage is 5000 to 25,000 IU/day. Higher dosages should be used only by clinicians skilled in the administration of vitamin A at these high levels, which may exceed 100,000 IU/day. I stay away from these higher doses for my patients and I recommend that you do, too.

Natural sources include beef or chicken liver, fatty fish, milk, egg yolks, and cheese. By the way, stay away from polar bear liver, which has 13,000 to 18,000 IU/g. Although you would be unlikely to find this at your local grocery store, even a spoonful or two of this stuff could put you on ice.

Beta Carotene

Beta carotene is helpful as an immune enhancer and antioxidant. Although it is a carotenoid and precursor to vitamin A, it is quite safe. You cannot get vitamin A toxicity from taking beta carotene. Even large enough doses to turn you yellow are safe. I have performed well-baby checks on quite a few infants who had a yellowish-orange tinge, not from jaundice, but from eating a lot of carrots, squash, and other carotene-containing baby foods.

The recommended daily dose, 15 mg, can be obtained entirely through the diet. When you think of eating beta carotene, think of eating **color**. Those lovely colors like orange, yellow, and red in our fruits and vegetables show they have lots of carotenoids: not only beta carotene but also other helpful carotenoids like lycopene, lutein, and zeaxanthin.

My wife loves to cook with color and dress up a plate with it. Her recipe for "farmer's chicken" (*pollo contadina*) features three colors of peppers (red, green, and yellow-orange), carrots, tomatoes, capers, white mushrooms, purple onions, and black olives on top of a tasty bed of brown rice. It looks too good to eat, though that has never stopped me or any of our guests!

So the bottom line here is to take your beta carotene in your diet by eating at least 5 servings of fruits and vegetables daily. In addition to the colored foods like squash (had to start with that, didn't I!), pumpkin, cantaloupe, tomatoes, carrots, and pink grapefruit, you can also get helpful carotenoids from potatoes and dark-green leafy vegetables like spinach or collard greens. In general, the darker the green, the higher the carotene content. You can also get significant carotenoids from legumes and grains. If you don't eat these foods regularly, it probably is worthwhile to take a beta carotene supplement with at least 25,000 to 50,000 IU/day.

Beta carotene cannot substitute for the use of vitamin A therapeutically. Like vitamin A, beta carotene is useful for eye function, and some studies show that eating foods high in it reduces strokes and heart attacks. A concern was raised in the CARET study (Beta Carotene and Retinol Efficacy Trial), which looked at the effects of beta carotene and vitamin A supplements on smokers. The rate of lung cancer actually was higher in the supplement group. Thus, it is not advisable to give these supplements to smokers (Omenn 1996).

However, the full range of carotenoids found in food, along with the antioxidant properties and immunity-boosting effects they produce, may still be protective against cancer. In fact, people who eat food containing high levels of beta carotene and the other carotenoids mentioned are generally healthier in terms of cancer, heart disease, and strokes.

The B Vitamins

The vitamins in this large group are present in common foods such as meat, fish, chicken, dairy products, legumes, nuts, peas, and dark-green leafy vegetables. Subgroups of people such as vegetarians; alcoholics; those with heart disease, GI surgery, or malabsorption; smokers; the elderly; and pregnant or nursing women have special need for supplementation but most of us get our RDA in food. Cooking food lightly and steaming instead of boiling vegetables help preserve their B vitamin content, because these vitamins are water-soluble.

The B vitamins and some related compounds are shown in the sidebar. The numerical system is a bit goofy because of the pattern of discovery of the chemistry of B vitamins, so to keep it easy, the names are often preferred.

The B Vitamins and Related Compounds

THE B VITAMINS

B_1—Thiamine

B_2—Riboflavin

B_3—Niacin

B_5—Pantothenic acid

B_6—Pyridoxine

B_7—Biotin

B_9—Folic acid

B_{12}—Cobalamin

"UNOFFICIAL" B VITAMINS

Biotin

Choline

Inositol

Para-aminobenzoic Acid (PABA)

Thiamine (B_1)

Thiamine is involved in energy metabolism and nervous system function, including memory. Thiamine is particularly well-known to be deficient in alcoholics. It is found naturally in pork, liver, fish, oranges, peas, peanut butter, whole grains, and other foods. The RDA is 0.3 mg for infants, 1.6 mg for nursing women, and 1 to 1.5 mg in other adults. Deficiency results in a condition known as beriberi, which is rarely seen in developed countries.

Alcoholics may need from 10 to 100 mg/day. At that dosage, thiamine is useful therapeutically for alcoholic psychosis. Thiamine also can be helpful in CHF, when it may be depleted by diuretics, and in some neurological conditions such as sciatica and trigeminal neuralgia when injected with vitamin B_{12}. Giving high doses causes a relative deficiency of vitamin B_6 or magnesium.

Riboflavin (B₂)

Riboflavin—ah, I recall it so well from reading the RDA lists on the cereal boxes when I was a child. It is involved in energy production via metabolism of carbohydrates. Supplemental levels range from 5 to 100 mg. The RDA is under 2 mg: 1.1 mg in children and up to about 1.8 mg in men and nursing women. Natural sources of riboflavin are primarily dairy products such as milk, cheese, yogurt, and ice cream. Those intolerant of milk products may be at higher risk of not getting enough vitamin B_2. Other rich sources are liver, fish, some vegetables, and baked goods made from riboflavin-enriched flour. Riboflavin deficiency is rare but can occur in pregnant and breast-feeding women, those taking birth control pills, athletes, the elderly, diabetics, and those taking antidepressants and drugs such as phenothiazines, doxorubicin (Adriamycin), or phenytoin (Dilantin).

Riboflavin regulates cell growth, helps the immune system, and improves the health of eyes, nerves, skin, nails, and hair. It may improve memory and reduce the tendency to develop cataracts and macular degeneration. In high doses of 400 mg/day, it has been used for migraine headache prophylaxis but may need to be taken for 3 to 4 months to be effective.

Niacin/Niacinamide (B₃)

Niacin (nicotinic acid) is also involved in energy metabolism as a component of the nicotinamide adenine dinucleotide (NAD/NADH) pathway. A related substance called *niacinamide* shares some, but not all, of niacin's clinical effects. The RDA is 5 to 13 mg for children and 16 to 20 mg for adults; part of that is converted from tryptophan in protein. Deficiency causes a condition called pellagra (characterized by dermatitis, dementia, and diarrhea) but unless you live in an impoverished area or are an alcoholic or a strict vegetarian or vegan, you are unlikely to be deficient. Natural sources of niacin include peanut butter, potatoes, rice, and whole grains. High-tryptophan foods that also help supply niacin through secondary conversion include tuna, turkey, chicken, and beef.

The most common clinical application of niacin is in lowering cholesterol. Dosages in the range of 1000 to 3000 mg/day have been reported to reduce total serum cholesterol as well as LDL and triglycerides, while increasing HDL cholesterol. A major drawback to using niacin for cholesterol is that it causes an uncomfortable flushing reaction. I walked into the lab one day to see one of my assistants sweating profusely and with a face red as a turkey in heat. She had been taking niacin for her cholesterol and was quite concerned about the sudden onset of this hot flash. Patients may get so anxious about this reaction that they go to the ER, thinking they are having a stroke or some other catastrophe, when actually the flushing is annoying and uncomfortable but not dangerous.

If the dose is gradually increased by 100 mg every few days, or if a patient takes an aspirin a half-hour before the niacin, the flush reaction will be prevented in many folks. Some people just cannot tolerate niacin but may be able to take a compound of niacin called inositol hexaniacinate. This useful compound, an inositol molecule (an unofficial B vitamin) with a niacin attached to each side of its six-sided ring, is much better tolerated. Dosages of 2 to 4 g/day are therapeutic, though lipid levels may take 3 or 4 months to stabilize.

Niacin is involved in normal brain function via tryptophan and serotonin metabolism. Thus it is used in certain psychiatric conditions such as depression, anxiety, and even schizophrenia and Alzheimer's disease. For depression, 500 to 1000 mg twice a day may potentiate the antidepressant effect of L-tryptophan. Higher doses (about 1000 mg 3 times/day) can be helpful in treating anxiety and even recent-onset schizophrenia.

Other common uses for niacin are for osteoarthritis (500–1000 mg 3 times/day); as a supplement in diabetes at a low dose (100 mg/day), in combination with chromium picolinate; for cerebrovascular insufficiency 200–500 mg/day; and for dysmenorrhea (100 mg every 2–3 hours). Some clinicians use niacin for intermittent claudication, dizziness, tinnitus, or premenstrual headaches. Its related compound, niacinamide, has been used for dermatological conditions such as acne and photosensitivity dermatitis, early Type I diabetes, and hypoglycemia. NADH has been used in Alzheimer's and Parkinson's diseases in limited studies.

Toxicity issues in the use of niacin (besides the skin flush) are that it can cause rhabdomyolysis if used with HMG-CoA reductase (lipid-lowering statin) drugs. Large doses can cause hypoglycemia or hyperglycemia in some diabetic patients. Liver function can be affected, and hepatitis may occur with doses greater than 3 g/day. This liver toxicity is seen more commonly with sustained-release niacin.

Pantothenic Acid (B₅)

Pantothenic acid is a bit of a lightweight among its **B**-rethren. It is a precursor for coenzyme A and is therefore a part of carbohydrate and fat metabolism. It has no RDA because apparently we all get enough of it (4 to 10 mg/day) from food, and there are no known deficiency diseases associated with it. Safe and adequate levels are from 2 mg in children to 7 mg in adults. It is present in most foods, especially such foods as whole grains, eggs, and dairy products. Alcoholics, because of their poor dietary habits, may become deficient in B_5, along with the other B vitamins.

Clinical uses may include for treating hypoadrenalism, encouraging wound healing, reducing postoperative ileus in surgical patients, and possibly treating allergic rhinitis (100 to 1000 mg b.i.d. or t.i.d. with an equivalent vitamin C dose). Its derivative, pantetheine, has been used in a dosage of 300 mg 3 to 4 times/day for hyperlipidemia, in *Candida*-related complex, or to treat a hangover.

Pyridoxine (B₆)

Pyridoxine is known to function in energy metabolism, nervous system function, cardiovascular health (via homocysteine metabolism), support of immune function, and as a coenzyme to convert proteins and carbohydrates into useable form. It has a low RDA (about 2 mg, depending to some extent on how much protein one eats), which varies from 1 mg in small children to 2.2 mg in nursing or pregnant women. Smokers, alcohol imbibers, those taking birth control pills, pregnant women (those who may have forgotten to take them!), nursing mothers, strict vegetarians, and those taking one of many drugs such as theophylline, hydralazine, or isoniazid all may require supplemental vitamin B_6 to prevent deficiency. Anemia and immune problems can occur with deficiency. Pyridoxine is naturally found in high-quality protein such as beef, liver, chicken, fish, pork, milk, and other dairy products. Bananas, avocados, potatoes, mangoes, and whole grains are the best plant sources; most other fruits and vegetables do not contain much pyridoxine.

My favorite use for vitamin B_6 is for any type of neuropathy. Although in my experience it works best for carpal tunnel syndrome at a dosage of 50 to 100 mg/day, some patients require 200 mg/day for a month. I don't give the higher dose longer than that because excess B_6 can *cause* sensory neuropathy or anemia. I also recommend it to good effect for other kinds of neuropathy, including diabetic neuropathy, often in combination with vitamin B_{12}. It can be given to patients with diabetes prophylactically.

I also use pyridoxine for patients with recurrent kidney stones. At a dosage of 10 to 50 mg/day, it can reduce the formation of calcium oxalate stones when given with magnesium (300 mg/day) and a mild diuretic such as chlorthalidone.

With the discovery of the effects of homocysteine metabolism on cardiac disease, it has been found that pyridoxine used with folic acid and cobalamin is useful in reducing cardiac risk. Its inhibition of platelet aggregation is also useful in atherosclerosis. Pyridoxine is helpful for the elderly and those who have trouble fending off infections; such conditions can suggest a pyridoxine deficiency. PMS, asthma, depression, menopausal arthritis, morning sickness, and chemotherapy-induced toxicity are other potential applications.

As noted above, high doses cause an irreversible sensory neuropathy. This side effect usually requires doses of over 500 mg/day but can occur with doses as low as 200 mg. Anemia is another potential problem with overdosing. Large doses also may increase the need for magnesium, zinc, some essential fatty acids, folic acid, and the other B vitamins.

Folic Acid (B$_9$)

Folic acid is involved in preventing chromosome breakage in DNA metabolism and is used in central nervous system function, immune function, and homocysteine metabolism. The RDA for this important vitamin is 200 µg but most authorities now recommend at least 400 µg. In fact, women of childbearing age should be certain to supplement their diet to get at least 400 µg/day of folic acid, because this amount has clearly been shown to prevent spina bifida and other neural tube defects in fetuses. The best natural sources are any kind of beans, spinach (see, Popeye was right!), beef or chicken liver, beets, and asparagus.

Deficiency of folic acid can cause a range of symptoms: anemia, weakness, sore tongue, heart palpitations, diarrhea, and others. Deficiency is common in alcoholics, those who use tobacco, and those with problems digesting and absorbing food. Pregnant and breast-feeding women need high levels. Therapeutically, 1 to 2 mg/day of folic acid along with B$_6$ and B$_{12}$ can remove damaging levels of homocysteine from the bloodstream to prevent atherosclerosis, stroke, and myocardial infarction. Studies have also found benefit in cervical dysplasia at doses of 10 mg/day, and in prevention of colon and cervical cancer and osteoporosis. Other conditions that respond to folate are glossitis and geographic tongue (zinc and B$_{12}$ are also useful for this) and megaloblastic anemia due to folate deficiency.

Before starting high doses of folic acid, it is wise to check the vitamin B$_{12}$ level and a CBC to prevent masking a B$_{12}$ deficiency. Many common drugs, such as sulfa, birth control pills, and cortisone, block the absorption of folate. On the other hand, it interferes with the function of other drugs such as the anticonvulsant phenytoin (which interestingly can also cause folate deficiency) and methotrexate. Increased folic acid may be required by those taking large doses of vitamin B_6, vitamin B_{12}, or zinc.

Cobalamin (B_{12})

Cobalamin, better known as vitamin B_{12}, is essential to the formation of red blood cells and the production of myelin in the nervous system. It also improves cardiovascular health by helping to remove homocysteine from the system, thereby preventing vascular damage produced by this amino acid. The RDA is quite low, from 0.5 µg in infants to 2 µg in adults, and up to 2.6 µg in pregnancy or lactation. This RDA is probably too low for those older than 50 years, who may not absorb this vitamin well because of loss of intrinsic factor or other absorptive difficulties. Those who smoke, are strict vegetarians, take antacids, or have had stomach surgery may also develop deficiency. Vitamin B_{12} deficiency results in tingling or numbness in the extremities, mood disorder, memory problems, dementia, and megaloblastic or pernicious anemia. Natural sources are primarily animal products such as beef (especially liver), other red meats, chicken, fish, clams, and dairy products. Absorption, not intake, is the most common problem. Those with vitamin B_{12} deficiency may supplement by taking it sublingually (1000 to 5000 µg), as an injection (1000 µg), or as oral supplements (100 to 500 µg). The injection or sublingual route is best for those who cannot absorb it because of intrinsic factor deficiency, surgery, or other GI absorption problem.

Vitamin B_{12} has gotten a bad rap as a placebo and as a marker of sloppy medical practice: "I'm tired, Doc. Could you get me a shot of B_{12}? It always picks me up." This was the refrain I got from a lot of my elderly patients very early in my medical practice. As a well-trained physician, I would order a CBC and tests for vitamin B_{12} and folic acid to demonstrate to them that this was an unnecessary intervention. The cost of these tests was enough to buy a 10-year supply of vitamin B_{12}, which comes in 30-mL vials for less than $10. They would give up on me in time and go to a less enlightened doctor who would give them their B_{12} shot.

I'm trainable. I decided that if these folks had been getting B_{12} for years from their old country doc without ill effects, and they felt better, and it was so dirt cheap, I was losing a lot of patient business and patient satisfaction by not giving this simple remedy. Only as I studied the matter further did I discover that many elderly people do indeed have trouble absorbing B_{12}. Because of biochemical individuality, some may need it even if their serum blood levels are normal. Don't try to tell that to Medicare, by the way; they will pay for B_{12} only if the serum level is demonstrably low in lab tests.

Besides using it as pepper-upper for vague complaints like fatigue, anxiety, depression, and insomnia, nutritionally oriented practitioners use B_{12} for neurological problems like neuritis, neuropathy, and neuralgia, usually in combination with thiamine and pyridoxine. It may be of some use for patients with dementia, childhood asthma, xanthelasma, acute viral hepatitis, and bursitis. It is very safe, even at high doses, so a dosage for subdeltoid bursitis or childhood asthma of 1000 to 3000 µg/day, though higher than usually given, is well tolerated. Excess cobalamin is excreted, and the liver can store several years' supply once the deficiency has been replaced. Of course, it is given for megaloblastic anemia.

Drugs that reduce gastric acid secretion, such as the proton-pump inhibitors, H_2-blockers, or other antacids, may impair absorption, as do potassium citrate, potassium chloride, colchicine, and some oral hypoglycemic agents. Problems with B_{12} absorption and utilization are aggravated by a deficiency of folic acid, iron, and vitamin E, and by large doses of vitamin C.

"Unofficial" B Vitamins

Biotin

Biotin is a coenzyme in oxidation reactions as well as in chain elongation of fatty acids. It is required for the utilization of fats and amino acids from foods. There is no RDA because gut bacteria manufacture it. There are some strange cases of deficiencies, however, such as egg-suckers (people who eat one or two dozen raw eggs a day; something in the raw egg white binds the biotin), those taking an antibiotic (which wipes out gut bacteria) for a prolonged period, or those on extremely low-calorie diets. Biotin comes from beef liver, brewer's yeast, egg yolks, whole grains, and nuts.

Biotin at a dosage of 2 to 3 mg/day can be helpful for hair and nail health. Some clinicians use large doses, such as 8 to 16 mg/day, to reduce blood glucose in diabetics. One report recommended 10 mg/day for dialysis patients, in whom it is thought to improve uremic neurological problems. A low dose of 10 to 15 µg may be useful for children with cradle cap or seborrheic dermatitis of infancy, because some infants may not yet have developed the gut flora to produce it themselves.

Choline

Similar to biotin, you can make choline, so there is no RDA. The dietary source from which it is derived, however, is phosphatidylcholine (lecithin), which comes from sources like eggs, red meat, liver, cauliflower, soybeans, rice, and cabbage. Choline is helpful for the metabolism of fats, and may be useful in reducing cholesterol. Lecithin is used to treat fatty liver, hepatitis, and other problems such as "hepatic diabetes" and toxic liver damage. It is also used for atherosclerosis, some forms of ataxia, blepharospasm, and possibly for Alzheimer's. I have seen it recommended for years as a "brain food" to stimulate memory and the proper function of the neurotransmitters (acetylcholine) in the central nervous system. Supplements are given at doses in the range of 500 to 1500 mg/day. Lecithin is also used for cholesterol problems.

Inositol

This B vitamin cousin is essential to neurotransmitter and cell membrane function. It has no known RDA. In the diet, it is found in organ meats, citrus, grains, nuts, fruits, and legumes. Therapeutic uses are limited and not well proven, but you will find it is sometimes used for liver problems, diabetic neuropathy, panic attacks, depression, and Alzheimer's disease.

Para-aminobenzoic Acid (PABA)

This agent is best known as a sunblock. It is made in the body from other compounds such as folic acid, and in the diet comes from liver (so many nutrients in liver, yet so few of us will eat it voluntarily!), whole grains, brown rice, and wheat germ. Nutritional clinicians have used it for many conditions, especially autoimmune and fibrotic disorders. Examples of clinical applications are vitiligo (100 mg 3 to 4 times/day for up to 18 months), Peyronie's disease, scleroderma, and dermatomyositis (1 to 3 g 4 times/day). It is also used (100 mg 3 to 4 times/day) to potentiate the effect of hormones like glucocorticoids and estrogens, perhaps allowing lower dosages to be used.

A concern about PABA is that it can interact with sulfa-containing antibiotics and drugs such as sulfasalazine and sulfamethoxazole. Large doses (12 g/day or more) may cause hypoglycemia, diarrhea, liver toxicity, nausea, rash, or fever.

Vitamin C

Unquestionably the best known, most widely used, safest, and most useful of all the vitamins, vitamin C is part of my prescription for just about every patient. Vitamin C is an important antioxidant and has been

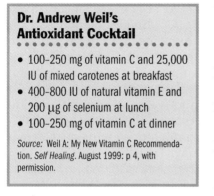

Dr. Andrew Weil's Antioxidant Cocktail • • • • • • • • • • • • • • •

- 100-250 mg of vitamin C and 25,000 IU of mixed carotenes at breakfast
- 400-800 IU of natural vitamin E and 200 µg of selenium at lunch
- 100-250 mg of vitamin C at dinner

Source: Weil A: My New Vitamin C Recommendation. *Self Healing.* August 1999: p 4, with permission.

widely studied. Nobel Prize winner Linus Pauling personally used up to 18 g/day. It is essential to tissue integrity and wound healing, enhances the immune system, and has antibiotic properties. Its clinical applications are many and varied. You can see from the sidebar how Dr. Andrew Weil (1999) uses vitamin C with other antioxidants. Suffice it to say that vitamin C is the "king of the road" of the vitamins.

Vitamin C is water-soluble and, according to recent studies (Balz 1999, Levine 1996, Levine et al 1999), the body's capacity to absorb it is limited and the body's tissues become saturated with a few hundred milligrams a day; any more than that is excreted in urine. The RDA is probably too low at 50 mg/day and perhaps should be closer to 200 mg/day, but this is a matter of debate and research. New recommendations probably will be between 100 and 200 mg/day. Clearly it is safe in doses of several grams daily, especially when used in treating various medical conditions. It is easily available in many fruits and green vegetables. Fresh fruits and vegetables usually contain more vitamin C than those that have been cooked, frozen, or prepared a few hours in advance. Eating the recommended 5 to 7 servings of fruit and vegetables a day will easily give the daily recommended amount of vitamin C.

Deficiency causes a condition called scurvy. You may have heard the story about the sailors on ships in the British Navy many years ago. Before refrigeration, on long voyages they subsisted on a diet of salted beef, hardtack, grog, and other staples that would last. Not knowing about vitamin C, they found that their gums bled, their teeth fell out, they bruised easily, they felt fatigued, and they had sore joints and other miseries. Someone found that adding limes to the sailors' diet prevented this condition, so a few barrels were packed on every ship and the sailors came to be known as "limeys." Scurvy is pretty rare now, but certain folks are more prone to a deficiency of vitamin C. I recommend it to all my diabetic patients as well as to smokers and those under stress. Geriatric patients, those with asthma or allergies, pregnant or breast-feeding mothers, alcoholics, and those going through major surgery may need more than usual. Aspirin use may also deplete vitamin C.

The clinical indications for using vitamin C are vast. The most common use is for viral infections such as colds and flu, in which it is common to take 500 mg or more up to 3 times/ day. It may also be useful for bacterial infections such as urinary tract infections and skin infections. It is useful in the prevention and treatment of atherosclerosis because of its antioxidant properties, lipid-lowering properties, and lowering effect on blood pressure. Diabetics have reduced cellular uptake of vitamin C, so I recommend a supplement not only for its beneficial effect on lipids but also for improved immune function, wound healing, and other common diabetic problems. Vitamin C also is used in asthma and other allergies. Because of its effect on collagen and other connective tissue, it can be helpful in spinal disc degeneration, osteogenesis imperfecta, Paget's disease of the bone, and rheumatological conditions such as gout and osteoarthritis. Though some claim it is valuable in the prevention and treatment of cancer, this has not been proven. The usual therapeutic dosage range is 500 to 3000 mg/day, though much higher doses are sometimes used.

Is there such a thing as too much of a good thing when it comes to vitamin C? Well, as usual, the answer to that question is "yes." The term for the maximum allowable dosage of vitamin C is "bowel tolerance." This varies genetically from person to person, but high doses (usually considered to be more than 4 g/day) will cause diarrhea or abdominal pain that can be relieved by reducing the dose, dividing it, taking the buffered forms, or taking it with meals. There are other concerns as well. Iron absorption is increased by vitamin C, which can adversely affect patients with hemochromatosis. Large doses may induce copper deficiency. About 1 in 300 people have a genetic defect in oxalate metabolism and may develop kidney stones if they take high-dose vitamin C, though this is controversial. It may interfere with the stool test for occult blood. And those who have been taking large doses have a risk of "rebound scurvy" if they suddenly stop.

Vitamin D

Vitamin D is involved in the metabolism and absorption of calcium. It is converted in the body into the active form by sunshine, being converted into vitamin D_3 or cholecalciferol. Some is present in food in the form of vitamin D_2 or ergocalciferol. The recommended or adequate dose is 200 to 400 IU or 5 to 10 mg in adults and children but 600 IU or 15 mg in older adults, whose skin doesn't convert it as well. Food sources include certain oily fish, shrimp, vitamin D–fortified milk, eggs, butter, and liver (there it is again). Deficiency of vitamin D can create rickets, a condition of poor bone development in children, though this is rare today. Vitamin D deficiency is a risk for people who are housebound, live in a northern climate, or otherwise don't get much sunshine, as well as the elderly; alcoholics; those with liver or kidney disease; strict vegetarians or vegans; and those taking steroids, cholestyramine, or certain anticonvulsants such as phenytoin and phenobarbital. Deficiency can weaken the immune system by affecting cellular immunity, and it may also be associated with colon and breast cancer.

Therapeutic uses include preventing osteoporosis and osteomalacia and treating psoriasis (1.25-dihydroxyvitamin D_3 orally or topically), scleroderma, and certain eye conditions such as keratoconus, retinitis pigmentosa, and night blindness. It is occasionally used to ameliorate hearing loss. It can be toxic in large dosages (2000 to 3000 IU/day), increasing the risk of atherosclerosis, kidney stones, and hypercalcemia. Some sources recommend a maximum of 1000 IU/day. I think this recommendation makes sense. You are unlikely to exceed it with diet alone (unless you guzzle cod liver oil or eat a few cans of sardines a day), but supplements can put you over the top. Like vitamin A, vitamin D can be toxic rather quickly. The best place to get it is from fortified milk, but use the low-fat or nonfat kind to reduce cholesterol intake. And don't forget to get some sunshine—but use your PABA sunblock. Things do get complicated, don't they?

Vitamin E

Vitamin E acts as an antioxidant, inhibits platelet aggregation, enhances the immune system, stabilizes cell membranes, and reduces cardiovascular risk. Another winner! Its main function is its ability to scavenge those nasty little free radicals. This fat-soluble vitamin has an RDA of 5 IU in infants, 10 IU in older children, and 12 to 18 IU in adults. This is much lower than the amount recommended by most nutritionally oriented physicians, who recommend 100 to 800 IU/day. Natural sources of vitamin E include some nuts and vegetable oils, wheat germ, avocados, asparagus, mangoes, and sweet potatoes. These foods are rather low in total vitamin E, however, and animal foods have practically none of it. The advantage of the food sources is that they have mixed tocopherols such as the gamma type and tocotrienols, which have independent health benefits as antioxidants and scavengers of different types of free radicals. The benefits of vitamin E require doses over 100 IU daily, so you would need to eat ½ pound of almonds, a few hundred sunflower seeds, multiple tablespoons of vegetable oil, or take supplements. The natural vitamin E (d-alpha-tocopherol) is the preferred supplement form. Though more expensive than the dl-alpha-tocopherol, it is more biologically active. If a person can't afford the natural or d-form, taking the less expensive dl-form in higher amounts will confer adequate benefits and certainly is better than not taking any. Because it is fat-soluble, poor absorption may result from conditions such as liver disease, inflammatory bowel disease, or cystic fibrosis, and from taking certain lipid-lowering drugs such as cholestyramine. The elderly also may need more to fend off infections.

Deficiency of vitamin E doesn't cause any clear clinical syndromes such as scurvy or rickets. Therapeutically, it is most useful in protecting against heart disease, however; some studies have shown 25% to 45% reduction of risk, although other studies have shown lesser effects or even no effect (Heart Outcomes Prevention Evaluation Study Investigators 2000, Stephens et al 1996, Reaven et al 1993, Stampfer et al 1993, Rimm 1993). It can raise HDL cholesterol levels in those with low baseline amounts. It is useful for intermittent claudication through its effects on lipid metabolism and oxidation. Because it affects the release of inflammatory mediators, it helps scleroderma, Raynaud's phenomenon, and other autoimmune diseases. Dupuytren's contracture and menopausal hot flashes are additional indications, and it can improve glucose metabolism in diabetics by preventing glycosylation of tissue proteins. Like vitamin C, I recommend it to all my diabetic patients. I have found doses of 400 to 1200 IU/day (integrated with a reduction of caffeine, chocolate, and stress) to be particularly useful for women with painful fibrocystic breasts. I also recommend it to those with eye problems such as macular degeneration or cataracts, and it may be helpful in Parkinson's disease and Alzheimer's disease. Studies show benefit in preventing several types of cancer such as colon cancer (in men, not women), oral and throat cancers, cervical and breast cancers, but not lung cancer in smokers (Albanes et al 1995, Alpha-tocopherol, Beta Carotene Cancer Prevention Study Group 1994). It has also been found to help some men with infertility. There doesn't seem to be a toxic dose; the usual dosage is 400 to 800 IU/day. Taking polyunsaturated fatty acids may increase the requirement for vitamin E. Vitamins A, C, and B_6 may enhance its effects, as do selenium and beta carotene. Because it is fat-soluble, it is better absorbed if you take it with some fat in your diet.

Vitamin E can interact with iron, so the two should not be taken together. It may reduce the severity of tardive dyskinesia related to phenothiazine use, and may enhance the effects of AZT and griseoful-vin. Taking it with warfarin may increase the tendency to bleed. I once took a small tumor off the neck of a patient who, though not on warfarin, was taking vitamin E along with ginkgo, aspirin, and garlic. All four substances prolong clotting times, so he kept oozing after I had removed the lesion. My lesson was to ask before a surgical procedure not only about blood thinners such as warfarin and aspirin, but also about over-the-counter agents like herbs and vitamin E. One concern is that excessive amounts of vitamin E may increase the risk of retinal bleeding in diabetics, but this may be offset by using vitamin K.

Vitamin K

Best known for its effects on the activation of certain blood-clotting factors, vitamin K also is required for the synthesis of the bone protein osteocalcin, so it also protects against osteoporosis. The RDA is 60 µg/day. It is found in some vegetables (including the green, leafy ones), green tea, liver (of course), and eggs. A deficiency might be expected to cause bleeding problems, and we routinely administer vitamin K to newborns to prevent bleeding, because their stores are low. Liver disease or alteration of gut flora (dysbiosis) due to prolonged antibiotic use can lead to a deficiency. So can inflammatory bowel disease and some cholesterol-lowering drugs such as cholestyramine and colestipol, because absorption is blocked.

The therapeutic use of vitamin K is to prevent bleeding resulting from deficiency, as in cirrhosis of the liver, or overvigorous use of heparin. It can also be used to prevent and treat osteoporosis. Injections along with vitamin C can be used for the nausea and vomiting of pregnancy, though I usually prefer B_6 for this indication. Chronic pain, including cancer pain, has been reported to respond to injections of 20 to 30 mg/day.

Chapter
13

Pharmacological and Biological Treatments

The work will teach you how to do it.
—Estonian proverb

This category of therapy includes a wide array of products used in an unconventional manner. Some are highly useful, safe, and effective and will soon be considered mainstream. I predict that glucosamine will be in this category. Many of them, however, are unproved, with claims based on testimonials but limited research and clinical studies. Others are controversial yet popular. Some are safe but not effective; others are potentially on the cutting edge of new therapies. Next to fad diets, pharmacological and biological therapies are probably the alternative therapies most prone to abuse and misrepresentation.

The list of therapies here bridges out from our discussions on nutriceuticals and includes chelation therapy and over-the-counter supplements such as dehydroepiandrosterone (DHEA), glucosamine sulfate and chondroitin sulfate, melatonin, glandular products, and dietary weight-loss products containing combinations of herbs and other supplements. More controversial yet are Coley's toxin, antineo-plastons, shark cartilage, hydrogen peroxide, bee pollen, and other products and procedures used for a wide variety of unconventional clinical indications. Although space prevents covering all of these in detail, I hope to cover the most common and useful agents.

It is important as you enter this field to be aware that some of the more unproved and controversial therapies are potentially dangerous and those who use them may delay using effective, proven therapy. Your professional license, reputation, and academic credibility may also be at risk with some of the more questionable therapies. Lest this have a chilling effect on your willingness to use these therapies, recall that many of today's conventional therapies were once nonconventional. Nonetheless, maintaining your objectivity and willingness to look at reliable studies as well as clinical observations will protect you and your patients from dangerous deceptions and costly fraudulent therapies.

▰▰▰ CHELATION THERAPY

Chelation therapy is based on the intravenous infusion of ethylenedi-amine tetraacetic acid (EDTA) to bind heavy metals in the bloodstream. Since its initial use about 50 years ago for removing lead, iron, copper, and other heavy metals, practitioners of chelation therapy have reasoned that it can remove calcium from atherosclerotic plaques. This is truly an area of heated disagreement. For years patients have been telling me about the benefits of chelation therapy on their heart, circulation, arthritis, vision, dementia, diabetes, and so on, but no major studies confidently support its benefits. Doctors doing chelation run the risk in some states of professional censure and even risk losing their licenses. When I asked a chelation therapy advocate about the scientific literature supporting this therapy, she sent me about 50 pages of Internet printouts mainly supporting the civil and legal rights of chelation therapists to include it in their scopes of practice. This outpouring is largely in response to the rather dim view some state medical boards take of chelation.

However, millions of patients have received this therapy safely. Early problems with high-dose EDTA were renal problems and cardiac arrhythmias, but lower doses of EDTA seem to have largely solved these problems. The therapy itself consists of an intravenous infusion of EDTA plus various vitamins from one to three times weekly for 20 to 30 sessions at a cost of roughly $100 per session. Though a few thousand dollars seems like a lot for a therapy largely supported by testimonials and anecdotes, many patients inexplicably feel better after these therapies. The cost is small compared with that of a cardiac bypass, which can cost 10 times as much or even more.

Though many of my patients have urged me to start administer-ing chelation, I have not done so, remaining both open-minded and skeptical. The accumulation of calcium in an atherosclerotic plaque is a late and relatively minor event compared to the buildup of scar tissue, fibrin, cholesterol, and other material in the plaque. The calcium doesn't really cause the problem with obstruction, plaque rupture, and vessel damage. Thus, removal of calcium doesn't entirely make sense as a mechanism of the imputed benefits of chelation. Though we may have a lot of placebo effect with chelation (especially if you don't want to admit you've been snookered out of a few grand), perhaps it has benefits not attributed to only calcium removal. Chelation of iron and copper, which stimulate free radicals known to be causative in atherosclerosis, may be an additional benefit. Most chelation therapists wisely advise healthy diet and exercise modification, which we also know to be helpful in athero-sclerosis.

Given the huge problem in this country with vascular disease, I am open to better research on therapies like chelation that can "bypass the bypass" and prevent the need for endarterectomies or other expensive, invasive, and risky vascular procedures. Certainly, I have been impressed by the enthusiastic claims of many of my patients who have undergone a series of chelation treatments. There are enough clinical and observational data that the National Center for Complementary and Alternative Medicine (NCCAM) is sponsoring research on this widely used therapy. Until there is real proof that it is unsafe, the prosecution of qualified practitioners is unwarranted. Given lack of hard evidence at this time, however, I can only advise it to patients for whom standard therapies are contraindicated or not desired. Nonetheless, you will find that patients will self-select and self-refer for this treatment. As always, keep an open mind, give them the information you do know, and avoid being confrontational. Who knows, maybe better studies really will prove it to work (Elihu et al 1998, Ernst 1997).

■■■■ CHONDROITIN SULFATE

Chondroitin sulfate is mainly used for osteoarthritis (Kerzberg et al 1987) and is extracted from shark and bovine cartilage as well as sea cucumber. Like glucosamine (see the following), chondroitin also contributes glycosaminoglycans to cartilage, but it is not as well absorbed as glucosamine primarily because of its higher molecular weight. Many arthritis formulations contain both chondroitin and glucosamine, though no study has shown that both together are any more effective than glucosamine alone. My recommendation is to use glucosamine alone instead of chondroitin or chondroitin-glucosamine combinations. Further research is now in progress to address this question.

■■■■ DHEA

DHEA is an endogenous steroid hormone produced in the adrenal gland as well as the ovaries and testes (Ebeling & Koivisto 1994). It is a stem or "mother" hormone from which other hormones are synthesized. It has received attention for its use in chronic fatigue, aging, immune disorders, and a variety of other conditions such as cancer, heart disease, diabetes, osteoporosis, and dementia. Interestingly, DHEA levels have been noted to decline with age, causing some clinicians to speculate that this is an "anti-aging hormone" (Yen et al 1995). Patients with chronic fatigue syndrome sometimes take this agent as an antidote to "adrenal depletion." The usual dosage ranges from 5 to 15 mg/day for women and from 10 to 30 mg/day for men. Observed side effects are hirsutism and acne, somewhat expected androgenic effects.

For the same reasons I am concerned about chronic use of melatonin, I think caution should be used in giving DHEA, a hormone with potentially powerful and widely distributed effects on the body. Its interaction with other hormones such as thyroid, corticosteroids, and the gonadal hormones needs to be better studied. Indeed, DHEA potentially can promote the growth of hormone-sensitive tumors and should be avoided by patients with a strong family history of such tumors and patients with established tumors of the prostate, breast, or ovary. Another study showed a paradoxical finding that men with *low* DHEA levels are more prone to cardiovascular-related death but women with *high* levels are more prone to cardiovascular death. Though DHEA may be useful clinically (Gaby 1996), my advice is to avoid using it until further research proves its safety and its efficacy.

▰▰▰▰ GLANDULARS

The extract of animal endocrine glands has had a long and useful history in medicine. Thyroid hormone replacement began and continues to be available as extract of bovine thyroid gland, although it has been supplanted by the more convenient and standardized dosing of levothyroxine. Glandulars derived from the liver, spleen, pancreas, and thymus, and from the adrenal and thyroid glands, are prescribed by chiropractors, naturopaths, and other alternative practitioners. Adrenal extracts have been suggested for chronic fatigue, asthma, eczema, psoriasis, and rheumatoid arthritis. Liver extracts are used for chronic hepatitis and chronic liver disease. Spleen extracts have been used in post-splenectomy patients and for autoimmune disease, infections, and cancer. Thymus extract likewise is used in recurrent infections, particularly viral infections, immune suppression from cancer treatment, allergy, and autoimmune disease. Thyroid extract primarily is indicated in hypothyroidism. Frankly, I have been suspicious of these products, even before the fear of "mad cow" disease became known. Except for thyroid, I have not used them in my patients. The potential for interference with the body's immune and endocrine systems is no less real than if we administered synthetic steroids or other hormones.

Nonetheless, they are widely used by some practitioners and you will encounter patients who are taking them. The safety, standardization, and potency of the extracts are critical to any effects they may have, so it is essential to know that the supplier follows good manufacturing processes. According to Pizzorno and Murray (1999),

"From the scientific data that currently exists [*sic*], there is enough evidence to support the use of orally administered glandular extracts." I remain a skeptic on the use of glandulars and look forward to more and better studies.

▰▰▰▰ GLUCOSAMINE SULFATE

A very useful agent is glucosamine sulfate, which is derived from shells of shrimp, crabs, and lobsters. It is an amino sugar that stimulates the manufacture of glycosaminoglycans, structural components of cartilage. The production of these structural elements declines with age, contributing to the development of osteoarthritis. Glucosamine sulfate supplementation is thought to offset this decline. Of the various forms of glucosamine available, only the sulfate form has been shown to be effective clinically, perhaps because the natural glycosaminoglycans contain sulfur.

The usual dosage is 500 mg 3 times/day or a single dose of 1500 mg/day for osteoarthritis. One of my patients claimed she had a positive effect from it but only when she took 3000 mg/day. One of its greatest advantages is that it does not have the gastrointestinal effects of commonly used anti-arthritic agents such as salicylates and nonsteroidal anti-inflammatory drugs (NSAIDs). Double-blind studies have found glucosamine to be more effective than placebo or NSAIDs, with a prolonged benefit compared to the NSAID after discontinuing treatment (McAlindon et al 2000, Muller-Fassbender et al 1994, Rovati et al 1994, Vaz 1982, Drovanti et al 1980). Although there is little direct anti-inflammatory effect of glucosamine, it relieves pain and inflammation of arthritis by rebuilding cartilage. It may take up to 4 to 6 weeks to reach full effect.

Although well tolerated, some mild gastrointestinal side effects such as heartburn, diarrhea, indigestion, or nausea may occur. Taking glucosamine with meals can reduce these effects. Some sources suggest being cautious with this agent in diabetic patients, but the minuscule amount of glucose in the usual dose is not significant. Those allergic to shellfish may develop a reaction to glucosamine because of its source.

▰▰▰▰ MELATONIN

Melatonin is a hormone manufactured in the pineal gland that affects circadian rhythms and the sleep-wake cycle. The primary use of this agent is to treat insomnia, particularly that associated with jet lag. For this problem, 3 to 5 mg can be taken in the evening after arriving at the destination (Petrie et al 1993). In some patients, particularly the elderly, a low melatonin level may contribute to insomnia and lower doses of 1 to 2 mg may be helpful (Haimov et al 1994, Singer et al 1996). I have some concerns about the use of melatonin on a long-term basis. As a hormone, it has global effects that may not be evident at this time. Claims for the use of melatonin in the treatment of cancer and multiple sclerosis require more study and it cannot be recommended routinely now for these purposes.

▰▰▰ PROBIOTICS

Would you believe taking bacteria can be good for you? Actually, we ingest billions of organisms daily in the air we breath, the food we eat, and the water we drink. Many foods such as yogurt, cheese, miso, sauerkraut, tempeh, beer, and wine depend entirely on bacteria or other microorganisms for their production. Probiotics are simply foods and supplements that contain live cultures of nontoxic, nonpathogenic, "friendly" bacteria. The best known and most useful of the probiotics are *Lactobacillus acidophilus* and *Bifidobacterium bifidum*. I recommend these, particularly for women who are prone to yeast infections (Hilton et al 1992), and especially if they are taking antibiotics. Many patients are aware of the effect of antibiotics on intestinal flora and take acidophilus regularly when they need to take antibiotics. Probiotics can be helpful prophylactically to prevent traveler's diarrhea (Scarpignato et al 1995), though at least one study did not support this use (Katelaris et al 1995). Although the most common side effect of these ingested bacteria is excess gas, they are sometimes prescribed to reduce gas in patients with excess flatulence.

Product quality depends on reputable manufacturers who know how to produce very high numbers of bacteria (hundreds of millions or a billion) as live, active cultures. Unless proven to be shelf-stable, most products require refrigeration, either before or after opening. Enteric coating can guarantee that the bacteria pass into the intestine unharmed by stomach acid. Taking the probiotic with a meal will help avoid degradation by stomach acids, although dairy products like yogurt produce their own buffering. Typical dosing after antibiotics is 15 to 20 billion organisms and can be started while the patient is still taking the antibiotic, but the dosing interval should be as far away from the antibiotic as is practical. The usual dosage of probiotics other than for post-antibiotic treatment is 1 to 10 billion cells of *L. acidophilus* or *B. bifidum* daily. As noted, higher amounts may cause flatulence.

I also recommend that patients taking antibiotics eat yogurt as a prophylactic against bacterial overgrowth and yeast infections. Some women with recurrent yeast infections have learned to recolonize the vagina directly by inserting a tampon dipped in commercial yogurt. The live bacteria in yogurt cause it to be better tolerated by lactase-deficient patients than other dairy products, because the bacteria secrete ß-galactosidase, which helps metabolize lactose.

SHARK CARTILAGE

If you have ever wondered why sharks don't get cancer, you are not alone. On the other hand, this question had never occurred to me until a book promoting shark cartilage for the treatment of cancer came out. Patients started asking whether the expensive capsules of shark cartilage could help cure their advanced cancers. As much as I wanted to encourage their hope, this is an unproved treatment. It is based on a reasonable assumption that shark cartilage may impair angiogenesis, the growth of new blood vessels, in tumors (Lee et al 1983). Impaired angiogenesis may be a problem if you need new vessels, however, such as if you have heart disease, have just had surgery, or are pregnant. Such patients should not take shark cartilage. An interesting study at the MD Anderson Cancer Center showed that, although not effective against lung cancer by itself, shark cartilage is a useful adjunct to chemotherapy and improves patients' response to and tolerance of a standard chemotherapy regimen (Richardson 1999). As we wait for more studies, I don't advise my patients to give up standard or proven therapy for cancer or arthritis in favor of shark cartilage.

Overall, shark cartilage seems to be quite safe. Make sure you take pure, white products. It is also one source of the chondroitin sulfate used for treatment of osteoarthritis.

OTHER THERAPIES

There are many other pharmacological and biological treatments. The bottom line on most of them is that there are some benefits but better studies are needed before they should be widely used. Here's a list of the more common ones and their alleged health benefits:

- **Androstenedione** is the steroid hormone made famous by the baseball slugger Mark McGwire. It is supposed to improve energy and muscle strength. I don't recommend it because it is a steroid hormone with unpredictable future effects involving the immune system, cardiovascular disease, or the development of hormone-sensitive cancers.

■ **Blue-green algae** is a seaweed product with all kinds of antioxidants, vitamins, essential fatty acids, proteins, amino acids, and phytochemicals. It is supposed to boost the immune system, reduce the risk of cancer and heart disease, treat arthritis, and so on. It is an expensive product that is probably not worth the price.

■ **Creatine** is used by athletes to improve performance. The literature I have seen recently does suggest some benefit in this regard, though the risks of increased injury, muscle cramping, and dehydration are widely described as well (Kelly 1997).

■ **Grape seed extract** is used as an antioxidant and contains bioflavonoids that can scavenge free radicals. It is used as an anti-aging agent and to prevent heart disease. The reasoning is that red wine, which contains many of the same constituents, is one factor that protects the French against the effects of their high-fat diets. Others have suggested, however, that their ingestion of large amounts of vegetables is the real protective agent in the "French Paradox."

■ **5-Hydroxytryptophan (5-HTP)** is a form of L-tryptophan that was taken off the market a few years ago after causing a number of fatalities from the eosinophilia myalgia syndrome (EMS). Both forms are involved in the serotonin pathway. I used L-tryptophan a lot in my practice for insomnia until a contaminated batch from Japan caused it to be withdrawn. 5-HTP is making a comeback as a treatment for depression, insomnia, fibromyalgia, and a variety of other disorders, even weight loss. The usual dosage is 50 to 100 mg 3 times daily; 100 to 300 mg before bedtime is the dose for insomnia. Starting with lower doses can prevent nausea. Vigilance for EMS seems prudent with prolonged use though. Because 5-HTP comes from a plant extract (the seed of *Griffonia simplicifolia*) rather than from the bacterial fermentation process used to make L-tryptophan, concerns about contamination are much less. I hope this one stays on the market.

■ **Pycnogenol** comes from pine trees and is also an antioxidant and free-radical scavenger. It has a wide array of claims for efficacy against aging, heart disease, cancer, arthritis, and other ailments. Though probably safe, it has limited scientific backing.

■ **S-adenosyl-L-methionine (SAMe)** is an interesting product that is widely marketed in Europe for major depression, osteoarthritis, inflammation, liver disease, and even schizophrenia. It has effects on folate metabolism and on the neurotransmitters serotonin and norepinephrine. It should not be used in bipolar disorder. When I first read about SAMe, it was on the cover of *Time* magazine. Anything that claims to do so much makes me a bit skeptical, and certainly more studies are needed. Nevertheless, this looks like a promising agent for several of the conditions for which it is recommended, especially depression and arthritis.

■ **Weight-loss aids** are always a booming business in this over-caloried country. Most of them contain ephedra, a sympathomimetic herb that suppresses appetite. Guaraná, a caffeine-like substance, is another common additive, as are a long list of minerals, vitamins, antioxidants, and other herbs. Both guaraná and ephedra are supposedly thermogenic, encouraging the burning of calories. Unfortunately, they achieve this effect by stimulating the heart rate and blood pressure. Chromium picolinate, which has some benefits in regulating carbohydrate metabolism, is often included (see Chap. 12). Some agents also include diuretics, which cause weight loss simply by depleting fluids. Overall, I am not enthusiastic about these agents, given their price, risk of side effects, and promise for a quick fix for long-standing obesity. Younger patients may tolerate them just fine, but sustained weight loss always involves lifestyle modification, dietary change, and often psychological support. When patients ask about these products, have them bring in the list of ingredients so you can make sure there aren't contraindications involving another medical problem such as coronary artery disease or hypertension.

Chapter 14

Bioelectromagnetic Therapies

Some things have to be believed to be seen.
—Ralph Hodgson

What lies behind us and what lies before us are tiny matters compared to what lies within us.
—William Morrow

BIOENERGETIC MEDICINE

Daniel Blodgett, MD

Bioenergetics is an approach to medical disorders from the viewpoint that the human body is surrounded and penetrated by various kinds of energy—electrical, magnetic, quantum physical, and subtle.

Conventional medicine concerns itself with health on the level of form, function, and chemistry. Viewing the body as having other dimensions involving energy requires a shift in perspective that some health-care practitioners find threatening, but it need not be. It offers the exciting possibility of healing on a more fundamental level. Our body is fed by intake of physical elements such as water, oxygen, minerals, proteins, fats, carbohydrates, and vitamins. Many ancient healing and religious traditions consider spiritual energy to be necessary for life to exist. This fundamental energy is known by various names, such as *chi* or *prana*, and its prime characteristic is the quality of love. When our energetic systems are open and unblocked, the free flow of this energy leads to a state of vibrant health of our physical, emotional, mental, and spiritual bodies.

Bioenergetic medicine attempts to modify disease processes by directing energy within or through the body rather than by using drugs or surgery. An example closer to the physical approach is the use of direct current flow of electricity through a nonunion fracture site to facilitate fracture healing. An example far from the physical approach is using a homeopathic remedy so dilute that no molecules of the substance used are likely to be in the water given to the patient.

Energy Healing

The concept of subtle energy has had slow acceptance into Western thought because it lacks a mathematical theory to explain it and an instrument to measure it. It is one of those things that have to be experienced to be believed. Subtle energy as a medium for healing has powerful effects but requires consciousness to direct the energy and to perceive the result. We are all familiar with the aura that certain people project, whether it be anger, sexuality, compassion, or confidence. On a subconscious level, we are all reacting to the energies of those around us. Energy healing is learning to be consciously aware of a person's energy field and helping the patient to reorganize it into a healthier and more integrated whole.

A wide variety of ways to do this have evolved in many different cultures. The level of sophistication used varies, as do the results. The method I learned at the School of Energy Mastery grew out of teachings of the theosophists, which developed in the first half of the 20th century. The theosophy beliefs in turn go back to ancient teachings of Hindu origin. The fundamentals involve different types of subtle energy moving through *chakras* located in seven areas of the body. Each chakra has a different set of tasks to do in supporting the human body to function efficiently and in harmony with the universe. Although different traditions may have other ways to view the types of subtle energy, for simplicity's sake it is practical to use *etheric, emotional, mental,* and *spiritual* energies.

Energy Exercises

As an exercise in learning, I invite you to close your eyes, take a few deep cleansing breaths, and scan the first or *physical layer* of your energy field. How does your body feel right now? Is it heavy or light, tight or loose, painful or relaxed, hungry or full? Focus your awareness into any areas that need attention and ask yourself, "What does my body need right now?" Many of us have learned to ignore the signals that our body sends us, so we persist in behaviors that cause us pain and ill health. The etheric (physical) layer of energy is like a blueprint that guides the physical body and assists it in tissue healing. People with clairvoyant sight usually report this layer of energy to be bright blue and highly organized.

Two simple exercises often help people to experience this layer directly. Hold your hands 8 to 10 inches apart and slowly bring them together with fingers open and palms facing. Most people are able to feel the interaction of the two fields as they touch as repulsion similar to two magnet ends of the same polarity brought together. The second exercise is to look at your fingertips held out in front of you against a white background. Hold the middle fingers about 1 inch apart and unfocus your gaze. Many people are able to see a blue haze around the fingers.

Now turn your attention to the *emotional layer*. This layer is in a state of constant flux as our emotions change. The colors in this field are varied and are seen by clairvoyants as swirling clouds. The next exercise is designed to help you learn where certain emotions are carried within your body. Close your eyes and recall the most frightening event of your life. As you relive the experience, notice the sensations in your body. Do you tighten up certain muscles, and if so, is it in areas that have recurrent pain? What is your breathing doing? How is the upper abdominal area? Is there a heavy or sinking feeling? What about the neck muscles? Do you tighten them or pull your head in like a turtle? OK—relax, take a few deep breaths, and let the emotion and any associated bodily sensations go.

Now imagine that you are in a moment when you felt a great sense of love. As you return to that time, feel your chest and heart area. Do you notice any sensations of expansion, lightness, soothing warmth, or pleasure? See if you get any sense of the feeling extending out from your body. The next time you are experiencing a strong emotion of any type, scan your energy and make note of what you feel and where. Check whether you have feelings in an area of your body that is not functioning as it should.

The *mental layer* may appear yellow and is highly organized. As you close your eyes and scan this layer, focus initially around the head. Does your mind feel alert or dull? Are your thoughts quiet or racing? Do you have recurrent intrusive thoughts that bother you? How well are you able to concentrate? Can you easily access information in your memory that you know is there? Do you habitually live in your mind and seldom venture out to experience your body or emotions? What thoughts about yourself or the world do you have that may be causing "dis-ease" in you now? An energy healer can help a person to access these often-unconscious thought forms and replace them with healthier thoughts of the person's own choosing. You can think of it as changing the software programming of the brain.

The *spiritual layer* is the most subtle. The best way to experience it is to focus your awareness over the top of your head. Close your eyes and ask to experience your connection to God or the Creator of the universe. Your beliefs about this may influence how this feels to you. If you have had an intensely religious or spiritual event in your life, recall it now and notice any sensations. Is there a feeling of love, peace, centeredness, or connection to all there is? I and many other energy healers believe that separation from the God energy is the ultimate source of all suffering and disease. Although physical healing may not be possible, being connected to this energy is a great source of comfort and hope to those who have illness. Numerous studies (Matthews et al 1993, 1995, 1997) have demonstrated that those with a belief in a higher spiritual power experience improved health and less morbidity than those without such beliefs.

Chakras

The chakra is described as a spinning wheel or disc of light that extends outwardly from the energy center located within the body, near the spine. Each of the seven major chakras has a traditional color and function. Table 14–1 shows the name, location, color, and function of each chakra. Different psychological issues are associated with each area. Pain or disease in an area controlled by a chakra is a clue to the healer about the likely emotional issues underlying the problem. Even if you do not study energy healing, knowing the issue that is most likely to be a source of a physical problem is helpful in asking questions of the patient.

Table 14–2 lists abuses that lead to deficiency or excess of energy in the affected chakra, the diseases commonly seen with energetic imbalances in each chakra, and healing modalities designed to promote healthy energy flow. A key point is that addressing the underlying energy of the disorder can lead to major improvements or resolution of the problem.

Although Western allopathic medicine may be useful or necessary in treating the disease, it seldom is able to return a person to a state of

Table 14–1   THE SEVEN MAJOR CHAKRAS

Name	Location	Color	Function
Seven	Extends upward from top of head	White	Wisdom, understanding
Six	Located behind forehead at pineal gland	Indigo	Thought, vision
Five	In throat area	Blue	Creativity, communication
Four	In heart area	Green	Love, intimacy
Three	In upper abdomen	Yellow	Power, integrity
Two	Just below navel	Orange	Connection, sexuality
One	Extends downward from sacrum	Red	Survival, body

Table 14–2 ENERGY IMBALANCES IN EACH CHAKRA: CAUSES AND HEALING MODALITIES

Chakra	Healthy	Abuses	Deficiency	Excess	Diseases	Healing
One	Healthy, sense of trust, grounded in reality, prosperity, ability to relax and be still	Trauma: birth, accidents, surgery, physical neglect, violence, extreme poverty	Underweight, fearful, anxious, chaos, lack of boundaries, undisciplined	Obesity, hoarding, greediness, fear of change, rigid boundaries	Diseases of bowels, anus, bones, teeth; eating disorders; frequent illness	Physical activity, massage, bioenergetic grounding, yoga, childmother relationship
Two	Experiences pleasure, healthy boundaries, moves gracefully, expressive emotionally	Sexual/emotional abuse, rejection, alcoholic families, denial of childhood feelings	Rigid body and attitudes, fear of change, no passion, sexual repression, excessive boundaries	Poor boundaries, bipolar, crisis junkies, seductive, manipulative	Low back pain, knee problems, disorder of genitourinary system, sexual dysfunction	12-Step program for addictions, dance/movement therapy, inner-child work
Three	Responsible, confident, disciplined, asserts needs, effective will	Shaming, physical abuse, authoritarianism, enmeshment	Low energy, weak will, poor self-discipline, unreliable, victim mentality, likes stimulants	Controlling, needs to be right, violent temper, likes sedatives, arrogant, hyperactive	Eating disorders, GI problems, diabetes, fatigue, hypertension, muscle spasms	Grounding exercises, physical exercise, deep relaxation, psychotherapy
Four	Compassionate, loving, peaceful, balanced, healthy immune system	Abandonment, loss, deaths, divorce, constant criticism, loveless upbringing	Antisocial, critical, cold, isolated, depressed, fears intimacy	Codependent, demanding, clinging, jealous	Asthma, chronic obstructive pulmonary disease, heart disease, breast disease, chest pain	Breathing exercises, journaling, forgiving self and others, psychotherapy to release grief

Five	Good listener, sense of rhythm, resonant voice, lives creatively	Lies, mixed messages, secrets, alcoholic families (don't talk, don't trust, don't feel)	Weak voice, tone deaf, introversion, inability to express feelings verbally	Talks too much, voice too loud, gossiping, interrupting, inability to listen	Disorders of throat, ears, voice, and neck; TMJ and thyroid problems	Loosening neck and shoulders, singing, chanting and toning, storytelling, silence (for excess), writing
Six	Good memory, perceptive, intuitive, sees patterns	Invalidation of intuitive and psychic experiences, what you see does not match what you are told, violence	Poor vision, poor memory, sees only black or white, denial of what is seen	Delusions, obsessions, nightmares, poor concentration	Headaches, eye problems, schizophrenia	Visual art, meditation, hypnosis, guided visualizations, dreamwork
Seven	Intelligent, aware, open-minded; wisdom, mastery, spiritual connection	Lies, forced religiosity, rigid education, invalidation of one's beliefs	Spiritual cynicism, apathy, rigid beliefs, learning difficulties	Confusion, dissociation from body, spiritual addiction	Coma, seizures, migraines, amnesia, brain tumors	Meditation, examining belief systems, cultivating inner witness, prayer, goal setting

healthy vitality where medication is no longer required. Once a disease has developed dense organ pathology, it is very difficult to reverse the process. Chronic obstructive pulmonary disease, congestive heart failure, renal failure, Alzheimer's disease, and cirrhosis are examples in which symptom control by powerful medications is needed. The greatest utility in energetic healing is intervening early in the process, when organ dysfunction is present but tissue pathology is minimal or absent.

Case Studies

Asthma

I treated one young man who had asthma. When he expressed an interest in an energetic approach to his problem, I was able to see that his heart chakra was narrowed down and that the cause was constant criticism by his authoritarian father. He had internalized his own inner critic, which constantly reminded him of his deficiencies as a person. The closed energy in the heart area was physically expressed by narrowing of the bronchial tree and frequent asthma attacks. When I brought this to his awareness and told him that he had a choice between criticizing or loving himself, he began choosing love. I had him say out loud an affirmation (I am worthy of love) 3 times a day for a week. He was given a daily breathing exercise that involved visualizing the golden light of love being breathed into his heart with each breath. I asked him to forgive his father and himself for having created this illness. He kept a journal recording his thoughts and emotions, with particular attention given to what seemed to trigger the asthma attacks. During the actual healing sessions with him, I guided him in releasing the stored-up anger and grief held in his chest. Over the course of 2 months, he was able to stop all his inhalers and feel what it was like to breathe freely. Even more important, he had learned how to love and accept himself and let go of the constant criticism that he had learned from his father. Additional ways to help this young man could have included homeopathy, flower essences, acupuncture, prayer, and other energetic modalities.

A Chaotic, Unproductive Life

A 40-year-old woman had difficulty in her life that centered on recurrent loss of her jobs. Although she had a good education in business, she could never seem to keep on track when attempting to bring a project to completion. Her personal life had always been chaotic and she drifted in and out of intimate relationships. When I talked to her about her life story and read her energy, it was clear that the problem was in her base (first) chakra. As a young child, she had lived with her single mother in a chaotic and impoverished home. Often her basic needs were not met, and she developed the survival strategy of living in a fantasy world created by her mind. As she continued this pattern into adulthood, the deficiency in the base chakra energy led to a major imbalance in her overall energy pattern. She suffered from frequent illnesses, was underweight, and had battled anorexia as a young adult. During healing sessions, we focused on the relationship with her mother. This woman had to learn how to nurture herself, because she had never experienced nurturing as a child. I recommended massage as a way to reconnect to her body in a positive way. She started an exercise program to build stamina and as a way to become more aware of her body's signals.

Every day she did a bioenergetic grounding exercise as a way of opening up the base chakra. I had her spend at least 1 hour every week in physical contact with the earth. She was to experience the "here and now" connection and was to offer gratitude to the earth for all the support it had provided in her life. We worked on a diet that would promote health and allow her to gain weight. When she noticed herself going into daydreaming or fantasy thoughts, she wrote them down. When we examined them together, we were able to identify recurrent thought patterns that kept her life in its chaotic and unproductive ways. Together we chose affirmations that she was to repeat to herself whenever she noticed herself going into her fantasy world. She was able to gain weight, have fewer illnesses, improve her job productivity, and start to gain a sense of mastery over her life. The healing process for her will be long, but she now has the tools to create the kind of life she has always dreamed about having.

It is apparent that self-responsibility is a key ingredient of this type of healing. Each person must be willing to stop being a victim and blaming others for how life has turned out. When we find the courage to really look within and experience ourselves as we actually are, we have already taken the first step on the road to healing. We then have the choice to change thoughts that keep us stuck and change behaviors that make us sick.

▅▅▅ REIKI

Linda Blakemore, RN

Reiki (pronounced *ray-key*) is an Eastern form of healing similar to the "laying on of hands" of Western society. Reiki is defined as *Rei,* universal mind or spirit, and *Ki*, the energy that sustains life. Thus Reiki is defined as spiritually guided, life-force energy. Reiki is a spiritually guided, hands-on healing practice. It is believed to have been practiced by Buddhist monks approximately 2500 years ago. The ancient Sutras of Buddhism describe an acquired ability to heal others, and the Buddha was described as having the ability to heal others instantly. A Japanese scholar, Mikao Usui, sought these gifts for many years. In 1916, during a mystical experience and after praying, meditating, and fasting for 21 days, he acquired the gift of instantaneous healing. At that time he also received information on how to teach or attune others with the use of four sacred symbols. He spent the rest of his life healing hundreds of people and attuning new healers. He became quite famous and opened two clinics in Tokyo before his death in 1926. He was able to open the natural channels of healing in others by "attuning" or drawing the sacred symbols (the same as those seen on Buddhist temple walls from 2500 years ago) into their chakras, or energy centers of the body, thus giving them the ability to heal themselves and others. Reiki was brought to the United States by Hawayo Takata, a Reiki Master from Hawaii (Petter 1997).

There are three levels of Reiki practitioners. Each level opens the ability to channel energy to the patient and practitioner. In the first level, the student receives a number of attunements during which the Reiki symbols are drawn into the chakras to open the body's natural energy centers. The student is taught about ethical principles of practice, the history of Reiki, and the energy flow through the chakras. Hand positions are taught for general overall balancing and for treatment of specific ailments. This course usually takes about 20 hours to complete and carries a first-degree practitioner level. The second-degree level course entails additional attunements, further opening energy channels to provide for a much greater flow of energy. Distance healing is taught to these practitioners. The third-degree Reiki practitioner is designated as a Master with a lifetime commitment to the principles of Reiki. The energy flow of Masters is limited only by their ability to open their channels. With each attunement, Reiki practitioners experience greater levels of healing, joy, prosperity, and wisdom for themselves.

A Reiki practitioner becomes a channel that brings forth universal energy through his or her hands and into the patient's body for healing. The practitioner's hands either lightly touch the patient's body or are held slightly over it. The energy is self-directed; it flows to the area of the body most in need of healing with the correct intensity to heal. Reiki has the ability to heal on many levels—physical, mental, emotional, or spiritual. Reiki is not a religion and is compatible with most beliefs. Many patients are comforted in that it requires no undressing and no touching of private areas of the body. The patient is treated with utmost respect and great care is taken to create an open, caring environment. Each patient's experience of Reiki energy is unique. Most patients report a peaceful sense of relaxation, bliss, joy, and love. They also report a removal or lessening of pain, anxiety, fear, and anger. Some will experience healing or lessening of disease after several sessions of Reiki. A few will see visions of color or angels, or may re-experience long-forgotten memories of childhood. Still others are able to access deeper levels of understanding within themselves to discover new solutions to the problems of their lives. Often released are emotional wounds that have led to "dis-ease," or lack of ease in the body. Reiki can and does create miracles for those who are ready to accept them.

Reiki is compatible with allopathic medical practice and has been shown to increase comfort level and decrease side effects in chemotherapy patients (Sell 1996). There are many testimonials of patients who have been helped or even cured by Reiki, but few scientific studies to date. Dr. Mehmet Oz of Columbia Presbyterian Medical Center in New York used subtle energy practitioners, including Reiki practitioners, in the operating room during open-heart surgery. None of the 11 heart patients treated with a combination of standard allopathic medicine and subtle energy treatment experienced the usual postoperative pain, depression, or rejection of their trans-plants (Rand 1998). Dr. Nancy Eos, a member of the teaching staff at the University of Michigan Medical School, was quoted as saying, "I can't imagine practicing medicine without Reiki. With Reiki all I have to do is touch a person. Things happen that don't usually happen. Pain lessens in intensity. Rashes fade. Wheezing gives way to breathing clearly. Angry people begin to joke with me" (Rand 1998). Also, Dr. Bettina Peyton, of Foote Hospital in Jackson, Michigan, has said, "Reiki's utter simplicity, coupled with its potentially powerful effects, compels us to acknowledge the concept of a universal healing energy" (Barnett et al 1996).

Today millions of Reiki practitioners around the world are working to achieve healing and peace for themselves and others. Some groups focus their energy on world peace and on bringing an end to human suffering (Reiki News, Summer 1997). People of today are searching for healing in all areas of their lives, and Reiki has the power to gently release life's burdens and allow life to be experienced with more joy. Although very few scientific studies have been completed, there are many testimonials of patients being helped and even cured by Reiki.

MAGNETIC FIELD THERAPY

Victor S. Sierpina, MD

The use of magnets and magnetic fields to heal the body is another fascinating bioelectromagnetic approach in integrative care. Externally applied pulsed electromagnetic fields have been used for some time in promoting the healing of nonunion fractures. More recently, the use of static magnetic fields in the form of locally applied magnets has become popular in sports medicine, arthritis, back pain, fatigue, poor sleep, and many other conditions. The data are not yet in on this form of healing, despite millions of dollars in sales of therapeutic magnets.

My dentist was the first to tell me about magnets, excitedly recounting how the application of a static magnet had reduced his chronic knee pain. With his hands and instruments in my mouth, he asked my learned opinion of this area of healing. After the visit I was able to discuss the matter with him further. Several of my patients with PhDs, MDs, and other advanced degrees have also given me exciting news about how magnets have helped their health problems, including foot pain, lumbago, headaches, and tennis elbow.

In a double-blind trial, Dr. Carlos Vallbona of Baylor School of Medicine has found the application of static magnets to be useful in substantially reducing pain in patients with post-polio syndrome (Vallbona 1997). He is not certain just how this happens. Suggested mechanisms include alteration of the flux of ions into and out of cells, effects on nerve tissue or neuropeptides because of the locally altered magnetic field, changes in circulation and clearance of local mediators of pain and inflammation, or effects on the pattern of injury current.

Some studies of the use of magnets have shown negative outcomes, however, and concerns have been expressed about noxious effects of magnets and magnetic fields. For instance, some suggest that positive magnets may stimulate cancer cells to grow in vitro and that living near high-tension power lines may be associated with higher rates of certain childhood malignancies (Bierman & Peters 1991). On the other hand, the Office of Alternative Medicine (OAM) found demonstrable therapeutic potential when it reviewed research into nonthermal, nonionizing electromagnetic fields in eight major new applications: bone repair, nerve stimulation, wound healing, treatment of osteoarthritis, electroacupuncture, tissue regeneration, immune system stimulation, and neuroendocrine modulation (Workshop on Alternative Medicine 1992).

You will find abundant anecdotal comments (some from magnet distributors) testifying to the benefits of using magnet inserts in your shoes, local magnets over trigger points, sleep systems including magnetic mattresses and pillows, magnetic jewelry, and more. We are initiating studies on magnets at the University of Texas Medical Branch after an initial pilot study showed pain reduction benefits for patients with osteoarthritis of the knees (Dr. Martha Hinman, UTMB School of Allied Health Sciences, personal communication, 1994). More and better studies like these are needed to prove safety and efficacy and to establish a mechanism of action of magnets in human health and healing. For now, I often hear about my patients' use of magnets after the fact. Enough of them have convinced me of their improvement that I am cautiously advising some of my chronic pain patients to consider their use, despite absence of conclusive scientific evidence.

▰▰▰ HEALING TOUCH

Connie Silva, RN, PhD

Healing Touch (HT) refers to multilevel energy-based skills designed to clear, balance, and harmonize the human subtle energy system with the use of touch. It is one of the energetic therapies that has been incorporated into the nursing profession within the past 20 years (Frost et al 1998). Some of the skills are designed as full-body techniques, whereas others address specific problems such as pain relief. A combination of techniques is used to realign the energies of clients with specific medical problems such as arthritis, back pain, and multiple sclerosis.

In 1989, Healing Touch was developed as a continuing education program for nurses, consisting of five workshops designated as Levels I, IIA, IIB, IIIA, and IIIB. At the completion of the five workshops and fulfillment of requirements, candidates are eligible for certification as HT practitioners. The first three workshops consist of 16 to 20 hours, during which participants learn energetic skills designed for specific conditions. The Level III workshops each requires 30 hours of participation. Participants learn to develop an energy-based plan for the client based on the energetic assessment and design a system of documentation.

The HT program originated from the private practice of Janet Mentgen, whose expertise in energetic concepts and techniques dates to years of study with different healers. In 1990, the program was endorsed for certification by the American Holistic Nurses Association. Because of its rapid growth, Healing Touch International has been the certifying body for HT since 1996 (Hutchison 1999). Certified HT practitioners can enroll in an instructors' course and become certified HT instructors.

Energy-Oriented Roots

Healing Touch, like Therapeutic Touch (TT) and many other energetic touch modalities such as Reiki, pranic healing, and jin shin, has its roots in ancient Eastern and Native American philosophies. The common element among these philosophies is that the source of energy in human beings is a life force that extends beyond the physical body and is "contiguous with the boundary of the environment." The field is electromagnetic in nature, is "in a continual state of flux," and varies continuously "in intensity, density, and extent" (Rogers, 1970, p. 90). Subtle energy-field interaction between the HT practitioner and the client is based on the belief that the human energy field consists of interpenetrating layers of energy that vibrate at different frequencies (Hutchison 1999). Through selected healing skills, the higher vibrational field of the practitioner aligns and harmonizes the client's unbalanced energies.

The Healing Touch Session

Some localized HT techniques can be administered in a session of a few minutes; full-body techniques may take an hour. A session may be held with the client sitting on a chair or lying on a massage table.

The HT practitioner follows five steps when administering HT:

1. "Centering" is the process of "bringing oneself to an inward focus of serenity" (Frost et al 1998, p. 174). The purpose of centering is to quiet the mind, eliminate anxieties and mental distractions, and focus attentively with full presence and therapeutic intent. A "universal source" of energy is visualized flowing through the practitioner's system. Throughout the session, the HT practitioner uses this fountain of universal energy through the palms of the hands to clear and modulate the client's energy.

2. The HT practitioner completes a comprehensive nursing history and performs a hand-scan assessment over the client's energy field. The palms of the hands are held 2 to 6 inches away from the client's field and moved from head to toes in a "gentle brushing" manner over the entire field. While scanning the energy field, some practitioners experience kinesthetic sensations such as coolness, heat, congestion, tingling, vibration, pressure, emptiness, and even pain. Hand-scanning information, along with observational data about the client (and intuitive feelings for some HT practitioners), determine the plan of care and HT techniques to be administered.

3. Movement refers to the third step of HT, "clearing or unruffling the field, with gentle brushing motions" of the hands, directing the congested energy down and out (Hutchison 1999). As in the assessment phase, the relaxed hands are held 2 to 6 inches from the body, with palms toward the client. The brushing motions may be "slow and sweeping or short and rapid" (Hutchison 1999, p 47).

4. The stillness of the hands constitutes the fourth step of HT—the balancing and modulating of the client's energies. The hands are placed over specific body parts, either held directly over the skin or in contact with it. The purpose is to transfer energy from the universal source via the practitioner's hands and allow for "repatterning" of the client's energy field. The HT practitioner continues to assess, unruffle, and balance the field throughout the session while in a centered state. The intervention phase is finished by holding the client's feet for a few minutes, a process referred to as *grounding*, to assist the client's return to a fully awake and alert state.

5. Evaluation is the fifth step of an HT session. The practitioner reassesses the field, observes client response, listens to feedback, and allows time for rest and integration of energy. The follow-up plan includes specific instructions for the day of the session, such as adequate fluid intake, and referrals to other health practitioners, particularly the primary health-care provider.

The goal of HT is to restore wholeness through realignment and harmony of subtle energies with the use of multilevel energy-based techniques. A successful session depends on the mental preparation and intent of the practitioner, data obtained from the nursing history and the hand-scan assessment, the practitioner's ability to raise his or her own vibrational level higher than the client's, and the client's openness to the process (Hess 1999).

▬▬▬ THERAPEUTIC TOUCH

Mary Anne Hanley, RN, MA

Therapeutic Touch (TT) is a scientifically based nursing intervention that has been used by professional nurses to support and comfort patients for more than 25 years. A contemporary interpretation of ancient healing arts, TT is a transpersonal healing approach during which the TT practitioner intentionally engages with the recipient energetically for the recipient's benefit. The goal of TT is to help or facilitate the recipient's innate healing processes rather than to effect a cure.

Developed by Dolores Krieger and Dora Kunz (Krieger 1979, Macrae 1987, Wager 1996), Therapeutic Touch differs from other like-named approaches, such as Healing Touch, in that TT is a specifically designed human-environment energy process. Healing Touch is a program of various skills and processes, one of which is TT. Therapeutic Touch has an extensive research base and has been studied by nurse researchers for the past quarter-century, with more than two dozen doctoral dissertations and several NIH-funded research projects. The breadth and depth of the TT research base was acknowledged by the first NIH consensus panel on alternative therapies in 1992.

Based on Rogers's (1970, 1994) nursing conceptual framework, the Science of Unitary Human Beings, which views human beings and their environment as open systems of energy in continuous mutual process, Krieger developed TT as one of the first clinical applications of this evolutionary nursing science. She proposed that the ability to help another person using TT is a human potential. Within the context of the mutual energy field process, the practitioner does not need to touch the recipient's body to accomplish a TT treatment, but the practitioner may (and frequently does) make physical contact, depending on the situation.

Technique

Therapeutic Touch is guided by a critical thinking and decision-making process. The phases of TT include (1) centering, (2) assessment, (3) intervention, and (4) evaluation. The novice practitioner carries out these phases sequentially, but with experience one can apply the phases simultaneously.

Centering—The process of bringing the body, mind, and emotion to a quiet, yet aware, state of consciousness. Meditation, breathing, imagery, or visualization are all approaches used to quiet the mind and to establish the practitioner's intention to help another. The practitioner maintains this state of quiet yet alert awareness throughout the TT treatment.

Assessment—Holding hands 2 to 6 inches from the recipient's body, the practitioner deliberately moves through the recipient's energy field from the head to the feet in a rhythmical and symmetrical manner. The practitioner may perceive sensory cues such as warmth, coolness, static energy, or tingling. The human energy field normally is dynamic, symmetrical, and balanced, and the practitioner attends to disruptions or disturbances in it.

Intervention—This phase is comprised of two types of energetic processes:

1. *Clearing.* Also called releasing or unruffling, this process is achieved as the practitioner uses the hands to move energy away from the recipient's field from the midpoint of the body using a smoothing or brushing movement. Clearing or unruffling facilitates the symmetrical flow of energy through the field. This phase releases excess energy and activates the recipient's healthy energy patterns.

2. *Balancing-Rebalancing.* This process includes directing, modulating, and projecting energy to facilitate patterning of energy and to reestablish order within the human energy field. The practitioner treats areas of perceived energetic congestion or deficit to mobilize energy or to modulate the flow of energy, using a principle of opposites. When the practitioner perceives congestion or heat, the treatment focuses on releasing the congestion or heat; when the practitioner perceives an area of deficit or coolness, the treatment intent is to direct energy to the area to correct the deficit or warm the cool area; when an energy imbalance is perceived, the treatment intent is to modulate energy to support or reestablish balance within the recipient's energy field.

Evaluation—As the final phase of the TT process, the practitioner reassesses the recipient's energy field, comparing the initial assessment with the outcome. As the practitioner gains experience, the evaluation process becomes continuous throughout the treatment, and treatment modifications are made as necessary.

Additional information about TT may be found in the references cited or by contacting the website of Nurse Healers–Professional Associates International, Inc. (http://www.Therapeutic-Touch.org).

Outcomes and Indications

The principal response to TT is relaxation, with signs of autonomic nervous system stimulation. Practitioners and recipients have noted changes in respiratory and heart rates with a generalized muscle relaxation. Therapeutic Touch has been useful in a variety of settings and has been used to manage pain (Meehan 1998), promote sleep and rest (Heidt 1991), relieve anxiety (Quinn 1984), and provide comfort and support to dying persons (Messenger 1994), among other clinical applications.

Nurse researchers have examined the effect of TT on a variety of client populations over the years. Examples of research include the effects of TT on the anxiety of hospitalized patients (Quinn 1984), postoperative pain (Meehan 1998), post-traumatic stress (Olson 1992), children with HIV (Ireland 1998), patients with burns (Turner 1998), grief and bereavement (Garrard 1995), and adults with arthritis (Gordon et al 1998). Such research studies have generally included one or more of the following comparisons: TT and mimic TT (choreographed movements that appear to be TT to the lay person), used as a placebo; TT and standard nursing care; TT and the use of narcotic analgesics; or TT and casual touch.

Although clinicians report positive outcomes of TT as an intervention, research findings have been equivocal. Several methodological limitations have been linked to the inconsistency of research findings, including the small number of subjects in the studies, restrictive time limits on the TT research treatments (for example, 5 minutes as opposed to 20 minutes of actual treatments), failure to describe and define the treatment adequately or to adhere to the Krieger-Kunz definition of TT, and failure to report demographic characteristics of the samples (Winstead-Fry et al 1999). These limitations are further complicated by the highly personal and subjective nature of the TT process. Qualitative methods have been used recently to gain a greater understanding and more thorough description of the lived experiences of TT recipients and practitioners in naturalistic settings. Researchers are continuing to refine methodological approaches to examining TT.

Case reports indicate that TT is effective in stimulating the relaxation response. It is believed that the relaxation response stimulates the recipient's unique ability for self-healing. Therapeutic Touch is used effectively as an adjunct with other mind-body interventions such as guided imagery and visualization. Meehan (1998) reported that TT may be synergistic with pain medications; recipients reported significantly longer duration of pain relief when medication and TT were used in combination.

The process of Therapeutic Touch contributes to the creation of a healing environment in which both the practitioner and recipient are open to change. Compassion, authenticity, and integrity characterize the TT process. What may be a relaxation response for one person becomes a life-changing event for another.

Case Study

Mel is 66 years old. He received his first TT treatment 12 years ago. His chief complaint was tightness and pain in his shoulders, and being unable to move his head. Using TT, I began to assess Mel's shoulders and back and perceived congestion in the area around his neck and along his spine. After clearing some of the congestion, I began to alternately clear excess energy and modulate fresh energy through these areas. I included light physical massage with the treatment. After the treatment, Mel reported that he felt less pain and his shoulders were not as tight. He felt relaxed.

The next day Mel arrived at my house. When I opened the door, he smiled, laughed, and said, "I am a believer! You did it!"

When I asked what I did, he replied, "I can turn my head! I haven't been able to turn my head for years! I got into my car this morning, and when I went to turn my body to look behind me, my head turned all by itself! I have full range of motion for the first time in years!"

Later, Mel's wife confirmed that he had not had full range of motion in his neck for several years and frequently experienced pain and muscle spasms in his neck and shoulders. Although his shoulders and neck may become tense or tight at times, he no longer experiences spasms and continues to have full range of motion.

▬▬▬ CONCLUSION

Victor S. Sierpina, MD

What are we to think of this assortment of sometimes subtle, sometimes metaphysical, and sometimes helpful energetic approaches? The National Center for Complementary and Alternative Medicine (NCCAM) now uses terminology that splits these approaches into two groups:

1. *Biofield medicine,* systems that use subtle energy fields in and around the body for medical purposes
2. *Bioelectromagnetics,* the unconventional use of electromagnetic fields for medical purposes

Many studies support the use of these therapies, though some urge caution, particularly in the use of bioelectromagnetic energy. One problem is that no generally accepted theory accounts for the phenomena of biofields or magnet therapy, either therapeutically or diagnostically. Yet both areas are finding increasing acceptance in clinical settings.

Further studies clearly are needed to characterize and systematize the nature of the biofield, to distinguish it from placebo or psychological healing, and to determine the safety and efficacy of magnets and externally applied magnetic fields. In the meantime, the nursing literature, the energy-healing and Eastern medicine literature, and the basic and clinical science research in these areas are provocative (Workshop on Alternative Medicine 1992). The goals of TT and HT, nursing interventions that have been adopted by other health-care professionals, are to support and facilitate healing and to promote health and well-being, even within illness, rather than to cure. Because all of these therapies are nondrug, noninvasive, and low-cost, the potential reward-to-risk ratio is great, and I recommend using them clinically while further studies are performed.

Chapter 15

Mind-Body Medicine

Separation of the mind and body is illusion. We as whole persons function as ecosystems responding to each stimulus in global ways.

—Wayne Jonas

Mind-body approaches are the "heart and soul" of integrative care. These approaches are not only effective but also inexpensive, easy to teach, and the gentlest and safest of all therapies. The term *mind-body* is a hybrid word that mirrors the profound duality in our thinking about health, arising from the thinking of the philosopher Descartes. Our conceptual split between mind and body resulted in the notion that mind and body are separate and do not affect each other in any significant way. Although this concept is curiously out of step with both religious and secular traditions, it has dominated Western scientific thinking for nearly half a millennium, ignoring long-standing human mind-body experiences such as meditation and monasticism, as well as altered states of consciousness resulting from prayer, fasting, chanting, yogic states, and others.

In his recent book *Reinventing Medicine*, physician-author Larry Dossey describes the evolution of modern medicine as traversing three phases (Dossey 1999). In Era I, the focus is on the purely physical aspects of health. Era II is the increasing use of the mind-body connection, using the mind to help heal the body. Era III is a combination of both the physical and mind-body with the added elements of nonlocal effects of consciousness, prayer, and positive intentionality in a truly whole-person system of care. Yet, throughout my medical work over the years, I have found that mind-body medicine has yet to come into its own in much of conventional care. Modern medicine does not consider the use of mind-body techniques such as relaxation, biofeedback, hypnosis, meditation, humor, and relaxing repetitive exercise such as tai chi, yoga, and aerobic exercise to be a highly valuable tool. Instead, it has been relegated to the area of "soft" therapy, valued lower than conventional approaches with drugs and surgery or seen as part of the nonphysical realms of psychiatry and psychology. On the other hand, Dr. Herbert Benson, the Harvard cardiologist who coined the term *the relaxation response*, believes that the area of mind-body medicine is not alternative

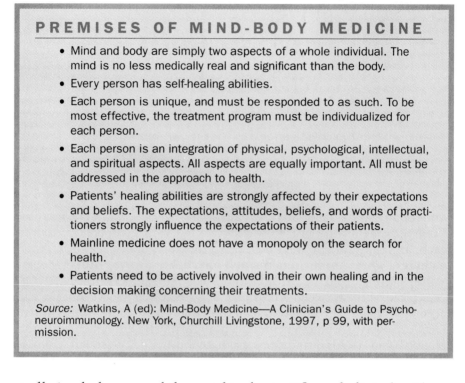

PREMISES OF MIND-BODY MEDICINE

- Mind and body are simply two aspects of a whole individual. The mind is no less medically real and significant than the body.
- Every person has self-healing abilities.
- Each person is unique, and must be responded to as such. To be most effective, the treatment program must be individualized for each person.
- Each person is an integration of physical, psychological, intellectual, and spiritual aspects. All aspects are equally important. All must be addressed in the approach to health.
- Patients' healing abilities are strongly affected by their expectations and beliefs. The expectations, attitudes, beliefs, and words of practitioners strongly influence the expectations of their patients.
- Mainline medicine does not have a monopoly on the search for health.
- Patients need to be actively involved in their own healing and in the decision making concerning their treatments.

Source: Watkins, A (ed): Mind-Body Medicine—A Clinician's Guide to Psychoneuroimmunology. New York, Churchill Livingstone, 1997, p 99, with permission.

at all simply because of the weight of scientific and clinical evidence that supports it (Benson & Stuart 1992, Benson 1998). Family medicine has adopted the biopsychosocial model as a paradigm of evaluation and treatment. This model encourages the more natural adoption of mind-body therapies into care, acknowledging the vital connection between biological health, psychological factors such as stress, and the importance of the patient's social support system (Engel 1977).

■■■■ STRESS AND PHYSIOLOGY

My first breakthrough in thinking about the intimate connection between mind and body came from studying both biofeedback and stress management when I was a second-year medical student. Biofeedback is a method by which we can train ourselves to become aware of our body's signals, often with the aid of an instrument. Observing changes in skin temperature or muscle tone, for example, allows us to learn to voluntarily affect physiological processes that are normally unconscious or autonomic. A person with headaches may observe a machine that gives visual or auditory feedback regarding skin temperature or muscle tension and thus may learn to correct and adapt his or her normal reactions so that the headaches are eliminated or modified by relaxation. After training, the person is able to continue the modified response without the equipment. Biofeedback has wide clinical application in control of pain, gastrointestinal disorders, headache, substance abuse, phobic reactions, and many other problems and is a clear-cut example of how the mind and body interact in illness and health. Many studies have been done that well support its efficacy.

When I was a medical student, I also offered to present a series of talks on stress management at a holistic health center. These led me to do extensive reading into the research on stress and its physiology. Walter Cannon (1939), Hans Selye (1956), and Herbert Benson (1975) all identified a set of clearly defined physiological reactions that characterize the body's response to stress. Endogenous catecholamines and steroids are released, including adrenocorticotropic hormone (ACTH), a hypothalamic-pituitary hormone; corticosteroids, adrenal cortex hormones; and epinephrine and norepinephrine, adrenal medulla hormones. The post-synaptic sympathetic tone is altered. Muscle tone increases, blood pressure rises, the heart beats faster, and more oxygen is consumed in an intricately orchestrated and adaptive response—the "fight or flight reaction."

This physiological reaction was very helpful for a primitive human who was being attacked by a wild animal or needed to fight an enemy to survive. It provided increased strength and energy for a quick response to a critical situation. For modern man, however, the stressors tend to be less acute and more cumulative: traffic jams, chronic job stress, financial or relational problems. When the same primitive reflexes take hold, they are not relieved by physical action. The effects on the body are predictable. Stress-related hormones and other physiological changes build up, causing conditions such as headache, gastric distress, hypertension, and heart disease. Learning that people can control this cascade of physiological responses through training in the "relaxation response" or other mind-body techniques was a major revelation for me.

An interesting counterpoint to the stress reaction is "stress hardiness." Some people have coping styles that help them adapt better to stress. Susan Kobasa (1990) described these people as having three characteristics: commitment, choice, and challenge. *Commitment* refers to an attitude of curiosity and involvement with whatever is happening. *Choice* refers to the belief that one can influence events, coupled with the willingness to act rather than be a victim of circumstances. *Challenge* is the belief that life's changes stimulate personal growth instead of threatening the status quo.

Another coping style that helps manage stress is termed *transformational*. This is the practice of reacting to stressful events by increasing interaction, exploring, controlling, and learning. This approach reduces stress by framing events in the context of continued personal growth and understanding.

On the other hand, a "regressive" coping style is characterized by backing away from stress and dwelling on one's own repetitive emotional reactions. This results in the opposite of stress hardiness and a state of helplessness in which the person fears and is threatened by change and feels powerless and alienated. A 30-year prospective study of Harvard alumni by George Vaillant found that those with a regressive coping style became ill four times more often than those with more mature coping styles characterized by such traits as humor, altruism, and sublimation (Vaillant 1977).

Author and psychologist Joan Borysenko (1987) encouraged the creation of new neuronal and psychological pathways to activate your inner healing potential, thereby increasing stress hardiness. These inner changes come from connecting to important values such as openness to love and hope, an attitude of forgiveness toward ourselves and others, an attitude of gratitude, and peace of mind. A greater ability to cope with stress comes not only from proper exercise and diet, but also from being of service to others, finding one's calling and following it with joy, and developing a deep sense of connectedness with others (Stienstra 1998).

■■■■ PSYCHONEUROIMMUNOLOGY

You can easily incorporate some areas of mind-body medicine into your practice and your self-care. One of these is psychoneuroimmunology. Although the word itself is a mouthful, psychoneuroimmunology is well worth your study. Hundreds of published studies have demonstrated the link between one's thoughts, emotions, and mental state and one's health. Mediators of the brain's effects on the immune system have been measured and identified as neuropeptides, hypothalamic and pituitary neuroendocrine signal molecules, and feedback cytokine molecules produced in the periphery. Interleukin, tumor necrosis factor, gonadotropins, ACTH, vasopressin, leukocyte-derived cytokines, and endorphins are among the substances involved in the bidirectional communication between the brain and the regulation of the immune system. The intestinal tract is lined with receptors for endorphins and cells that create neuropeptides. These include such hormones as cholecystikinin, vasoactive intestinal peptide, glucagon, and gastrin. The term "gut reaction" may refer to the release of these substances, which are made by both the gut and the brain and which are immunologically active as well as psychoactive. Likewise, the autonomic nervous system has effects on inflammation and lymphoid tissue

(Figure 15–1). Effects have been documented in vitro and in vivo on cellular and immune function, including effects on the common cold, bacterial and viral infections, and cancer.

The basic science in the area of psychoneuroimmunology (PNI) is fascinating and provocative. The clinical applications and implications are vast. The *psych* (study of the mind), *neuro* (study of the brain), and *immuno* (study of the immune system) components of this field offer us powerful new tools to affect our health. If thoughts and dreams can affect our physiological reactions, if stress and emotional experiences modify our adaptability to change and our risk of infection, cancer, and other disease, it is reasonable and necessary to explore the possibilities of using the mind to heal the body.

Carl Simonton, a cancer specialist, and his colleagues first made this field popular by describing techniques of visualization that he used to

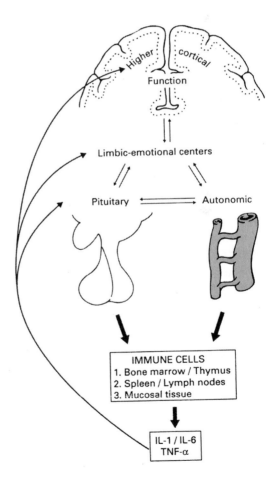

Figure 15–1   Bidirectional communication between the central nervous system and the immune system. Cytokines from the immune system communicate information to the brain, regulating its function, and the brain talks back in a bidirectional flow of cytokines, hormones, and peptides. IL-1 = interleukin-1, IL-6 = interleukin-6, TNF-α = tumor necrosis factor-α. (From Watkins, A (ed): Mind-Body Medicine—A Clinician's Guide to Psychoneuroimmunology. New York, Churchill Livingstone, 1997, p 6, with permission.)

enhance his patients' abilities to respond to treatment for cancer (1978). He taught relaxation techniques and had his patients picture their own white blood cells as powerful sharks pursuing a weak and confused school of fish, the cancer cells. He also helped to identify that in the year or two preceding the onset of cancer, many patients had experienced a major life stressor, depression, or traumatic event. In Simonton's view, these events weakened the ordinary immune surveillance that our healthy cells perform to rid our bodies of the frequently occurring mutations and abnormal cells that become cancer.

If the mind can affect even cancer, it should not be surprising that psychoneuroimmunological effects have been described in infectious diseases such as HIV infection as well as in heart disease, hypertension, allergy, gastrointestinal disease and aging. Studies have shown that death of a spouse causes significant immunosuppression 2 to 6 weeks later (Bartrop et al 1977), that traumatic marital separation is more immunosuppressive than bereavement (Kiecolt-Glaser et al 1987, 1988), that highly stressed people are more prone to upper respiratory infections (Cohen et al 1991), and that stress before examinations reduces immunocompetence in medical students (Kiecolt-Glaser et al 1986). I encourage my patients to use approaches of relaxation and imagery to boost their immune systems, and I build them into the treatment plan of every cancer patient and many others. Negative thinking, it seems, does affect us not only psychologically but also at a molecular and cellular level. Positive, optimistic, happy images and humor all create a sunny and healthful internal climate that stimulates optimal immune function (Figure 15–2).

■■■■■ THE RELAXATION RESPONSE

I have mentioned the relaxation response frequently throughout this book because it is so vital to our clinical practice of alternative and integrative care. A short session of instruction in the relaxation response, often taking 5 minutes or less, can teach patients to start to take control of their own health, to reverse automatic stressful reactions to daily events, and to control and reduce disabling physical and psychological symptoms.

Dr. Herbert Benson, a cardiologist and leader in this area, started by measuring the physiological effects of stress in healthy, volunteer subjects and how those effects were altered by meditation (Benson 1972, 1975). He discovered that the process of meditation decreases many of the physiological reactions to stress by a method not specific to any

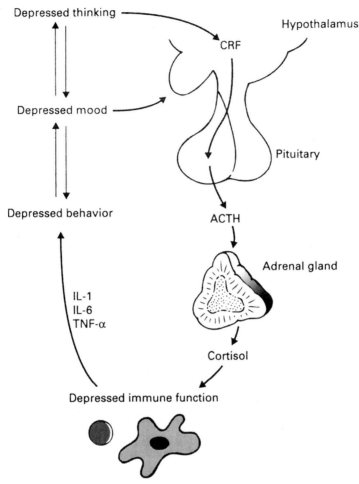

Figure 15–2   **The relationship between thought, mood, behavior, and immune function. Depressed thinking and mood can alter the autonomic and neuroendocrine output from the brain, potentially modulating immunity. Similarly, immunity and depressed behavior can alter CNS function, thereby altering autonomic and neuroendocrine activity. (From Watkins, A (ed): Mind-Body Medicine—A Clinician's Guide to Psychoneuroimmunology. New York, Churchill Livingstone, 1997, p 16, with permission.)**

particular discipline or religious practice. His initial research was done using volunteers from a transcendental meditation group, but the effects of the relaxation response can be achieved by many techniques:

■ Diaphragmatic breathing
■ Meditation

- Body scan
- Mindfulness
- Repetitive exercise
- Repetitive prayer
- Progressive muscle relaxation
- Yoga or tai chi stretching
- Imagery

Breathing exercise is essential and includes altering the rate and depth of breathing and using diaphragmatic rather than chest-type breathing. In diaphragmatic breathing, we relax our abdominal muscles and allow our breath to enter all the way to our lower belly. This permits deeper and more complete breaths; slower, deeper breathing generates a more profound sense of relaxation.

Slow, deep breathing also involves an important mental focusing aspect that is central to the relaxation response. The basic components of the relaxation response are a mental focusing device and a passive attitude to distracting thoughts. The steps of practicing the response are:

1. Pick a focus word, image, or prayer, rooted in your own beliefs:

   - The Lord is my Shepherd; Come, Lord; Our Father; Lord Jesus, have mercy on me; Hail Mary
   - Shalom, Sh'ma Yisroel ("Hear, o Israel"), Echod ("One")
   - Allah, Om, Maranatha ("Come, Lord"), Abba ("Father")
   - Neutral words like *one, peace, love, calm, let go, ocean, relax*

2. Sit quietly in a comfortable position.
3. Close your eyes.
4. Relax your muscles.
5. Breathe slowly and naturally, repeating your focus word.
6. Assume a passive attitude.
7. Continue for 10 to 20 minutes.
8. Practice the technique once or twice daily.
9. When distracting thoughts arise, let them go with a return to your focus word, attention to your breathing, or a phrase such as "Oh, well" or "Next." (Adapted from Benson, 1992, pp. 33–65.)

Commonly in my practice, I see patients bothered by stress-related illness or illness that causes stress, such as polysomatic syndrome, headache, fatigue, irritable bowel syndrome, exacerbation of asthma, reduction of immunity, frequent upper respiratory infections, heart disease, cancer, ulcers, anxiety, depression, or insomnia. Rather than prescribing a sedative drug for stress, I will have these patients lie on the exam table for a few minutes while I teach them the simple techniques of diaphragmatic breathing coupled with a focus word. I encourage them to practice these techniques regularly as a means to generally improve their health, to overcome anxiety or other mental distress, to manage pain or stress, or otherwise to reduce the risk of developing or worsening disease. I often write down the name of one of Dr. Benson's books on a prescription pad and encourage the patient to buy it and learn more about the practice on their own at home.

▰▰▰ OTHER MIND-BODY APPROACHES

Stress-Management Training

A variety of programs offer stress-management training. Although they vary in emphasis, they commonly use some of the relaxation techniques described above, as well as exercise, time management, and attitudinal adjustment. This kind of training has been included in corporate and organizational wellness programs for a couple of decades now and continues to be a methodical and practical way to help employees and others to learn to cope better with the stresses of life. The benefits, both physical and psychological, are similar to those described for the relaxation response and psychoneuroimmunology.

Mindfulness Meditation

Mindfulness meditation is a subset of relaxing meditation therapies and has also been incorporated in Benson's work. Jon Kabat-Zinn (1990), drawing from the traditions of Zen and other Buddhist meditation, has developed training programs using this technique to help persons suffering from stress-related problems or stress-causing problems. In short, this approach involves teaching us to be fully present in the moment, to notice our surroundings in a heightened way, and to be mindful and aware of our feelings, physical sensations, and the interplay of our environment. Practical applications of mindfulness can involve "minis," moments of relaxation throughout the day that do not require a 10- or 20-minute session. During each of these moments, one can apply four aspects of mindfulness:

1. Focus your attention on momentary experience as a means to elicit the relaxation response.

2. Pay full attention to the sensations of your body, with breathing the primary focus of mindfulness.

3. Be mindful of emotions that arise and their impact on the body.

4. Be mindful of your thinking process.

Mindfulness can be used in many ways to reduce stress during the workday:

■ As you awaken, bring attention to your breathing. Instead of letting your mind spin off into yesterday or today, take mindful breaths. Focus on your breathing, and sense the effects of breathing throughout your body.

■ Instead of hurrying to your usual routine, slow down and enjoy something special about the morning: a flower that bloomed, the sound of birds, the wind in the trees.

■ When stopped at a red light, pay attention to your breathing and enjoy the landscape around you.

■ While sitting at a red light, desk, or keyboard, become aware of the subtle signs of physical tension. Take some mindful breaths to relax and release tension.

■ Walk mindfully to your car. See and appreciate something new in the environment. Enjoy walking without rushing.

■ As you go to sleep, let go of today and tomorrow, and take some slow, mindful breaths.

We can take advantage of such mindful moments at any time, letting go of the past and the future, and bringing our attention to the present moment. As an exercise, try eating an orange mindfully: Take a moment to appreciate its origin. Look carefully at its color, texture, and shape. Notice the wonderful smell as you begin to peel it. See, as if for the first time, how the orange is formed into sections. Then gently break it apart, slowly eating one section at a time, enjoying each bite.

Traditional Exercises

Types of Asian exercise such as *tai chi* and *yoga,* which incorporate deep breathing, repetitive movement, meditation, and self-awareness, are other techniques that fit into the mind-body classification. The long traditions associated with these practices—both in the martial art and spiritual cultivation aspects—have always assumed a unity of mind and body. Being centered on the breathing, training the body, and being aware of the spiritual dimension all blend to make these exercises both physically helpful and deeply relaxing. Benson's term *remembered wellness* comes to mind here: the body, once taught to relax deeply, can more and more easily return to this state in the course of an ordinary day. It remembers the deep relaxation and flexibility of yoga or tai chi until everyday acts become imbued with the ease, centeredness, flexibility, and relaxation that these practices teach. I find that both of these types of exercise are particularly useful for geriatric patients because of their gentle physical demands, but they also are valuable for anyone suffering from stress-related problems because of the power to learn to become calm that is obtained through their practice.

Support Groups

Support groups are another powerful mind-body intervention. Though we have long appreciated the effect on health of family and community support, it was not until David Spiegel studied the effects of support groups on breast cancer patients that we were aware of specific effects on cancer (Speigel 1991). His CommonWeal program brought women suffering from breast cancer together for regular group support sessions. Although they regularly reported an improvement in the quality of their life and a decrease in fear, isolation, and loneliness, the stunning statistical finding was that the women participating in the support group actually lived longer. This increased longevity may be another psychoneuroimmunological effect or it may result from other factors. In any case, the benefits of such support groups for addiction, cancer, and other conditions remain a fascinating area for potential research and clinical application in an integrative model of care.

Hypnotherapy

Hypnosis and hypnotherapy once were mainstream medical interventions, but they were shunted aside in favor of developments in physical biomedicine. Though still not considered as integral to whole person care by most physicians, the use of hypnosis can be helpful in many physical conditions and psychological afflictions. The induction of a trance state by certain words or symbols creates a state of enhanced suggestibility in the patient. In this state, underlying unhealthy assumptions, inner traumas and fears, or negative expectations may be reversed. By suggesting an alternative outlook and response, hypnotherapy can help a person with a fixed fear or physical condition to react differently. For example, I have had several patients with profound anxiety about surgery. Anxiety and its subsequent catecholamine release makes patients more prone to negative outcomes from surgery or anesthesia. After several hypnosis sessions, they successfully underwent necessary procedures with less apprehension, changing not only their expectations but even their physiology.

Interactive Guided Imagery

The kind of visualization I described earlier in cancer patients has been modified into a form called *interactive guided imagery* by Dr. Martin Rossman (1987). He allows patients to develop their own images and visualizations rather than using those suggested by a therapist. This method helps the patient to communicate with the symptom and identify methods of relieving the distress. Images patients create themselves can be much more powerful for the individual. For example, one 14-year-old boy with cancer, having grown up with the movie *Jaws*, was not reassured by the shark imagery already described. As a country boy from Florida, however, he was impressed with the determination and survival instincts of the catfish, which will walk across a road to a new pond to find adequate water during a drought. For this boy, the catfish was a more potent inner image than a shark and he used it successfully to help combat his tumor.

Once, as a medical student, I used this technique to calm and relieve the pain of a man suffering from a kidney stone. Narcotics had not relieved his pain, so I sat with him, laid my hand over his flank, and led him through a breathing and visualization process. We traveled experientially together to a beach lined with palm trees, where the gentle lapping of the azure waves synchronized with his breath. As he slowed his breathing, he changed his focus from his pain to the word "ocean" and mentally and psychologically entered that beach scene. He gradually drifted peacefully into a painless sleep. I left quietly, reverentially, with the profound wonder of a student who had seen for the first time the power of mind-body medicine at work.

Spirituality and Prayer

Spirituality and prayer are a significant subcategory in the National Center for Complementary and Alternative Medicine (NCCAM) classification of mind-body medicine. I have discussed these at length in Chapter 4.

Humor

Journalist Norman Cousins made the therapeutic use of humor famous when he reported in the *New England Journal of Medicine* that he had been cured of a life-threatening illness by using laughter therapy employing humorous television shows and movies (Cousins 1976,

1979). This unique approach markedly reduced his need for pain medication. When he eventually recovered from what was considered an incurable condition, he took a position at the UCLA Medical School to encourage education and research into mind-body medicine.

Journaling

Journaling—recording one's thoughts, dreams, and reflections—can be therapeutic for both physical and psychological problems. A recent study found that the writing down of previous stressful and traumatic events relieved symptoms of both asthma and rheumatoid arthritis (Smyth 1999). This is a cost-effective, easily prescribed approach that can be readily adapted to any clinical setting and to many conditions.

Dance, Music, Art

Dance therapy, music therapy, and art therapy are other mind-body interventions with deep ethnic and cultural roots. They have been found useful in fields as varied as depression and recovery from stroke. More study is needed to define their clinical effectiveness, but they are safe and their cost is low (Graham-Pole 2000).

CONCLUSION

There are many more mind-body therapies than we have space to consider here. Conventional practice seldom uses them in caring for patients with physical problems, so I hope this chapter has given you some ideas for broadening your own practice. If we listen carefully to patients' fears and complaints, to their inner images and choice of language, and if we pay attention to their signs and symptoms of stress-related problems, we can adapt potent techniques from the field of mind-body medicine to expand our options for whole-person care. This may be the easiest, most cost-effective, and most empowering thing we can do for our patients.

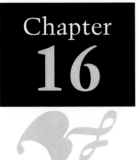

Chapter 16

Hands-on Healing Techniques

By his deeds we know a man.

—African proverb

To do is to be.

—Socrates

To be is to do.

—Plato

The way to do is to be.

—Lao Tsu

Doo-be-doo-be-doo.

—Frank Sinatra

CHIROPRACTIC

Lew Huff, D.C.

Historical Perspective

Chiropractic is a branch of the healing arts concerned with health and the prevention of disease. Chiropractors consider a person to be an integrated being but give special attention to spinal biomechanics and musculoskeletal, neurological, vascular, and nutritional relationships. The central concept in chiropractic thought is that disturbances of the body's structural and functional interrelationships may induce or aggravate disturbances in other organ systems or body areas. Proper structure and biomechanical integrity are important for the maintenance of homeostasis and resistance to disease. An impaired nervous system may diminish the body's defenses and its ability to adapt to internal and external stress and environmental changes, making it more susceptible to disease.

Historically, chiropractors have occupied a unique place among alternative healers. The use of osseous and soft-tissue manipulation dates back to ancient Egypt, Japan, China, and North America. Hippocrates and Galen both wrote about manipulation and its therapeutic effects. "Bonesetters" were popular in Europe and the United States in

226

the early 19th century. Early American bonesetters and osteopaths may have influenced early chiropractic ideas.

Chiropractic officially began in 1895 when Daniel David Palmer, the Father of Chiropractic, began to experiment with manipulative procedures in his office in Davenport, Iowa. Over time, chiropractors began to refine manipulative skills and organize manipulation into a viable health-care delivery system. Unlike other unorthodox medical movements of the 19th century, chiropractic not only survived but flourished, in part because chiropractors tapped into the vitalist and spiritualist tracts popular in those days.

Modern Chiropractic

Today's chiropractic doctor is well trained in diagnosis, treatment methods, consultation, and referral to other health care providers. The emphasis of patient management is on spinal and extremity manipulation, physical medicine modalities, rehabilitation, and nutrition.

Chiropractors may become board certified in subspecialties such as orthopaedics, sports medicine, nutrition, or neurology. Certification programs exist in various manipulative techniques and acupuncture.

Basic Chiropractic Principles

Chiropractic was founded on principles that focus on prevention and the use of nontoxic, natural therapies. The basic premise of chiropractic is that the body has a natural tendency to heal itself, and clinicians must identify and treat the *cause* of disease, not the symptoms. Chiropractors believe that each person should be viewed as an integrated whole, not as a set of symptoms, and also that prevention is the best cure.

Referral

Problems appropriately referred for chiropractic care might include musculoskeletal disorders such as low back pain, sciatica, facet syndrome, strain-sprain injuries, uncomplicated disc herniation, piriformis syndrome, spondylolisthesis, headaches of spinal origin, carpal tunnel syndrome, and TMJ. Patients with uncomplicated low back pain especially may be candidates for chiropractic care if the symptoms are prolonged or are poorly controlled with medication.

Contraindications to manipulation include fractures, dislocations, neurological complications, bone pathology, spinal motion instability, systemic diseases, or infection. A chiropractor detecting any of these conditions would refer the patient to other appropriate health care providers.

Referral to another provider also would be warranted for most patients if a 4- to 6-week trial of manipulation failed to produce signs of improvement. The Rand Studies (Shekelle et al 1991), U.S. Agency for Health Care Policy and Research (AHCPR) Guidelines (Bigos et al 1994), Quebec Task Force (Spitzer et al 1987), and Royal College of General Practitioners (Waddel et al 1996) all indicate that a 4- to 6-week trial of manipulation is appropriate. If there are no signs of improvement, the patient should be re-evaluated or referred to an appropriate medical specialist. Intensity of pain, duration of pain, the age of the patient, and the number of prior episodes may lengthen the treatment time.

Studies on Chiropractic

In recent years, independent researchers and various government agencies have conducted studies that focus on the efficacy, appropriateness, and cost-effectiveness of chiropractic care. The AHCPR, in its Clinical Practice Guideline #14, and the U.S. Department of Health and Human Resources endorse spinal manipulation for acute low back pain. Statistics show that more than 90% of all manipulations in the United States are performed by chiropractors.

The Manga Report (Manga et al 1993), funded by the Ontario Ministry of Health in Canada, overwhelmingly supported the efficacy, safety, scientific validity, and cost-effectiveness of chiropractic for low back pain. This report found that manipulation by chiropractors was more effective and safer than the medical management of low back pain. The Royal College of General Practitioners report of 1996 (Waddell et al 1996) found that manipulation provides pain relief, higher activity levels, and greater patient satisfaction than medical treatment for back pain. Other supportive studies are listed in "Studies That Support Chiropractic Care," and in an excellent review of chiropractic by Kaptchuk et al (1998).

Risks and Complications

Any medical procedure has risks and possible complications, and chiropractic manipulation is no exception. A thorough exam with an eye on risk factors helps to minimize those risks. Certain neuropathies; cauda equina syndrome; the presence of inflammation, infection, or malignancy; and frank herniation with positive neurological signs are contraindications for manipulation. A few cases have been reported of cerebral vascular accidents following manipulation of the cervical spine and of cauda equina syndrome following manipulation of the lumbar spine. With proper screening, these risks are greatly minimized. The Royal College of General Practitioners (Waddel et al 1996) stated, "The

STUDIES THAT SUPPORT CHIROPRACTIC CARE

Wight Study of recurring headaches, 1978
New Zealand Commission, 1980
Florida Worker's Comp, 1988
Washington HMO Study, 1989
Rand studies, 1990, 1994
Utah Worker's Comp, 1991
Oregon Worker's Comp, 1991
Virginia Comparison Study, 1992
Manga Report, 1993
Saskatchewan Clinical Research, 1993
Royal College of General Practitioners, 1996

Source: Adapted from *Studies on Chiropractic.* Published by the National Board of Chiropractic Examiners, 901 54th Ave., Greeley, CO 90634. Phone 907-356-9100.

risks of manipulation are very low in skilled hands." Nevertheless, the practitioner must be aware of these risks and inform the patient of them before treatment.

Tips on Choosing a Doctor of Chiropractic

Beware of clinicians who make extravagant claims of success or who insist on treatment plans that involve months or years of care. Word of mouth is the best way to find a qualified, skilled chiropractor, but if this is not available, you can contact the American Chiropractic Association or the local chapter of your state chiropractic association. Another source of referral is the state licensing agency, which can tell you if the clinician is currently licensed and if there are any complaints or actions pending against him or her.

What to Expect on the First Visit

Chiropractors are trained extensively in skillful history taking, examination, and special testing. A careful history will be followed by a thorough exam. The clinician will then focus on the patient's area of complaint or concern and will decide whether x-rays or other special tests will be needed. If the patient is a candidate for chiropractic care, the treatment plan will be explained and an estimate made of the duration of the treatment. Typically, a 4- to 6-week trial of care will be initiated; if no signs of improvement are noted, the patient will be reassessed or referred to another health care provider.

Conclusion

Chiropractic is now the third-largest primary health-care delivery system in the Western world, after medicine and dentistry, and the largest drugless health care system in the world. Today chiropractic is taught and practiced throughout the world and has earned broad acceptance. It has moved away from its early years of sectarian dogma into a position as the orthodox nontraditional approach to health, a sort of "orthodox unorthodoxy." Modern chiropractic appeals both to the scientific community, owing to recent studies illuminating the efficacy of spinal manipulation, and to those with holistic health and New Age sensibilities.

▬▬▬▬ MASSAGE THERAPY

Victor S. Sierpina, MD

Common Indications for Massage Therapy*
• • • • • • • • • • • • • • • • • • •

Anxiety
Arthritis
Attention deficit/hyperactivity disorder (ADHD)
Colic
Depression
Eating disorders
Fibromyalgia
Headaches
Immune deficiency
Lymphedema
Musculoskeletal problems
Pregnancy and childbirth
Prematurity of infants
Premenstrual syndrome (PMS)
Sexual dysfunction
Sprains, strains, acute and chronic injuries
Sports injuries
Stress

*The most important indications are shown in boldface type.

After chiropractic, massage therapy is probably the best known of the hands-on techniques. In recent years, a substantial body of research has supported the use of massage in various applications. For instance, newborn premature babies gain weight better if massaged. No major professional athletic team is without a massage therapist to return injured players to the field or court as quickly as possible. Massage is a safe and highly effective technique for handling certain chronic ailments, and it may be unparalleled for managing stress (see "Common Indications for Massage Therapy").

The range of benefits and applications of massage are so vast that they touch virtually every field of medicine and health care in some way. Recognized as core to medical treatment since the time of Hippocrates, massage arises from a number of traditions. These include shiatsu or other systems that use acupressure points and meridians, Swedish massage, neu-

Contraindications for Massage Therapy
. . . .

Bleeding disorders

Blood clots

Broken bones

Dislocated joints

Enlarged liver or spleen

High fever

Open wounds

Peptic ulcer

Phlebitis

Pregnancy (unless therapist is specially trained)

Severe psoriasis

Skin infections

Some kinds of cancer, especially massage directly over malignant tumors

Uncontrolled hypertension

romuscular massage, deep-tissue massage, sports massage, myofascial release, and others. Swedish massage, which is based on traditional European methods and Western concepts of anatomy and physiology, uses five techniques: effleurage (gliding strokes), petrissage (kneading), friction (rubbing), tapotement (percussion), and vibration.

We require students in our Alternative and Integrative Therapy to have a massage as part of their course of study. I never hear a complaint about this requirement. I explain to students that reading about massage will never give them the feel for the experience that having one does. Every primary care provider and specialist needs to become familiar with referral for massage. You should learn the general types of massage and its indications and contraindications (see "Contraindications for Massage Therapy"). Listen to what your patients report about their experiences with massage and specific massage therapists so you can learn which are the best-qualified therapists in your community. As with other referrals, it is essential to know the practitioner to whom you are referring your patients. Most states require licensure, which acts as a significant marker of adequate training and ethical conduct. Well-trained therapists will be aware of the important indications and contraindications for massage. I generally leave the specific type of massage up to the therapist and the patient to decide together, though I usually have some initial ideas of which type of treatment is reasonable before I refer.

■■■ POSTURAL AND STRUCTURAL RE-EDUCATION THERAPIES

Victor S. Sierpina, MD

The underlying concept of this kind of therapy is the re-education of the body through movement, touch, and relief of structural and functional stress. The best known are the techniques of Alexander, Feldenkrais, Trager, and Rolf. A skilled therapist helps the patient experience a healthy alignment of the posture, improved coordination and balance, and heightened awareness of proper body mechanics.

The Alexander technique had an interesting origin. It was developed by an actor who concluded that his voice loss was due to poor postural habits. Alexander practitioners address problems of the head, neck, and shoulders as well as other chronic conditions such as breathing problems, myalgia, rheumatism, and even anxiety, stress, and hypertension. They help their clients retrain their kinesthetic sense by a series of exercises during which the light touches of the practitioner teach them to use their bodies with less stress and tension. It is popular among people in drama and other performing arts.

Feldenkrais, a physicist, developed a concept called "awareness through movement," in which the trained practitioner guides students to increasing awareness of their actions. By words and gentle touch, the student is guided to become aware of existing movement patterns and optional ones as well. The term "functional integration" refers to the coherent organization of choices for functional movement patterns. The hands-on aspect in the Feldenkrais method is to teach and communicate rather than to manipulate the student directly. The student does the work of shifting awareness and altering movement, form, and posture in response to the suggestions of the practitioner. The Feldenkrais method has a wide array of applications; it is used for developmentally challenged children, neurological and orthopaedic physical therapy, pain management, the performing arts, and even animal rehabilitation.

The Trager method was developed by a Hawaiian physician who had been a boxer. This system uses gentle shaking and rocking of the joints to ease movement and to release chronic patterns of tension and misalignment. The bouncing, compressions, stretching, and elongations stimulate clients to experience new degrees of freedom in their movement. A meditative aspect called "menastics" is included, which helps clients to enhance their enjoyment of the free movement and flexibility of the body parts. Trager is used for neurological and orthopaedic problems, chronic pain, headache, and other chronic illnesses associated with abnormal movement patterns, such as multiple sclerosis, chronic lung disease, and cerebral palsy.

Rolfing, or "being Rolfed," is a well-known system of structural integration that focuses on treating fascial injury, tension, and misalignment. Unwinding or stretching injured and thickened fascial layers back to their normal condition is thought to allow the associated bones and muscles supported by the fascia also to return to their normal positions. A condition is created in which healing and normal functioning can return. The technique involves stretching the fascial sheaths through sliding pressure. It has been used in a variety of conditions such as cerebral palsy, anxiety, stress, low back pain, and whiplash.

OSTEOPATHIC MEDICINE

Lisa Nash, DO

Osteopathic medicine is a unique *philosophy* of health care. This form of American medicine was originated by Dr. Andrew Taylor Still in 1874. Both the philosophy and its interpretation have evolved over time. Dr. Still was dissatisfied with the effectiveness of 19th-century medicine. He believed that many of the medications of his day were useless or, even worse, possibly harmful, so he had little use for pharmaceuticals. A large portion of Dr. Still's knowledge of the human body was based on mechanical principles, in keeping with the information available in his time. We now have come to appreciate a broader conceptualization of the philosophy. Some very modern concepts (preventive medicine and the biopsychosocial model, for example) were first practiced by osteopathic physicians and taught in osteopathic medical schools.

Dr. Still was a pioneer of preventive medicine. He emphasized the importance of keeping fit and eating properly. He believed that helping patients take more responsibility for their own well-being should be one of the medical profession's primary goals. Osteopathic physicians take a whole-person approach to care and look for underlying causes for disease, recognizing that these may be physical, emotional, mental, or spiritual. In keeping with this holistic approach to care, most osteopathic physicians enter primary care fields, often in small towns and rural and other underserved areas. Osteopathic specialty physicians also practice in all recognized fields of tertiary medicine.

Osteopathic philosophy is based upon four key principles:

1. **The body is a unit;** the person is a unit of body, mind, and spirit.
2. **The body is capable of self-regulation, self-healing, and health maintenance.** Dr. Still believed that the body itself produces all the chemicals needed for healing and self-regulation and that by helping this process, we can promote healing.
3. **Structure and function are reciprocally interrelated.**
4. **Rational treatment is based on an understanding of the basic principles of body unity, self-regulation, and the interrelationship of structure and function.**

In keeping with the founding principles of osteopathic medicine, the role of the musculoskeletal system is considered more significant than in traditional allopathic medicine. Musculoskeletal abnormalities are referred to as *somatic dysfunction,* defined as "impaired or altered function of related components of the somatic (body framework) system:

skeletal, arthrodial, and myofascial structures, and related vascular, lymphatic, and neural elements" (Ward 1997). Osteopathic manipulative medicine (or osteopathic manipulative treatment, OMT) is the system of treatments practiced by osteopathic physicians to deal with somatic dysfunction. There are at least 13 groups or types of techniques. Some of the most commonly employed are HVLA (high velocity, low amplitude), muscle energy, soft-tissue techniques, and myofascial release techniques. Craniosacral manipulation is the cranial osteopathy approach based on the concept that the skull bones can shift slightly and affect spinal fluid pressure and other neurological mechanisms. It has been used increasingly in recent years for a number of neurological conditions, including traumatic brain injury.

OMT is useful and beneficial for the treatment of patients of all ages, newborn to geriatric, and for a wide variety of disorders. These techniques may be used to treat both acute and chronic conditions (which may have acute exacerbations). They may be used alone or in conjunction with other forms of treatment such as medications or surgery. OMT is useful in conditions such as pregnancy, to provide relief of discomfort in the low back and pelvis when medications are best avoided. For some conditions (such as somatic dysfunction of the lumbar spine induced by lifting a heavy object with poor technique), response to treatment may be very dramatic, with complete resolution of the dysfunction and associated symptoms immediately after a single treatment. Other conditions may require a series of treatments, each tailored to the findings of repeat examination and response to previous treatment, with improvement or resolution of symptoms being achieved over time.

Besides treating musculoskeletal complaints and abnormalities, OMT is also commonly used to relieve symptoms and abnormalities associated with a variety of other disorders, such as asthma, sinus complaints, and migraines, to name a few. Appropriately applied OMT promotes healing in many situations by promoting the normal flow of blood and lymphatic fluid.

Just as there are appropriate *indications* for specific forms of OMT, there are also *contraindications*. For instance, high velocity–low amplitude thrust techniques should not be used on a patient with cancer known to be metastatic to bone.

Focused training in the role of the musculoskeletal system and OMT are special components in the education and medical practice of osteopathic physicians. First articulated in the founding principles of osteopathic medicine, this enhanced understanding remains a vital component and reinforces the overall concept of the whole-person approach to medicine taken by today's osteopathic physicians.

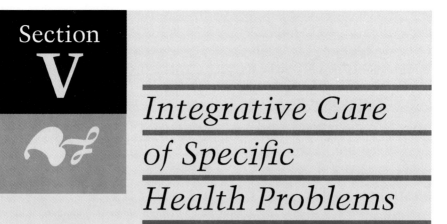

Section

V

Integrative Care of Specific Health Problems

Knowing is not enough, we must apply. Willing is not enough, we must do.
—Johann von Goethe

One learns by doing the thing; for though you think you know it, you have no certainty until you try.
—Sophocles

Many common problems in primary care can be helped with simple, natural, alternative approaches. Using both text and tables, the chapters in this section summarize many of the most common primary care problems and illustrate their treatment using an integrative approach. Particularly with major illnesses such as cancer and heart disease, I still consider conventional therapies such as medication the primary treatment and the standard of care. I use them regularly with my patients. They are mentioned briefly in these chapters but are better covered in standard texts. Even with the most serious disorders, however, alternative therapies can play an important adjunctive and complementary role, and they are the focus of these chapters.

One feature deserves a bit of explanation. Often in the course of a day, a colleague pulls me aside or calls to ask for a "curbside consult" regarding alternative therapy options for a patient. This kind of informal consultation occurs daily in clinics and hospitals. Providers tap each other's knowledge and expertise about the care of a patient without the formal process of a written referral and evaluation. The "Curbside Consults" in these chapters give a synopsis of the basic approach I might take and the advice I would give if asked about integrating alternative therapies into a treatment plan. The recommendations are listed in the order that I usually prescribe them. These "Consults" are not meant to be comprehensive but rather are intended to suggest my priorities in the integrative evaluation and treatment of patients. I hope they will help you to select an approach from the many options listed in the text and tables, so you can get a good start in using alternative therapies.

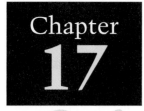

Chapter 17

Anxiety and Depression

Clearly, anxiety and depression are common complaints in any primary care practice. By some estimates, 75% or more of complaints brought to the health care setting have a predominant psychological component. Stress, anxiety, and depression are not only widespread, they are often concealed diagnoses. By this I mean the patient is more likely to complain of a somatic symptom—headache, backache, fatigue, indigestion, chest discomfort or palpitations, and so on—than to claim to be anxious or depressed.

As thorough clinicians, we must be diligent in ruling out serious organic pathology when a patient presents with a physical complaint. But the psychological dimension should always be included in the differential diagnosis of any physical symptom. When test after test comes up negative, and the patient seems not to be responding to standard treatment or doesn't fit the profile of any well-defined clinical syndrome, you should consider anxiety, depression, or stress-related disease. Though I have already discussed stress in Chapter 15, I mention it here because stress is clearly associated with many illnesses, either being caused by the illness or contributing to its occurrence. Likewise, illness can cause both anxiety and depression. A person with a new diagnosis of cancer or heart disease commonly will react in this way, for example.

Standard therapy for anxiety and depression includes psychopharmacological agents and counseling or

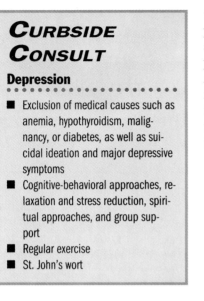

therapy. In severe cases, particularly if patients are at risk of injuring themselves or others, medication and hospitalization are absolutely necessary. As the brief cases in this chapter will illustrate, however, therapies other than medication, such as mind-body techniques, herbs, or movement, often prove useful.

Case Study: Anxiety

Sally V. is a 37-year-old who presents with frequent palpitations, shortness of breath, and feelings of impending doom. She has been seen several times in the ER and has been diagnosed with "hyperventilation." Chest x-rays, EKGs, CBC, and blood tests for electrolytes, thyroid, and so on have all been consistently normal. As you examine this thin white woman, you notice a slight click in mid-systole on her cardiac exam. Other than an anxious appearance and a voice to match, you find nothing else remarkable. You inquire as to her home and work life, her spiritual practices, and her family relationships. Nothing seems out of order, but she says these attacks of panic and anxiety have gone on for several years and seem to be getting worse. Her previous doctor had tried a number of medications, including alprazolam, amitriptyline, clonazepam, and hydroxyzine. She had also taken a beta blocker and sleeping medication (zolpidem), and had been referred for counseling and hypnotherapy.

She reports to you that the medications made her very drowsy and unable to function. She never followed up the referral for counseling and hypnotherapy because the doctor, shoving the referral slip across the desk to her, had told her rather abruptly that there was "nothing wrong" and it was "all in her head." She is eager to get rid of these disabling symptoms, which have interfered with life at home and on the job. She knows there is something wrong and cannot be persuaded that it is "mental" rather than physical because, after all, her heart beats irregularly, she is short of breath, and she has numbness of her mouth and fingers when the episodes occur.

What Is Your Approach?

It is clear that the patient has had several fairly extensive evaluations in the ER, so a lot more testing will not be either productive or cost-effective. You do order an echocardiogram and a 24-hour Holter monitor because of the cardiac symptoms and the systolic click. You suspect mitral valve prolapse based on the presence of the mid-systolic click and its associated anxiety symptoms. The echo does show a slight mitral valve prolapse but no significant mitral regurgitation. Holter monitoring shows only occasional premature atrial contractions, which are unassociated with symptoms reported in the patient diary of feeling short of breath and scared, with heart pounding and some numbness around the mouth and hands. You confer with Sally regarding the results of the tests and your recommendations.

What Are Your Recommendations?

Because the patient has a mild case of mitral valve prolapse, the use of a low-dose beta blocker may be helpful. Because she had problems with this medication previously, you choose to start with a very low dose (for example, atenolol, 12.5 mg/day). You also teach her some deep-breathing exercises that she can do whenever she starts to hyperventilate. You teach her "relaxation response" techniques not only to help her relax during her anxiety/panic spells but also to "down-regulate" her sympathetic system on a regular basis (Benson & Stuart 1992). Additionally, you recommend that she enroll in a regular aerobics class and avoid tobacco, sugar, caffeine, and alcohol.

She returns to your office in a month. Though her palpitations haven't returned and she has not been to the ER, the night before last she almost went there because of shortness of breath. She practiced her deep-breathing exercises and decided she could wait until her office visit for medical care. She has started jogging instead of taking aerobics because the aerobics class meets at a time inconvenient for her work schedule at the travel agency. Overall, she feels better but still struggles with "being on the edge" of feeling tense and worried a lot.

On further inquiry, you find that she is marginally involved in her local church. You ask whether the church has been a source of support to her in the past, and she responds affirmatively. You suggest that the social and spiritual support may be useful for her current condition (Koenig et al 1993). Additionally, you recommend the use of some supplements and herbs, to which she readily agrees. Your prescription includes magnesium, 200 mg twice a day; valerian, 300 mg three times a day (Robbers, 1999); and some chamomile tea at bedtime.

She returns in another month, beaming. "This is the best I've felt in years. My husband says I'm like a new woman!" she exclaims. When you ask what has been happening, she says she feels a lot calmer and in better control of her body with the breathing exercises, has started to pray and meditate with a church group, and is continuing to watch her diet and exercise regularly. She hasn't even thought about going to the ER this month and wonders about stopping the atenolol.

Case Summary

This patient presented with a very typical picture of hyperventilation and anxiety. The mitral valve prolapse, which had been associated in the past with anxiety, may or may not have been related. The medical workup was negative and a diagnosis of anxiety was clear. Because of the failure to respond to standard therapy, an integrative approach of herbs, exercise, low-dose medication, and mind-body and spiritual approaches seemed reasonable. It might have taken this patient several months to obtain a positive response to the variety of lifestyle changes and other prescriptions offered to her.

A summary of alternative approaches to anxiety is listed in Table 17–1.

Case Study: Depression

Julia H., a 32-year-old, married African-American woman, comes to your office with complaints of low mood. She says that she has developed low energy, is awakening early in the morning, and has lost much of her interest in her normal activities, including food, hobbies, work, exercise, and sex. She denies feeling suicidal and has no personal or family history of mental disease. Her relationship with her husband is loving and supportive. Further inquiry reveals no major life stressors such as a new baby, marital problems, or loss of a loved one. She readily admits to job-related stress; a recent promotion at her law firm has forced her to work longer hours. She likes the work, however, and sees this promotion as positive because one of her life goals is to become a partner in the firm.

A physical examination is negative for any significant abnormal findings; blood work for anemia, thyroid disease, diabetes, and renal or liver disease is within normal limits. Based on the history, physical, and lab testing, you make a diagnosis of mild to moderate depression. The patient accepts this assessment with equanimity but has fears about taking antidepressant drugs. "I don't think it's that bad," she tells you. "Isn't there something else we could try besides medication?"

What Would You Recommend?

The best-studied and best-evidenced treatments for depression are St. John's wort (Ernst 1998), exercise (Glemister 1996), and prayer or religious practice (Hertsgaard et al 1984, Koenig et al 1994). She tells you that since her job promotion, she has reduced her regular aerobic workouts from 4 times a week to maybe once. She is active in her

Table 17–1   ALTERNATIVE THERAPIES FOR ANXIETY

Therapy	Best Evidence*	Probably Useful†	Least Evidence‡
Herbals	Valerian (150–300 mg t.i.d.; 1–3 mL of tincture t.i.d.) Kava kava (45–70 mg kavalactones t.i.d.) St. John's wort (300 mg t.i.d.)	Chamomile Hops Oats (oat straw) Passion flower Peppermint Skullcap	Aromatherapy
Diet and Nutrition/ Lifestyle	High-potency multi-vitamin Exercise Eliminate caffeine, alcohol, tobacco, sugar	Flaxseed oil (1 T/d) Magnesium (200–300 mg t.i.d.) Niacinamide (500 mg q.i.d.) Phosphatidyl choline (4 g t.i.d.)	
Mind-Body Interventions	Biofeedback Cognitive-behavioral therapy Deep breathing Group therapy Hypnotherapy Meditation Relaxation response Spiritual healing	Dance Music Qi Gong Tai chi Yoga	
Pharmacological and Biological Treatments			
Bioelectromagnetic Therapies	Craniostimulation Energy healing		Electrosleep
Alternative Systems of Care	Acupuncture Ayurveda	*Homeopathic:* Gelsemium (30C t.i.d.–q.i.d.) Argentum nitricum (6C t.i.d.–q.i.d.) Ignatia amara (6C t.i.d.–q.i.d.)	
Hands-on Healing Techniques	Massage	Chiropractic	Craniosacral therapy

*Therapies with the highest degree of scientific support for efficacy and safety
†Therapies that are often helpful but that do not have the highest degree of supporting evidence for efficacy and safety
‡Therapies that may be useful but that have limited scientific evidence for efficacy and safety

Table 17–2 ALTERNATIVE THERAPIES FOR DEPRESSION

Therapy	Best Evidence*	Probably Useful†	Least Evidence‡
Herbals	St. John's wort (300 mg t.i.d., 0.3% hypericin)	Ginkgo biloba (80 mg t.i.d.) in elderly	St. John's wort and 5-HTP in combination Damiana Yohimbe Aromatherapy
Diet and Nutrition/ Lifestyle	Exercise Relaxation, stress reduction Thiamine (1–10 mg/d) Niacin (500–1000 mg b.i.d.) Pyridoxine (50–100 mg/d) Folic acid (800 µg/d) Vitamin B_{12} (800 µg/d) Vitamin C (500–1000 mg t.i.d.)	S-adenosyl-L-methionine (SAMe) (200 mg b.i.d.–400 mg q.i.d.) *Avoid in bipolar disorder.* 5-HT (hydroxytryptophan) (100–200 mg t.i.d.) Flaxseed oil (1 T/d) Iron replacement Vitamin E (200–400 IU/d)	Inositol Phenylalanine Phosphatidylserine Tyrosine Detect and treat food allergy Restrict caffeine and sugar
Mind-Body Interventions	Cognitive-behavioral therapy Spiritual approaches, prayer	Tai chi Qi Gong Hypnosis Meditation Biofeedback	
Pharmacological and Biological Treatments			DHEA Neural therapy
Bioelectromagnetic Therapies	Light therapy (for Seasonal Affective Disorder)	Magnetic brain stimulation Energy healing	
Alternative Systems of Care	Acupuncture	Ayurveda	*Homeopathy* (not commonly used except for postpartum depression): *Each t.i.d. for 2 wk:* Sepia (30C) Ignatia (30C) Pulsatilla (30C) Natrum muriatricum (30C)
Hands-on Healing Techniques	Massage	Craniosacral therapy	

*Therapies with the highest degree of scientific support for efficacy and safety
†Therapies that are often helpful but that do not have the highest degree of supporting evidence for efficacy and safety
‡Therapies that may be useful but that have limited scientific evidence for efficacy and safety

church as a youth leader and says that she derives personal strength from her faith and the church community. In fact, she feels a little guilty about being depressed and thinks that perhaps if her faith were stronger, she wouldn't feel this way. You reassure her that life stress can sometimes upset the neurotransmitters that affect mood. You recommend that she try to restart her aerobic workouts at least 3 times a week because of the benefits of endorphin release, personal satisfaction, and social contact that this activity can provide. In addition, you recommend the use of St. John's wort. You advise her to take 300 mg t.i.d. of the standardized 0.3% hypericin–containing extract and advise that it will take a few weeks, perhaps as long as a month, before she feels back to herself.

She returns in a month in a considerably brighter mood. You approvingly note that she has lost a couple of pounds, and she attributes the loss to the regular workouts. She feels the St. John's wort is also helping and notes no side effects from it except for some mild GI distress, which has resolved. Her interest in life and her regular activities has returned. Though her work situation is still quite demanding, she feels better able to handle it. You recommend a follow-up visit in 3 months to monitor her progress. At that time, she still is doing well, and you recommend trying to discontinue the St. John's wort. When she comes in for follow-up a couple of months later, your medical assistant smilingly brings in a lab slip with a positive urine HCG. Your happy patient is pregnant! As you order her prenatal labs and give her a pregnancy instructional packet and prenatal vitamins, you muse (to yourself) that apparently her interest in sex has returned!

Summary: Depression

In addition to St. John's wort and exercise, there is a long list of less well proven but often useful therapies for depression, which appears on Table 17–2. Before using them, be sure the patient is not psychotic or suicidal. Close follow-up is essential.

Chapter 18

Arthritis

With the aging of the population, we clinicians will encounter chronic problems such as arthritis even more often. The standard therapies can be quite useful in treating arthritis, but many have long-term risks and toxicities, and most of them do not fundamentally affect the disease process. (An exception is the conventional therapy for rheumatoid arthritis, which does have a marked effect on the progression of the autoimmune aspects of the disease and its clinical manifestations.) The conventional approach for osteoarthritis, for example, is to recommend weight loss, the use of acetaminophen in doses up to 4 g/day for pain control, and the use of nonsteroidal anti-inflammatory drugs (NSAIDs). Weight loss is always a challenge. Taking acetaminophen at this dosage entails some risk of liver toxicity and is merely masking symptoms. NSAIDs, though useful for inflammation, also have risks (especially in the elderly), such as gastrointestinal bleeding and potential effects on the CNS, heart, liver, and kidneys. Their cost, particularly for the newer agents, also can be a problem for elderly people on fixed incomes.

CURBSIDE CONSULT

Arthritis

- Weight loss, regular exercise, physical therapy, lifestyle modification
- Glucosamine, ginger, capsaicin, acetaminophen
- Flexibility exercises such as tai chi or yoga
- Vitamin C, avoiding the nightshade family of foods and other food allergens
- Acupuncture, magnet therapy
- Manual therapies: chiropractic, osteopathic, massage

Case Study: Osteoarthritis

John W. is a 62-year-old retired engineer who comes to your office complaining of knee pain. He used to play football and suffered some injuries to his knees while he was in college. He further injured his right medial meniscus on a ski trip to Colorado a few years back. John is about 25 pounds overweight, which he attributes to a rich diet and inactivity since retirement. Both his knees have bothered him for several years, but they seem to be getting worse lately. He has joint pain when he climbs stairs, if he tries to jog, and at night. Weather changes also make his knees hurt more. He has been taking 1 gram of acetaminophen up to 4 times a day with some relief, but when his knees are acting up, it doesn't help very much.

His past medical history is significant for hypertension, a bleeding peptic ulcer, a hiatal hernia with episodic gastroesophageal reflux, and an appendectomy. Physical exam shows a portly gentleman, about 5' 9" tall and 215 pounds, BP 138/88. Cardiovascular, lung, and abdominal exams are normal. A musculoskeletal exam shows Heberden's nodes on the distal phalanges of both hands, some tenderness at the right first metacarpophalangeal joint, and tenderness of both knee joint lines without effusion or ligament instability. You review lab tests and x-rays ordered at his last visit. The blood work showed normal renal function, blood glucose and electrolyte levels, negative antinuclear antibody (ANA) and rheumatoid factor (RF), and normal erythrocyte sedimentation rate (ESR) of 7 mm/hr. X-rays of both knees revealed eburnation, joint space narrowing, and osteophyte formation consistent with mild to moderate osteoarthritis.

What Is Your Plan of Care?

Because of John's history of GI problems, including bleeding, NSAIDs are not a good option for controlling his pain. It might be possible to use a combination of misoprostol and an NSAID to protect the stomach while helping with the arthritis pain, or to use the new COX-2 agents, which have fewer GI side effects. He is reluctant to take either agent, however, because of the severity of his prior bleeding ulcer episode, which required a blood transfusion of 3 units. You decide to explore other options. John's knee problems prevent him from being as active as he would like, and he attributes his weight problem to this inactivity. You recommend some non–weight-bearing exercise to help him lose weight, offering him such choices as swimming, cycling, water aerobics, and the gentle exercise of tai chi. You tell him about local classes and explain that these exercises not only will help him with weight loss but also will protect his knees from further damage by strengthening the muscles and ligaments in his legs and back. They also should have positive effects on his blood pressure, stress level, and general sense of well-being.

Next, you recommend that he start taking glucosamine sulfate, 1500 mg/day (Muller-Fassbender et al 1994, Rovati et al 1994). You advise him that it may take 4 to 6 weeks to see the full effect in reducing his knee complaints. You also tell him about the benefits of hot and cold applications and the use of capsaicin cream over the affected joints, and you tell him that continuing to wear the copper bracelet you see on his wrist might help.

At the next visit, he reports good improvement in his knee

symptoms and a reduction in his use of acetaminophen to a couple of times a day at most, mainly before a rainstorm or other weather change.

A year later he comes in for his annual physical and says his knees are doing fine. In addition to the therapies you prescribed, he read some of the material you gave him about arthritis and decided

Table 18–1 ALTERNATIVE THERAPIES FOR ARTHRITIS

Therapy	Best Evidence*	Probably Useful†	Least Evidence‡
Herbals	Boswellia (150–400 mg t.i.d.) Capsaicin (topically) Ginger concentrate (500 mg t.i.d.)	White willow (60–120 mg/d salicin; 1–2 mL t.i.d. tincture)	Aromatherapy Devil's claw Horsetail Sea cucumber Yucca
Diet and Nutrition/ Lifestyle	Weight loss Exercise Vitamin C (500–1000 mg t.i.d.) Vitamin E (400–800 IU/d)	Vitamin B_3 (niacinamide) (1–3 g/d); check liver enzymes Boron (6 mg/d) Omega-3 fatty acids (fish oil) (3 g/d)	Eliminate solanine from diet (found in nightshade plants: tomatoes, white potatoes, peppers, egg-plant, tobacco) Copper bracelet or supplement D-phenylalanine Pantothenic acid Zinc
Mind-Body Interventions	Cognitive-behavioral therapy	Biofeedback Qi Gong Relaxation Social support Tai chi Yoga	Guided imagery Meditation Music
Pharmacological and Biological Treatments	Glucosamine sulfate (500 mg t.i.d. or as single dose) S-adenosyl-L-methionine (SAMe) (400 mg t.i.d.)	Chondroitin sulfate (400 mg t.i.d.)	DMSO Chelation therapy Shark and bovine cartilage
Bioelectromagnetic Therapies		Static magnet therapy Pulsed electromag-netic fields Transcutaneous electrical nerve stimulation	

Table 18–1   ALTERNATIVE THERAPIES FOR ARTHRITIS *(Continued)*

Therapy	Best Evidence*	Probably Useful†	Least Evidence‡

Alternative Systems of Care	Acupuncture
	Acupressure
	Ayurveda
	Traditional Chinese medicine
			Homeopathic:
			Gout:
			  Nux vomica (6C)
			  Belladonna (6C)
			  Calcarea fluorica (6C)
			  Colchicum (6C)
			Osteoarthritis:
			  Rhus toxicodendron (6C t.i.d. for 2 wk)
			  Ledum (6C q.i.d. for 2 wk)
			  Belladonna (6C q.d. for 2 wk)
			  Apis millifica (6C t.i.d. for 2 wk)
			Rheumatoid arthritis:
			  Rhus toxicodendron (6C t.i.d. for 2 wk)
			  Bryonia (6C q.i.d. for 2 wk)
			  Ruta graveolens (6C q.i.d. for 2 wk)
			  Pulsatilla (30C t.i.d. for 2 wk)
			  Arnica ointments and gels

Hands-on Healing Techniques	Physical therapy	Massage Chiropractic Osteopathy	Craniosacral therapy Rolfing

*Therapies with the highest degree of scientific support for efficacy and safety
†Therapies that are often helpful but that do not have the highest degree of supporting evidence for efficacy and safety
‡Therapies that may be useful but that have limited scientific evidence for efficacy and safety.

to try acupuncture as well (Ernst 1997, Christensen et al 1992). A friend recommended a local acupuncturist who did a series of about 10 treatments, which John felt gave him even more improvement. The acupuncturist supported your recommendation about tai chi, and he is going to a weekly class at the YMCA and is practicing daily, besides using his exercycle. Although John's osteoarthritis is a chronic problem, this approach has benefited him in safe and reasonable ways. With regular exercise, weight loss, and supplementation, he may go for many years with minimal impairment of his lifestyle because of the arthritis and postpone or avoid the need for joint replacement surgery.

See Table 18–1 for a summary of alternative approaches to arthritis.

Chapter 19

Asthma

Asthma, a condition characterized by coughing, wheezing, mucus production, and shortness of breath, is on the rise, particularly in children. There are a number of theories as to why this is happening. The fact that children who are breast-fed less often develop asthma later in their life suggests that diet and exposure to foreign proteins in infancy may set up an immunological reaction that leads to asthma. Other factors such as increased environmental pollution, food allergy and additives, exposure to smoking and indoor pets, housecleaning practices, and even the whooping cough vaccine have all been associated with asthma. For many years, emotional stress has clearly been found to trigger asthma attacks. A psychospiritual interpretation even associates asthma with unexpressed grief. In the Ayurvedic tradition, asthma is related to digestive problems, adding weight to the argument that diet, food allergy, and certain foods can contribute to asthma.

Asthma is broadly categorized as extrinsic asthma, due to allergy, and intrinsic asthma, due to other factors such as stress, exercise, and infection. One of my first steps in any asthma treatment program is to reduce exposure to likely or known allergens. This approach should be tried for every asthmatic patient but must be customized to each individual. Highly potent sensitizers for allergic reactions include animal danders, proteins in saliva on pet hair, and dust mite proteins. Thus, I recommend that my patients with asthma keep pets, especially cats, outdoors. If animal lovers protest, I urge that they at least keep the animals out of the

CURBSIDE CONSULT

Asthma

- Maximal benefits of standard therapy such as inhalers; regular use of peak flow meter for self-monitoring; influenza and pneumonia immunizations
- Environmental control measures to minimize exposure to allergens, smoke, and pollution
- Detection and elimination of food allergies
- Regular physical activity, deep-breathing exercises
- Supplements such as vitamins B_6, C, and E, beta carotene, magnesium
- Herbals such as quercetin, licorice
- Onions and garlic in diet

bedroom so that allergen exposure is reduced for several hours a night. Dust mites occur in ordinary household dust and can be reduced (again focusing on the bedroom areas) by regular mopping or vacuuming, removing carpeting and rugs from the bedroom, or applying a mild chemical treatment to the carpets. Covering mattresses and pillows with plastic, eliminating feather pillows, and removing large collections of dust-trapping stuffed toys are other environmental measures to reduce asthma. Air-conditioning may help some asthmatics by filtering out airborne pollens, especially during the spring and summer allergy season.

Food allergy may be a factor, so I attempt to reduce dairy, wheat, and food additives in the diets of children with recurrent allergy manifestations and asthma. A systematic rotation diet, which eliminates suspected offending foods one by one, may be the only practical way to determine which foods are triggering an allergic reaction. Reducing dairy, wheat, or additives reduces mucus formation and allergic reactions in some patients. Cutting sugar also seems to help some children to produce less mucus, which tenaciously plugs the respiratory tree and exacerbates asthma. Reducing salt intake also may reduce bronchial hyperreactivity. Smokers in the household need to move outside (permanently?) to smoke, though the smoke on their clothing and exhalation when they return indoors can still create respiratory problems, especially for smaller children.

The overall concept here is to raise the allergic threshold. The goal is to reduce the body's exposure to allergens and irritants for even parts of the day or night. Then the triggering factors for an asthmatic attack are less likely to precipitate attacks as frequently and intensely. This approach can also help patients with allergic rhinitis.

It is important to recognize that asthma can be a life-threatening disease. Many advances in pharmacotherapy have reduced the death toll, and these proven and effective prescriptions should not be disregarded in favor of solely naturalistic approaches, except perhaps in milder cases. The standard of care includes the use of home nebulizers, cromolyn, steroid and beta-agonist metered-dose inhalers, and newer agents such as leukotriene antagonists. Immunizations for influenza and pneumonia also are indicated and are helpful in selected populations.

Every chronic asthmatic needs to have a peak flow meter at home. This simple hand-held device allows day-to-day monitoring of the forced expiratory peak flow. A reduction of 15% of the flow from the usual baseline signals the onset of an exacerbation of asthma, even in the absence of worsening clinical signs and symptoms. This can alert the patient or parent that an increased dosage of the maintenance therapy, rescue therapy such as a nebulizer, or a call to the health care provider is needed. Such a monitoring program can spare many unnecessary ER visits and hospitalizations.

For moderate to severe asthmatics, an integrative approach necessarily will involve medications. Ancillary and environmental measures, however, can lessen the frequency and severity of attacks, reduce the need for and expense of medications, and improve the quality of life for the asthmatic child or adult. Let's look at such an integrated approach in a case study.

Case Study: Asthma

His mother brings Terrell D., a 10-year-old African-American boy, into your office for a checkup of his asthma. He was in the ER Saturday night for a flare-up that did not resolve with the use of a metered-dose inhaler with a spacer device or his home nebulizer, which administered a mixture of saline and albuterol. His mother is concerned because Terrell's asthma seems to be getting worse with age, rather than better, as she had been told it would do by a well-meaning family member. Additionally, the ER doctor, having seen Terrell several times for similar episodes, has recommended that he see an allergist or pediatric asthma specialist to start on inhaled steroids. Mrs. D. is upset and uncomfortable with the idea of inhaled steroids for Terrell because she is concerned about potential effects on growth and development and other side effects she has read about.

What Questions Would You Ask?

Certainly, you would like to gather as complete a history as possible about Terrell's asthma, including age of onset, precipitating factors, hospitalizations, medication use, any other medical problems, presence of smokers in the house, any social problems, and family history. Mrs D. reports that Terrell was hospitalized with bronchiolitis a couple of times in his first year of life, and she was told that he had asthma when he was about 2 years old. He has been using beta-agonists off and on in both liquid and inhaled form since early childhood. Changes in the weather, high pollen counts, colds, and smoke exposure all seem to bring on the attacks. He was hospitalized with pneumonia when he was 5 years old and has had several admissions in the past for flare-ups of asthma that have not responded to ER treatment. He has had eczema but no other medical problems. He is an average student and is a little small for his age. His father, who does not live with him, is a two-pack-a-day smoker. He sometimes visits on the weekends and has done so since the divorce a couple of years ago. There are several pets in the home: a cockatiel who stays in his cage, two cats who wander the house at will, and a Labrador retriever who mostly stays outside. Terrell's diet is what

Mrs. D. considers normal, though he seems to drink a lot of milk and soft drinks. Several of Terrell's cousins, an aunt, and his sister have asthma or hay fever, though not as bad as his.

What Do You Expect to Find on Physical Examination?

Terrell is a smallish 10-year-old, in the 10th percentile for height and weight. He appears comfortable today, though he seems apprehensive as you examine him. His tympanic membranes are clear with a normal light reflex, his nasal turbinates are covered with pale to blue mucosal tissue, and he has a watery nasal discharge. He has large tonsils and anterior cervical adenopathy. His lungs are clear today except for a slightly prolonged expiration phase. His heart sounds are normal, but a grade II systolic murmur is noted. His chest wall is thin and somewhat bony, but he is not using accessory muscles for respiration.

What Do You Recommend?

It seems that Terrell's asthma and accompanying allergic rhinitis have both intrinsic and extrinsic components. His is a long-standing condition with a clear-cut genetic tendency. Environmental factors also are likely to play a role. You decide to try a multipronged approach.

Noting Terrell's anxiety, you inquire about the yoga class you recommended to Mrs. D. some months back to help her manage her own stress. She reports enjoying it, and you recommend teaching Terrell some of the deep abdominal, diaphragmatic breathing that she has learned. You tell her that this will help him to relax and also will improve his lung capacity when he is having breathing problems. You cite some studies showing that asthmatics attending yoga classes have improved outcomes, which have been attributed to improved breathing mechanics, effects on endogenous glucocorticoid production, and changes in autonomic tone (Gore 1982). Mrs. D. needs no convincing and agrees to teach Terrell the breathing exercises.

Next you inquire about allergens and find that the cats sleep in Terrell's bedroom and that he has a feather pillow, but that the rug and stuffed toys were removed some time ago on the recommendation of the allergist. After some resistance, Mrs. D. agrees to keep the cats out of Terrell's bedroom and to replace the allergenic feather pillow.

You ask about Terrell's use of the peak flow meter you provided some time back. They admit that they haven't used it regularly, so you patiently explain the benefits and have your nurse demonstrate its use.

At this point, you may have made as much progress as you can in a single visit. At the next visit, in 2 weeks, however, you suggest some nutritional supplements that may be helpful, including vitamins B_6 (Collipp 1975), C (Bucca 1990), and E (Panganamala et al 1982), magnesium (Haury 1940 and Skobeloff 1989), and quercetin. Mrs. D., an avid fan of health food store products, agrees readily to using these supplements, which she has read about in *Prevention* magazine. She is glad you suggested them but was reluctant to ask you about them, fearing you might think she didn't know what she was talking about.

You ask if Terrell likes garlic and onions, which can help clear bronchial secretions (Dorsch 1985 and Vanderhoek 1980), and recommend increasing the use of those while decreasing his intake of dairy products and soft drinks. You remind Mrs. D. that calcium is essential to healthy, growing bones but is available from other foods besides dairy products, such as sardines, salmon, and green leafy vegetables. Sunshine will help Terrell convert vitamin D so that the calcium can be used.

Mrs. D. reports that she has been keeping the cats out of the bedroom, that she has cleaned the floor more regularly to minimize dust mites, and that she has made her ex-husband smoke outdoors when he visits. Terrell seems to like the yoga breathing exercises and seems more relaxed. He even is doing better at school.

At his next visit, in a couple of months, you give him a flu shot and refill his inhaler and nebulizer medications. You note with pleasure that his use of the inhalers has gone down, and Mrs. D. reports that he only needed the nebulizer once, after his father took him out to the amusement park and smoked cigarettes in the car on the way there and back. The smoke brought on an attack, and they found that Terrell's peak flow had dropped almost 20%. The nebulizer helped, however, and coupling that with some deep breathing, Terrell was able to avoid going to the ER. He is taking the supplements and is tolerating them well. Mrs. D. asks if you would suggest anything else, and you add oral vitamin B_{12}, 1000 µg daily (Simon 1951), and licorice (not the candy, but rather 250-mg capsules of the dry powdered extract, *Glycyrrhiza glabra*, 3 times/day). You explain that B_{12} reduces sulfite-related reactions and licorice is an anti-inflammatory and expectorant. Terrell is using the peak flow meter regularly and he and his mother are happy to see the daily values creeping gradually to the normal range for his size and age.

You don't see him again until spring, when he comes in for a sports physical. They report that he had a good winter, with only one visit to the ER for an asthma attack, much better than the winter before. In fact, Terrell wants to join the cross-country team. You examine him and clear him for this sport, explaining the benefits of running to him and his mother. You also advise that during cold weather, when the pollen count is high, or prior to a heavy workout, he may need to increase the dose of his inhaler before exercise. He also may need to take some additional quercetin, or even add an antihistamine.

Before leaving, Terrell smiles and gives you a "high five."

Table 19–1 ALTERNATIVE THERAPIES FOR ASTHMA

Therapy	Best Evidence*	Probably Useful†	Least Evidence‡
Herbals	*Atropa belladonna* Capsaicin *Ephedra sinensis* (12.5–25 mg t.i.d.) Quercetin (400 mg a.c. t.i.d.) *Glycyrrhiza glabra* (1–2 g t.i.d. pow- dered root; 2–4 mL t.i.d. extract; 250–500 mg dry powdered extract t.i.d.) Grape seed extract (50–100 mg t.i.d.) Guaiac wood (guafe- nisin 600 mg b.i.d.)	*Gingko biloba* (60 mg b.i.d.) *Tylophora asth- matica* (200 mg b.i.d.)	*Coleus forskohli* (50 mg t.i.d.) *Lobelia inflata* Coltsfoot (poten- tially toxic)
Diet and Nutrition/ Lifestyle	Avoid sulfites, aspi- rin, tartrazine, biogenic amines Environmental con- trol Vitamin C (10– 30 mg/kg/d in divided doses)	Carotenes (25,000– 50,000 IU/d) Essential fatty acids (fish oils, omega-3 fatty acids) Magnesium (200– 400 mg t.i.d.) Vitamin E (200– 400 IU/d) Zinc (15–30 mg/d) Food allergy identifi- cation & avoid- ance (milk, egg, wheat) Green tea (*Camellia sinensis*) Onions, garlic Reduced sodium intake	Treat hypochlor- hydria Probiotics Selenium (200 µg/d) Vitamin B_6 (if on theophylline: 25–50 mg b.i.d.) Vitamin B_{12} (sulfite- sensitive children: 1000 µg/d or IM weekly)
Mind-Body Interventions		Biofeedback Hypnosis Yoga breathing tech- niques	Treat depression Stress management
Pharmacological and Biological Treatments			Anti-*Candida* diet DHEA

Table 19–1   ALTERNATIVE THERAPIES FOR ASTHMA *(Continued)*

Therapy	Best Evidence*	Probably Useful†	Least Evidence‡
Bioelectromagnetic Therapies			Electrical stimulation
Alternative Systems of Care		Acupuncture African herbs Ayurvedic herbals Chinese herbals Homeopathy	
Hands-on Healing Techniques	Massage		Chiropractic Osteopathy

*Therapies with the highest degree of scientific support for efficacy and safety
†Therapies that are often helpful but that do not have the highest degree of supporting evidence for efficacy and safety
‡Therapies that may be useful but that have limited scientific evidence for efficacy and safety

Case Summary

As this case illustrates, the integrative treatment of asthma is a multifactorial program. Environmental measures, dietary intervention, supplements, herbs, and mind-body approaches such as deep breathing exercises all may be used to maximize the response to therapy. Immunizations for influenza and possibly pneumonia are helpful. Regular use of the peak flow meter to monitor progress also empowers patients to control and take responsibility for their asthma. They become your treatment partners by using the peak flow information to become aware of times when medication may need to be adjusted. Encouraging asthmatics, particularly children, to participate as fully as possible in sports and other activities builds self-esteem and confidence and improves their overall pulmonary conditioning.

Table 19–1 summarizes alternative approaches to asthma.

Chapter

20 *Cancer*

Cancer is no more a disease of cells than a traffic jam is a disease of automobiles. Both traffic jams and cancer are problems of the ecology—of an entire organism, in the case of the city, of the whole person, in the case of cancer.

—R. D. Smithers, former president of the British Cancer Council

Along with cardiovascular disease, cancer is a leading cause of death in our society. Despite legions of researchers, countless publications in both clinical and basic science, billions of research dollars, and decades of study, the treatment of most cancers—particularly common ones such as lung, breast, and colon cancer—remains unsatisfactory. Moreover, according to Michael Lerner, noted authority on alternative medicine and cancer, "There is no cure for cancer among any of the alternative therapies" (Lerner 1994).

With that comment, you might ask why this book includes a chapter on integrative approaches to cancer. One reason is that you as a health care professional should be familiar with the most common alternative therapies employed by patients. When frightened and desperate, patients may succumb to any type of charlatanism or hope for cure, no matter how poorly supported by evidence. Your role is to advise and support them while steering them away from unproved, expensive, or dangerous therapies or any therapy that delays proven treatment or is contraindicated. Another important reason to discuss alternative approaches is that some of them do offer promise of benefit, as documented by scientific studies. Though they may not *cure* cancer, they are useful in the adjunctive support of cancer patients, im-

CURBSIDE CONSULT

Cancer

- Mind-body approaches, including imagery and visualization, relaxation, group support
- Adequate management of depression, anxiety, and pain
- Spiritual practice, including prayer, church attendance, meditation
- Plant-based diet high in antioxidants and fiber, with supplemental vitamins C and E, selenium, beta carotene, therapeutic mushrooms such as shiitake and maitake, and possibly soy
- Physical approaches including regular moderate exercise, yoga, or tai chi; massage, therapeutic touch

proving the quality of their lives or even prolonging them. In this chapter, I will list the best-studied therapies and discuss an approach to the care of the cancer patient that is holistic, compassionate, and beneficial.

PREVENTION FIRST

Later parts of this chapter will detail many alternative approaches that are applicable to cancer care. The truly wise clinician, however, encourages patients to follow the kind of lifestyle that will prevent cancer in the first place. Many of these, such as avoiding smoking and excess alcohol, are obvious, but there is evidence that we need to teach our patients other types of interventions (Table 20–1). Clearly certain foods help prevent cancer: the carotenoids, cruciferous vegetables such as broccoli, dark-green leafy vegetables, and, generally, high-fiber and whole-grain cereal diets are high on the list. Other foods that have been shown to be helpful in prevention include tea, legumes, soy, nuts, fruits, whole-grain barley, yogurt, and garlic. Antioxidants from unprocessed foods, spices, and herbs show greater benefit than extracted micronutrients. Chlorinated water may be associated with colon cancer, and pickled, smoked, or overcooked meats may all contribute to cancer and are best avoided (Wirth 1999).

Physical activity reduces several types of cancer. Aspirin can reduce colon cancer. Many mind-body therapies also have been associated with cancer prevention.

CANCER CARE

Mind-Body Interventions: A Mainstay

Over the years, I have evolved an approach for cancer patients that is individualized but also includes some basic, general interventions. Although supplements, diet, herbs, and other such therapies can be useful adjuncts in the care of the cancer patient, I center my initial recommendations on a mind-body approach. The mainstays of this approach, supported by years of research, are listed in Table 20–2.

The diagnosis and treatment of cancer are highly stressful life events. However, research by Simonton and others (1978) found that a majority of their cancer patients had suffered some major life stressor within the 18 months *preceding the diagnosis of their cancer.* Because stress has been shown to reduce immunocompetence (Amkraut 1975), I encourage all of my cancer patients to regularly practice a mind-body

Table 20–1   NUTRITIONAL AND LIFESTYLE FACTORS INFLUENCING THE RISK OF VARIOUS TYPES OF CANCER

Type of Cancer	Vegetables	Fruits	Carotenoids in Food	Vit. C in Food	Fats	Meat	Salt & Salting	Alcohol	Obesity	Physical Activity	Smoking Tobacco
Mouth & pharynx	⇓⇓⇓	⇓⇓⇓		⇓				⇑⇑⇑⇑			⇑⇑⇑⇑
Nasopharynx							⇑⇑⇑⇑‡				⇑⇑⇑
Larynx	⇓⇓	⇓⇓		⇓				⇑⇑⇑⇑			⇑⇑⇑⇑
Esophagus	⇓⇓⇓	⇓⇓⇓	⇓	⇓				⇑⇑⇑⇑			⇑⇑⇑⇑
Lung	⇓⇓⇓	⇓⇓⇓	⇓⇓	⇓	⇑⇑*			⇑		⇓	⇑⇑⇑⇑
Stomach	⇓⇓⇓	⇓⇓⇓	⇓	⇓⇓⇓			⇑⇑⇑				
Pancreas	⇓⇓	⇓⇓		⇓		⇑					⇑⇑⇑⇑
Liver	⇓							⇑⇑⇑⇑			

Colon, rectum	⇓⇓⇓		⇒		⇑*		⇑⇑	⇑	⇑	⇓⇓⇓	⇐
Breast	⇓⇓	⇒⇒	⇒		⇑*	⇑	⇑⇑	⇑	⇑	⇒	⇐⇐⇐
Endometrium	⇒	⇒	⇒		⇑†	⇐	⇐	⇐⇐⇐			
Cervix	⇒	⇒	⇒	⇒							⇐⇐⇐⇐
Kidney	⇒	⇒				⇐	⇐⇐	⇐⇐			⇐
Bladder	⇓⇓	⇒⇒	⇒⇒								⇐⇐⇐⇐

⇓⇓⇓ = Decreases risk, convincing evidence
⇓⇓ = Decreases risk, probable
⇓ = Decreases risk, possible
⇑⇑⇑ = Increases risk, convincing evidence
⇑⇑ = Increases risk, probable
⇑ = Increases risk, possible
Source: American Institute for Cancer Research

*Both total fat and saturated or animal fat
†Saturated or animal fat only
‡Salted fish

Table 20–2 ALTERNATIVE APPROACHES TO CANCER PREVENTION

Therapy	Best Evidence*	Probably Useful†	Least Evidence‡
Herbals	Antioxidant herbs: hypericum, eleutherococcus, rhodiola, leonurus, aralia, valeriana, echinopanax, schisandara, panax, ginseng	Astragalus membranaceus Ginseng	Garlic
Diet and Nutrition/ Lifestyle	Antioxidants in unprocessed foods, e.g., fruits, vegetables Glutathione, lipoic acid, dietary omega-3 fatty acids Low-fat, high-vegetable, high-fiber diet Abstention from tobacco, excess alcohol Selenium	Vegetarian diet, cruciferous and green leafy vegetables, fruit, nuts, legumes, green tea, garlic (stomach cancer), cumin, rosemary (breast cancer), turmeric, saffron, yogurt, tofu Avoid chlorinated water, pickled or smoked foods, overcooked food like beef or pork Moderate exercise Soy	
Mind-Body Interventions		Getting rid of anger, negative emotions Stress management Treatment of depression, feelings of helplessness, hopelessness Encouraging a fighting spirit Imagery, biofeedback, hypnosis, meditation Yoga, Qi Gong Spiritual approaches, prayer, faith healing	

*Therapies with the highest degree of scientific support for efficacy and safety
†Therapies that are often helpful but that do not have the highest degree of supporting evidence for efficacy and safety
‡Therapies that may be useful but that have limited scientific evidence for efficacy and safety

relaxation technique such as meditation, prayer, deep breathing, yoga, tai chi, or another method of their choosing. I also recommend coupling active imagery with these relaxation techniques. This imagery is the positive visualization of the successful response of the body in handling the cancer and in receiving the maximum amount of benefit from treatment. Depression and anxiety are addressed and managed with mind-body approaches, counseling, herbs, or medication (see Chap. 17). Cancer support groups have been shown to improve the longevity of women with breast cancer (Spiegel et al 1989), so I recommend enrollment in one of these as soon as is practical.

I also recommend some books, writing out their titles on my prescription pad, a symbolic and powerful method of emphasizing my support of them as a real part of the treatment, just as any prescription would be. I particularly suggest the works of O. Carl Simonton, such as *Getting Well Again* (1978). Simonton is a radiation oncologist who has championed the use of imagery and relaxation in cancer. Of course, another well-known author is Bernie Siegel, a surgeon who has written a number of excellent books on this topic, starting with *Love, Medicine, and Miracles* (1986). Dr. Siegel has investigated the lives of many cancer patients in an attempt to discover the underlying factors differentiating those who do well from those who do not. I prescribe these readings with the intent of encouraging patients to look to the positive things they can think and do in the face of this diagnosis and of supporting them during their treatment. I do not diminish the value of any other conventional therapy or alternative therapy they may choose, unless I believe it will be unnecessary or harmful, but I emphasize the things they can take an active part in doing.

The Vital Quartet

The approach I take is supported by the work of Michael Lerner (1999), who, after reviewing the entire range of alternative cancer therapies, concludes that a "vital quartet" of approaches should be applied in every case. These are:

1. Spiritual
2. Psychological
3. Nutritional
4. Physical

Whether someone follows a strictly conventional therapy program or pursues an alternative treatment method, these four elements will help support them. I agree with Lerner's contention that although we hope to cure our patients' cancer, improving and maintaining function, controlling pain, and helping patients find healing in their illnesses are high priorities.

The spiritual dimension can involve prayer, faith healing, helping patients to find meaning, and encouraging them to connect or reconnect with religious or community practices and find a deeper connection with their personal spirituality.

The psychological dimension incorporates psychoneuroimmunology, psycho-oncology (coping skills for cancer patients), stress reduction and stress management, social and group support, imagery, and encouraging healthy personality adaptations such as a "fighting spirit" or sometimes even denial.

Nutritional support during cancer treatment often takes the form of vegetarian-type diets, which are rich in antioxidants and put less stress on the digestive system than high-fat or even high-protein diets. Other nutritional approaches include unconventional diets like the Block, Livingston-Wheeler, Gerson, or Hoxsey diets; wheat-grass therapy; and macrobiotics. Supplementation with micronutrients such as selenium and certain vitamins is also common. For a detailed discussion of these nutritional approaches, see Michael Lerner's book *Choices in Healing* (1994). The conventional medical practice of oncology has been reluctant to recognize the benefits of nutritional approaches to cancer; likewise, there is a gap between practitioners of some diet therapies for cancer and mainstream professionals.

The physical dimension involves pain relief and relaxation, as well as maintaining functional status through regular exercise, massage, Therapeutic Touch, and even chiropractic; manipulation may be safely done on those with cancer by skilled practitioners, although the risk of pathological fractures must always be kept foremost in mind.

Advising Patients with Cancer

Consider integrating some of the therapies in Table 20–3 into your patient's treatment plan. Above all, offer hope—if not of cure, then at least of care and healing. Avoid pronouncements such as, "You have X months to live" or, worse yet, "I give you X weeks, months, years. . ." as if the matter of life and death were really in your hands. Many patients take these prognoses, even when framed as statistical averages, as a death sentence and give up hope. On the other hand, imparting some sense of the inevitability of the impending death is necessary when the time grows short, so that the family can get financial affairs in order, contact other family members, and start a grieving process. To start the grieving process too soon, however, is a danger. If the patient doesn't die "on schedule," the family is left with the ambivalent feelings of already having grieved and dealt with their loss while the patient is still alive and with them, requiring their continued support and attention. This can be draining and exhausting, although an excellent hospice team will ameliorate it (see "The Role of Hospice"). In any case, communicating about the prognosis is a delicate and critically important task. A practitioner who knows the patient and family well and is trusted and respected by them is in the best position to do it well.

Table 20–3 ALTERNATIVE THERAPIES FOR CANCER TREATMENT

Therapy	Best Evidence*	Probably Useful†	Least Evidence‡
Herbals		Mistletoe (bladder) Yew (paclitaxel)(breast) Hoxsey Astragalus membranaceus Polysaccharide krestin Chlorella PC SPES Capsaicin	Chaparral (toxic) Pau d'arco Essiac tea Evening primrose oil
Diet and Nutrition/ Lifestyle		Mushrooms: maitake, shii-take (colon), enokitake	Whole grain barley Macrobiotic diet Gerson diet Hippocrates wheat-grass diet Livingston Wheeler Kelley-Gonzalez nutritional programs Vitamins A, C, E (contro-versial)
Mind-Body Interven-tions		Getting rid of anger, nega-tive emotions Support groups (breast) Group therapy (melanoma) Stress management Treatment of depression, feelings of helplessness, hopelessness Encouraging a fighting spirit Imagery, biofeedback, hyp-nosis, meditation Yoga, Qi Gong Spiritual approaches, prayer, faith healing	Intuitive, psychic approaches
Pharmaco-logical and Biological Treat-ments			Antineoplastins (brain) Shark cartilage Bovine tracheal cartilage Hydrazine (cachexia, lung) Ozone therapy, hydrogen peroxide Livingston therapy Immunoaugmentive therapies Melatonin

(Continued)

Table 20–3　ALTERNATIVE THERAPIES FOR CANCER TREATMENT *(Continued)*

Therapy	Best Evidence*	Probably Useful†	Least Evidence‡
Bioelectro-magnetic Therapies			Nordenstrom electrical stimulation Therapeutic Touch
Alternative Systems of Care		Acupuncture, acupressure, moxibustion for relief of pain, nausea, side effects of cancer treatment	Chinese herbal remedies Ayurveda *Homeopathy:* Gelsemium (anxiety: 6C 2–3×) Ipecac (nausea: 30C 3–4× q 15–30 min) Nux vomica (nausea/vomiting: 6C t.i.d.–q.i.d. for 1–2 d) Cadmium Sulfuricum (vomiting, exhaustion: 30C t.i.d. for 1–2 d)
Hands-on Healing Techniques		Massage and gentle manipulation for pain control, immunostimulation, relaxation	Laying on of hands

*Therapies with the highest degree of scientific support for efficacy and safety
†Therapies that are often helpful but that do not have the highest degree of supporting evidence for efficacy and safety
‡Therapies that may be useful but that have limited scientific evidence for efficacy and safety

When a cancer patient asks me about prognosis, I usually say something to this effect: "No one can tell you exactly how long you will live. That is in the hands of a Higher Power. Your will to live, your personal strength, and your family support are all important factors in the treatment of this cancer. Let's work together on a treatment plan for you. There are things I think you can do to improve the quality and the quantity of your life from here on. These are . . . ."

Case Study: Breast Cancer

Diana L. is a 55-year-old professor of business in a local graduate school. A routine mammogram showed several abnormal calcifications in her right breast, and stereotactic needle biopsy revealed that these suspicious calcifications were a result of an intraductal cell carcinoma.

THE ROLE OF HOSPICE

One word of advice. Be willing to stop. Yes, I said *stop*. Sometimes the most compassionate and competent care is to advise the patient when a therapy, be it conventional or alternative, is no longer working. This has to be done carefully so that patients do not misperceive that you are abandoning them. But when the side effects, cost, and risks outweigh the marginal benefit of a therapy, it is often incumbent on the primary care practitioner to recommend stopping the treatment. In my experience, some oncologists tend to persist to the end with their therapies and will often continue even if the patients themselves do not want to or are exhausted from the side effects. You need to be brave and wise and show good judgment in terminating further useless therapy.

It is only at this point that the considerable services of the hospice movement can be employed to manage the palliative care. Hospice care is an interdisciplinary team approach that supports patients and their families, usually at home, during the dying process of a terminal disease. Visiting nurses, social workers, counselors, and others are involved in helping to keep patients comfortable. They provide medications, medical supplies, nutritional advice, and monitoring in the comfort of patients' own homes, although most hospices have some dedicated beds in the hospital for patients who must be out of the home.

Use hospice treatment early, rather than late, in terminal cases. Hospice experts report that nationally the average hospice involvement is about 2 weeks. This is a major professional mistake. The use of hospice in the last *several months* of a terminal patient's care is enormously beneficial to the quality of palliative care, pain control, and the emotional and spiritual issues facing the patient and family during this difficult time. Your role as a primary care provider is to involve hospice early, stay involved yourself, and make the best efforts you can to prolong living but not to prolong dying.

Her medical history is significant only for migraine headaches. She has been married twice but never had children, saying that she never really had time for a family. She exercises 3 or 4 times a week in an aerobics class or at home, has never smoked, and gave up alcohol several years ago because it seemed to aggravate her headaches. Her diet is low in fat, and though she is not a vegetarian, she eats little red meat and has either fish or chicken only about 3 times a week. In addition to her migraine medications, sumatriptan and butalbital, she has been receiving hormone replacement therapy with estrogen and progesterone since her menopause 6 years before. Her sister and an aunt have had breast cancer. Her review of systems is entirely normal and she is feeling well, with no complaints other than some stress about impending surgery and treatment for her malignancy.

The physical exam shows a well-developed African-American female looking younger than her stated age. Her vital signs are normal, with a BP of 120/80, pulse 70, temperature of 37°C, weight 130 pounds, and height 5′ 4″. HEENT exam is normal. Her lungs are clear and her heart sounds are normal. She has rather large breasts for her size but no palpable masses, nipple discharge, skin changes, or axillary adenopathy. There is a healing puncture site in the outer quadrant of the right breast where the needle biopsy was done. The rest of the exam is unremarkable.

At this time, Diana is asking for a referral to a surgeon and an oncologist. Because she has read up on her condition, she thinks a modified radical mastectomy may be done and asks you about the options for reconstructive surgery and whom you would recommend to perform it. In the meantime, while she is preparing for surgery, she strongly desires to engage in several alternative approaches and wants to discuss them with you. Her husband is in the waiting room, and you invite both of them into your office for a consultation.

Diana is enthusiastic about using mind-body therapies. She adopts a personal plan that includes several modalities. She practices daily meditation and prayer. A colleague recommends a hypnotist, who prepares a tape that includes Diana's choice of music to assist in relaxation and imagery. She also participates in a breast cancer support group. There, women all across the breast cancer spectrum, from early diagnosis to long-term cure to recurrence, are able to encourage Diana and support her while sharing their stories and what they have experienced and learned.

An equally important aspect of creating confidence and reducing anxiety for her was in her choice of specialty physicians. She scheduled visits with several surgeons, oncologists, and even the anesthesiologists at two major medical centers to get acquainted with them and to make sure she felt comfortable with their attitudes as well as their skills and knowledge. Ultimately, she chose her physicians based on their willingness to answer her questions and provide the latest and best surgical techniques for this kind of cancer, including reconstructive surgery, and on her intuitive sense of whether she resonated with them emotionally.

Having reviewed the literature on nutritional support, Diana maintained her highly healthful semi-vegetarian diet. She added more fruit and vegetable juices, soy shakes, green tea, and supplemental vitamins C and E, beta carotene, and selenium, as well as some Chinese herbs and mushrooms prescribed by a traditional Chinese medical practitioner.

She also received acupuncture for general immune support, improved tissue healing, and pain reduction. The Chinese practitioner also gave her some Qi Gong exercises. Diana's sister, a nurse, recommended some friends who applied Therapeutic Touch treatments over several sessions.

After her surgery, a modified radical mastectomy with reconstruction, she took a lengthy time away from work to recuperate physically, emotionally, and spiritually. During that time, she continued many of the preoperative interventions, including the support group, dietary changes, Qi Gong, prayer, and meditation.

She recently came in for an annual well-woman exam. She is back to work and in the full swing of her life. Although she realizes that after only 1 year she is not yet in the clear, the cancer has been, as for many people, a major transformative event in her personal life, marriage, and work. Many patients with cancer eventually see it as having helped them make needed changes in their lives, emotionally and spiritually as well as physically. "I just wish I didn't need to get cancer to reach these realizations," Diana says, recounting past resentments toward her mother and husband that she had been carrying, which she needed to let go as part of her healing journey.

Case Summary and Comments

Does an integrative approach work? One thing that struck me, as it might have you, about this case was the sheer number of interventions Diana chose as part of an integrative plan of care. This makes the scientific study of a holistic and integrative approach to cancer care difficult. If Diana survives beyond the 5-year mark that is considered a benchmark for breast cancer cure, which of the interventions she tried contributed to a positive outcome? Was it an excellent surgical technique, some component of her diet, the improved immunocompetence of her cells related to the mind-body interventions, prayer, or some other factor? From her point of view, of course, none of this matters. What matters to her and her family is that she has survived and grown from the experience. The clinical scientist, though, finds this multiplicity of interventions and therapies messy to study, and indeed they are, requiring a whole-science approach that may use nonlinear dynamic modeling and other advanced research and statistical methodologies.

Though the combination of standard therapy with nutritional, emotional, mind-body, herbal, and other approaches may seem like a lot of work and a major change in lifestyle, such a combination is not unusual. Cancer has a way of getting folks' attention, and the introduction of a variety of approaches over a few weeks or months is a healthful way of coping with the shock of this diagnosis. The more involved patients become in making positive, personal choices and changes in their lives as a result of the cancer, the more quality of life they experience, whether the cancer is cured, in remission, or recurrent. Several studies (Greer et al 1982, Bahnson 1980, Fawzy et al 1993) have found that the involved cancer survivor often does better in all realms—body, mind, and spirit—than the dejected or passive patient who simply does what the therapist, doctor, or specialist tells them to do, with little or no involvement of their own. Bernie Siegel's work (1986, 1993) also emphasizes that what he calls "the exceptional cancer patient" and "survivor" is often very deeply involved, emotionally and spiritually, in the process of recovering from cancer.

▬▬▬ CONCLUSION

What I have found is that cancer patients, more than anything, want to be listened to, to have their fears addressed, to be empowered by having choices, and above all, not to be abandoned by their health-care team when hope of a physical cure seems to be gone. They seek reassurance that you will be with them, control their pain, help them through their therapies, and be a trusted guide and friend when they have questions. Both professionally and personally, I have grown more in the care of terminal cancer patients than in any other area of my practice. I have worked closely with patients in their final stages, with the hospice team (see box), and with the family, making house calls, managing pain, providing emotional and spiritual support, and attending the last rites and funerals. Several times I have been present at the exact moment of their death and have found it to be a deeply profound moment in the development of my caring, compassion, and humanity.

When conventional cancer therapy has not had the desired outcome, we often face desperate patients and families, who are afraid and are willing to grasp at straws and spend their money unnecessarily on therapies that are promised as cures. Without doubt, the area of alternative cancer therapies is large and heterogeneous, and the evidence for many therapies is marginal. Your role as an integrative practitioner is to review the evidence of what is truly helpful in the alternative realm and what is not. Such therapies as mind-body approaches and nutritional changes offer safe and low-cost opportunities for adjunctive support. Many other therapies may require huge investments of patients' time, money, and failing reserves with little proof of efficacy. As you advise patients with cancer, be sure to include your preferences as well as theirs in the final prescription. Be willing to admit that you might not know much about some therapies, but share what you do know and encourage patients to read and study to find what is best for them. In the meanwhile, develop for yourself a core approach that involves a blend of effective mind-body, nutritional, and supplemental therapies, group support when appropriate, and the kind of spiritual support the person desires. Blend these with the best of known and proven conventional cancer therapies.

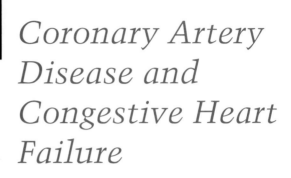

Chapter 21

Coronary Artery Disease and Congestive Heart Failure

In the United States, heart disease is still the leading cause of death. Lifestyle factors contribute significantly to this statistic. A motto for the U.S. health care system might be "a cardiac cath lab in every town, and a fast-food restaurant on every corner." Our lifestyle choices drive an ever-escalating cycle of technology and remedies for heart disease, which continues to occur at alarming rates. In addition to the omnipresent fast-food restaurants with their high-fat, high-sodium food, we are plagued by lessened but continuing tobacco use, sedentary lifestyles, obesity, stress, and other risk factors. The Centers for Disease Control surveyed the actual causes of death in the United States and estimate that 50% of the total deaths per year are from preventable, nongenetic causes. Topping the list of culprits were tobacco, sedentary lifestyle, diet, and alcohol, which together accounted for nearly two-thirds of preventable deaths.

Paradoxically, as we manage to prolong our patients' lives through better management of coronary artery disease (CAD), we see increasing incidence and prevalence of congestive heart failure (CHF) secondary to CAD. Because of aggressive and effective medical intervention, many people are surviving myocardial infarctions (MIs) rather than dying of acute arrhythmias and massive heart failure. Interventions such as thrombolytic therapy, antiarrhythmics, close monitoring in critical-care units, angioplasty, and revascularization have helped cardiologists and cardiovascular surgeons to preserve myocardium and prolong and improve the quality of life after MI. Eventually, however, the compensatory mechanisms of the heart muscle and the volume control mediated through the kidneys are exceeded, and CAD patients frequently develop progressive CHF.

Also contributing to the genesis of CAD are the effects of stress, exhaustion, fatigue, emotional distress, and excess effort (Nixon et al 1997, pp 42–47; Brezinka et al 1996; Greenwood et al 1996). These risk factors intersect to affect not just the anatomy of the coronary vessels but also the healthy function of the whole person. You have certainly heard of the "type A" personality, the hard-driving, time-conscious, ambitious person who seems to accomplish much in life but who is more prone to coronary disease (Friedman et al 1959). This behavior and its associated cardiac risk can be changed and reduced by counseling (Friedman et al 1986). Other evidence suggests that the coronary atheroma, the fixed stenosis of the "culprit artery," is not the whole picture in accounting for the clinical appearance of the coronary syndrome (Nixon et al 1997, p 55). Vasospasm and vasoconstriction can occlude an otherwise normal artery and lead to infarction (Fukai 1993). These vasoactive effects are the end result of stress and may occur in the absence of anatomical obstruction. It is well established that even small atheromatous plaques can be associated with a major cardiac event whereas larger stenoses may cause no symptoms at all (Mayou et al 1994; Nixon et al 1997, pp 54–55). What is the difference?

Historical, sociological, and physiological studies point to the central role of exhaustion and fatigue in negatively affecting human performance. Studies of battle fatigue and the "effort syndrome" show that the limits of our functional capacities and homeostatic mechanisms, however robust, decrease logarithmically when once exceeded. Cardiac function is damaged by a variety of factors and mechanisms: loss of sleep, abnormal neuroendocrine arousal, hyperventilation with hypocapnia resulting in multiple metabolic changes, increased hemostasis, decreased fibrinolysis, persistent catecholamine stimulation, excessive vasoactivity, and endothelial damage. Even poor self-esteem, disordered emotions such as unresolved anger (Wenneberg et al 1997), and the inability to relax and be at ease are all cited as contributors to the cascade of events leading to a cardiac event. These influences are mediated via physiological, cellular, and neuroendocrine pathways and are causative, not merely associated or coincidental factors.

The person who is overstressed, working his or her hardest to achieve goals defined by society as valuable but failing to rest, reflect, and recreate, is at high risk for heart disease. Depression clearly affects cardiac risk negatively, whereas other markers of life satisfaction, social support, stress management, and self-efficacy reduce it (Barefoot et al 1996, Frasure-Smith et al 1993, Greenwood et al 1996, Cousins 1983). Even persons with the classic cardiac risk factors— hypertension, hypercholesterolemia, diabetes, and so on—were less prone to CAD if they could answer in the affirmative these two questions:

1. "Do you like your work?"
2. "Are you a happy person?"

Clearly, more is going on with heart disease than the purely anatomical concerns about blocked arteries, high cholesterol, and plaque formation. Cardiologists these days may attribute a cardiac event to the aftermath of a plaque rupture, and no doubt this is part of the picture. But the reason it ruptured *at that time*, what made the person particularly susceptible to vasospasm, clot formation, and coronary occlusion, are best addressed by mind-body medicine.

In designing an integrative approach to CAD and CHF, keep in mind that "the best medicine is teaching people not to need it." Prevention of these conditions is a far greater societal and professional imperative and challenge than treating them. The simple economics of a recent study speaks volumes, estimating a $30,000 saving for each person following the Dean Ornish regimen of a 10%-fat diet, stress management, and cardiac support versus the conventional therapy of revascularization surgery (Kostreski 1999). The approach used by Benson and others in teaching patients the "relaxation response" as a means of quieting an overactive sympathetic system is another highly cost-effective, low-technology approach to both prevention and rehabilitation of cardiac disease (Benson 1996; Ornish et al 1983; Nixon et al 1997, pp 65–67). We would be well-advised to integrate such approaches into our thinking and practices.

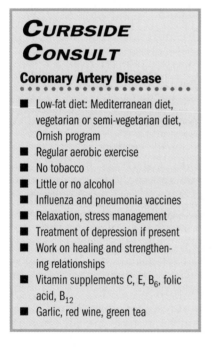

CURBSIDE CONSULT

Coronary Artery Disease

- Low-fat diet: Mediterranean diet, vegetarian or semi-vegetarian diet, Ornish program
- Regular aerobic exercise
- No tobacco
- Little or no alcohol
- Influenza and pneumonia vaccines
- Relaxation, stress management
- Treatment of depression if present
- Work on healing and strengthening relationships
- Vitamin supplements C, E, B_6, folic acid, B_{12}
- Garlic, red wine, green tea

CORONARY ARTERY DISEASE

Case Study: Coronary Artery Disease

George B. is a successful 55-year-old executive at a local oil refinery. He comes to your office complaining of episodes of chest pain that occur with exertion and stress and are relieved by rest. He has noticed these episodes over the last couple of months. He describes them as a squeezing pain in the center of the chest, which lasts 3 to 5 minutes and does not radiate to the arm, neck, or jaw. They have been coming more frequently, and although they go away by themselves, George is realistically worried because his closest friend at work recently suffered an MI, requiring hospitalization and cardiac bypass surgery. Since his friend's infarction, George has had to work harder to complete the tasks in his department and is spending less time with his family. He also has neglected his favorite hobby, deep-sea fishing, which he used to do nearly every week.

A recent health screening showed his total cholesterol to be 267. His past medical history was remarkable for hyperlipidemia, a herniorrhaphy, and recurrent attacks of bronchitis. He was recently divorced, has a 35-pack-year smoking history, and has 3 to 5 drinks of alcohol per day, sometimes more on the weekends. When asked about his diet and exercise pattern, George grimaces and reports that although he has been trying to reduce his fat intake, he often has to eat on the run at work and grabs a pizza, hamburger and fries, or other fast-food for both lunch and dinner. He usually has 3 or 4 cups of coffee with cigarettes and a Danish for breakfast. As for exercise, "Who has time?" he says.

His father suffered an MI in his early 50s, and his older brother had coronary artery bypass grafting (CABG) at age 62. Pertinent positives in the review of systems are dyspnea on exertion after one flight of stairs or walking three blocks, which he attributes to smoking and being out of shape; occasional GI upset, especially on Mondays; episodic erectile dysfunction; and cramping in the legs after walking a few blocks.

He is an overweight, white male, 5′ 11″ tall and 230 pounds. His BP is 110/75 and pulse, 76. He displays nicotine stomatitis, a grade-1 right carotid bruit, and no jugular venous distension. His lungs reveal bilateral crepitations, and breath sounds are slightly decreased. The cardiac exam shows a regular rate and rhythm, normal S1 and S2 without murmur or gallop. His abdomen is obese but without organomegaly. Grade-1 bruits are noted over both iliac and femoral arteries, and the distal pulses in his legs are decreased to +1 at the popliteal, posterior tibial, and dorsal pedis sites. There is no peripheral edema, clubbing, or cyanosis. An EKG is within normal limits. Lab testing is normal except that his total cholesterol is 252, with an LDL of 212, an HDL of 28, and normal triglycerides.

What Is Your Diagnosis?

There is little doubt in your mind that George is suffering from angina pectoris. He has multiple risk factors, a stressful lifestyle with poor diet and little exercise, and a strong family history of heart problems. His angina symptoms are classic: exercise-induced chest pain relieved by rest. The normal EKG is not reassuring in the face of the history; the EKG often can be normal in CAD prior to infarction. In addition, he has chronic obstructive pulmonary disease (COPD), peripheral vascular disease (PVD) with intermittent claudication and impotence, obesity, and hyperlipoproteinemia with a poor risk ratio (high LDL/ low HDL). He may also have alcohol abuse syndrome, with alcoholic gastritis after weekend binges.

What Are Your Recommendations?

The standard of care would demand that you order a cardiac stress study for George. This could be one of several types of exams: an exercise treadmill test using the classic Bruce protocol, a stress echocardiogram, a pharmacological stress study such as a dobutamine stress echo, or a nuclear scintigraphy, thallium scan. The choice of tests is determined to some degree by the expertise in your local hospital facility but also depends on what would produce the best information about George. Because of his poor exercise tolerance due to deconditioning, obesity, COPD, and PVD, you feel that the dobutamine stress study will yield the best results. As expected, it is abnormal. It shows poor perfusion in several arterial runoffs, indicating ischemic heart disease.

Now what?

The cardiologist and you confer with George. Though a cardiac catheterization might reasonably be offered to George because of his age and condition, the three of you decide on a trial of medical management. The cardiologist recommends the use of a beta blocker, a long-acting nitrate, and sublingual nitroglycerin for anginal episodes, as well as a lipid-lowering statin drug. He also advises George to quite smoking and drinking, and to lose weight.

I think this "standard of care" plan is necessary but not sufficient. At this point, a clinician trained in integrative health care can bring together additional resources for George. We can further reduce his risk of suffering further anginal episodes, lessen his probability of MI, and lower the chance that he will need further invasive studies and procedures such as cardiac catheterization, stent placement, angioplasty, or bypass surgery.

From what you have learned so far in this book and elsewhere, what other options could be recommended for this 55-year-old man with known CAD, in addition to standard medical treatment?

Let us start with lifestyle, but let's be realistic. George has been at least 40 pounds overweight for 15 years or more, has smoked all his adult life, has been through a lot of stress with divorce and work problems, and has no clue as to a healthy diet and exercise program.

Thus, the cardiologist's well-intentioned advice to lose weight and quit smoking and drinking is likely to fall on deaf ears or, even worse, create a sense of helplessness and hopelessness as George tries to make multiple changes in his unhealthy lifestyle. You must *listen* to George and show that you understand and acknowledge his feelings, which are likely to include fear, confusion, and frustration. Recommend changes that you think he realistically can make, a little at a time.

He says, "I really don't want to go through what my brother did with his bypass, so I'll do whatever it takes to get my heart well. But I feel so down right now, what with the divorce, my buddy's heart attack, and work stuff and all. I just don't know if I have the energy to do much. What do you recommend?"

Because it is clear from studies that stress (divorce is one of the top stressors) can lead to cardiac problems and also that depression is a risk factor for heart attack, you decide to tackle these first. Although you have a number of supplemental measures in mind, your first priority is getting George out of his depression so he can work on the many lifestyle changes ahead of him (Barefoot et al 1996, Frasure-Smith et al 1993). To do that, you prescribe bupropion, an agent that is useful in depression and also for quitting smoking. You also recommend some graded exercise, not only because of its beneficial effects on cholesterol, obesity, and collateral coronary circulation, but also because of its proven effects on depression and stress. You advise George to start slowly by taking a 10-minute walk each day, either before work or at lunchtime. He can gradually increase that over the next few weeks to walking 20 minutes most days (Dunn et al 1999). You also explain the importance of the medications you and the cardiologist have recommended and suggest a baby aspirin and perhaps a little garlic in the diet to decrease platelet aggregation (Phelps et al 1993, Warshafsky et al 1995). You advise George either to limit alcohol to one or two drinks of red wine daily (Pace-Asciak et al 1996) or to quit drinking completely.

When he returns in 2 weeks, his affect is improved and he says he has more energy. He is walking about 4 times a week, following the low-cholesterol diet your hospital nutritionist provided, and has cut his smoking to about 3 cigarettes a day. He has had only one brief chest pain episode, when he was running to catch a plane at the airport. You check his pulse, blood pressure, and EKG and find nothing worrisome. You also order a liver function panel and lipid profile. He asks you what else he can do.

Seeing that he is making some positive lifestyle changes, you feel it is reasonable to suggest supplements and herbs. He agrees, and you advise that besides the aspirin and prescription medications, he should start taking a vitamin-B complex, explaining that the B vitamins are often low in people who smoke or are under a lot of stress. You also advise 500 mg of vitamin C twice a day (Balz 1999, Hallfrisch et al 1994), but you don't recommend the vitamin E that you would ordinarily suggest for a patient with CAD (Rimm 1993, Stampfer et al 1993) because of the concern that in smokers it may be associated with a higher risk of lung cancer (The Alpha-Tocopheral, Beta Carotene Cancer Prevention Study Group 1994). Also, you explain that vitamin E has recently been shown not to be effective in high-risk cardiac patients like him (Yusuf et al 2000). Finally, you recommend ginkgo biloba, 60 mg twice a day, to improve peripheral and cardiac circulation and decrease platelet aggregation (Blumenthal 1998).

You don't see George for another month but are glad to see that he has lost some weight, has quit smoking, has reduced his alcohol intake as recommended, and is continuing to exercise regularly. He would like to consider even more exercise. He hasn't been having chest pains. His cholesterol level is now 198, with an LDL of 120. You recommend that he attend the nearby Mind-Body Cardiac Rehabilitation Program, where, in addition to basic information about heart disease, they will give him an exercise prescription, teach him how to breathe properly, and instruct him on stress management and relaxation techniques.

Over the next several months, George continues to be pain-free but is still preoccupied about his brother's surgery and his father's cardiac death. Although he is doing reasonably well, you realize that he is still at relatively high risk for a future cardiovascular event and that his concerns about his family history are realistic given his other risk factors. George comes in for a recheck when he has another episode of chest pain after a stressful business meeting. You give him some literature on several cardiac rehab centers that specifically address making major lifestyle changes and you encourage him to consider one of Dr. Dean Ornish's programs. You explain that while he is there, he will learn to eat and cook a very low-fat diet and will learn the value of relationships, relaxation, and exercise in cardiac health. He feels he has learned many of these things at the Mind-Body Rehab, but he admits that his social life isn't very healthy and he has been slipping a bit on his diet. His cholesterol has rebounded to 240.

Just after receiving some final divorce papers in the mail, George suffers a ''coincidental'' angina attack, and he decides to schedule a medical leave. He goes to the Ornish program in an adjacent state for a multiweek program. On returning, he has lost 15 pounds, feels more energy, and is enthusiastic about his new lifestyle plan. Over the next several months, you find that he is doing well and is able to discontinue his antilipemic medication and nitrates and wean off the beta blocker without any ill effects. A year after his Ornish program, you see him at a

Table 21–1   ALTERNATIVE THERAPIES FOR CORONARY ARTERY DISEASE

Therapy	Best Evidence*	Probably Useful†	Least Evidence‡
Herbals		Ginkgo biloba (40 mg t.i.d.) Garlic (900 mg/d or 1 clove) Curcumin (400 mg t.i.d.) Green tea (3–5 c/d)	Khella (250–300 mg/d) Eleutherococcus (Siberian ginseng) (2–3 g/d) Gugulipid (25 mg/t.i.d.)—lipid-lowering agent
Diet and Nutrition/ Lifestyle	Exercise Stop tobacco, caffeine, alcohol Low-fat diet/dietary antioxidants Ornish program Vegetarian diet Vitamin C (1g/d) Vitamin E (400–800 IU/d) Vitamin B_6 (50–100 mg/d) Vitamin B_{12} (800 μg /d) Folic acid (800 μg /d)	Resveratrol (red wine) and other bioflavonoids Consumption of nuts Selenium (100–200 μg/d) Pantethine (300 mg t.i.d.)	Evening primrose oil (3-6 g/d)
Mind-Body Interventions	Relaxation and stress management Screen and treat for depression Guided imagery	Cognitive-behavioral therapy Social support Anger/hostility management Meditation Tai chi Yoga	
Pharmacological and Biological Treatments			Chelation therapy
Alternative Systems of Care		Acupuncture Traditional Chinese medicine Ayurveda	

*Therapies with the highest degree of scientific support for efficacy and safety
†Therapies that are often helpful but that do not have the highest degree of supporting evidence for efficacy and safety
‡Therapies that may be useful but that have limited scientific evidence for efficacy and safety

local theater and you chat briefly. "I'm doing great," he says. "I want you to meet my new fiancée; her name is Hope."

Case Summary

George's situation is far from unique. He fits the typical profile of a coronary patient with high risk from his genetics, lifestyle, and psychosocial profile. In developing a personalized plan for him that extends beyond the standard of care, you have engaged his active involvement in his own care and risk reduction, using safe, well-documented, and natural approaches. A summary of the alternative and integrative measures that are useful in CAD is outlined in Table 21–1.

■■■■■ CONGESTIVE HEART FAILURE

When I was a medical student and resident, CHF was most frequently the result of untreated or undiagnosed hypertension or valvular heart disease from rheumatic fever. The recognition and early treatment of these conditions have changed the epidemiology of CHF, which now is primarily due to the long-term effects of CAD. The standard of therapy for CHF has also evolved. Instead of the traditional digoxin and diuretics, first-line therapy now consists of angiotensin-converting enzyme (ACE) inhibitors and diuretics, then sometimes low-dose beta blockers or digoxin as third-line agents. As these measures fail, however, we often find that we are running out of options; 5 years after diagnosis, most CHF patients have breathed their last breath. Are there alternative and integrative approaches that may be helpful? Let us examine a case in which we use an integrative approach to the problem of CHF.

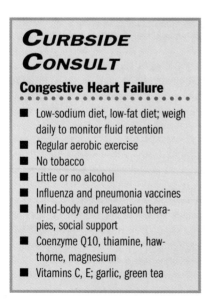

CURBSIDE CONSULT

Congestive Heart Failure

- Low-sodium diet, low-fat diet; weigh daily to monitor fluid retention
- Regular aerobic exercise
- No tobacco
- Little or no alcohol
- Influenza and pneumonia vaccines
- Mind-body and relaxation therapies, social support
- Coenzyme Q10, thiamine, hawthorne, magnesium
- Vitamins C, E; garlic, green tea

Case Study: Congestive Heart Failure

Monica L. is a 64-year-old retired certified public accountant. She smoked heavily much of her life and had hypertension, hypercholesterolemia, diabetes mellitus type 2, and a strong family history of heart disease. She was forced to retire at age 59 from her position as a partner in a CPA firm because of a series of three MIs. She has had an angioplasty twice, three-vessel bypass surgery, and several admissions over the past 2 years for CHF. Each time she was admitted to the hospital, her complaint was a progression of fatigue, dyspnea, peripheral edema, and difficulty sleeping. She has responded to medical management, including an ACE inhibitor, high-dose diuretics, and a recently added low-dose beta blocker, but her status remains precarious. Stress, dietary indiscretions, or even a respiratory infection can easily tip her into an acute exacerbation of CHF requiring hospitalization. Her cardiologist follows her closely, but as her primary care provider you also see her regularly.

She sees you 2 weeks after her latest hospitalization. As you are taking the interval history and reviewing the discharge summary, she tells you about her feelings of discouragement and frustration with the chronic and progressive disease. "Sometimes I wish I'd just had a heart attack and died in my sleep. This back and forth to the hospital, the shortness of breath, fatigue, and just not being able to do anything is really getting to me. Isn't there something else we can do?"

She hands you some material she found in a health magazine and several pages downloaded from the Internet. The articles are touting the benefits in treating heart failure of several supplements. You review her articles and her medication list. During her recent hospitalization, her diuretics were increased again with the addition of metolazone, a powerful loop diuretic. The maximum dose of ACE inhibitor has been reached, worsening her renal function. The cardiologist and you had decided to add digoxin. Her bradycardia of 58 and BP of 98/55 limit further increases in the beta blocker. Her diabetes and hypercholesterolemia are reasonably controlled with medication. With her ejection fraction running below 30% (normal 50%–75%), you recognize that even limited improvements in her cardiac function will be helpful, though her long-term prognosis is rather poor.

What Are Your Recommendations?

You recommend hawthorn at an initial dose of 100 mg t.i.d., coenzyme Q10 at 150 mg/day, thiamine at 100 mg/day, and supplemental magnesium 300 mg/day (Baggio et al 1994; Morisco et al 1993; Leuchtgens 1993; Tauchert et al 1994; Gottlieb 1989, 1990; Leslie et al 1996). Besides continuing to take aspirin, you advise that she add garlic, vitamin C, and vitamin E to her diet (Rapola 1997). When she expresses concern about the number of pills being added to her current regimen of half a dozen drugs, you suggest that she add one agent a week, starting with hawthorn, then CoQ10, and finally the vitamin and mineral supplements. She agrees to this graded approach and feels encouraged at the prospect of improvement.

You continue to see her regularly. You advise her to monitor her weight daily on a bathroom scale to note any fluctuations in fluid overload. You give her detailed instructions on a low-sodium diet and warn her that even one high-sodium meal (she loves delicatessen food, especially kosher pickles) might be enough to precipitate a problem with sodium overload and fluid retention.

In the fall you administer her flu shot, double-check that her pneumonia vaccine is current, and renew her medications. Over the preceding 3 months, she has not had any additional hospitalizations, is sleeping better, and has more energy. Although not back to her old self, she is happy that she can at least go for short walks in the park with her son and granddaughter and that she can even climb a flight of stairs at the senior center without extreme breathlessness. Her exercise tolerance is still limited, but you encourage regular walks, even 10 minutes at a time, to keep her active and mobile. She is pleased and says it is nice to hear of something that she *can* do instead of all the things she is forbidden to do because of her CHF.

Table 21–2 ALTERNATIVE THERAPIES FOR CONGESTIVE HEART FAILURE

Therapy	Best Evidence*	Probably Useful†	Least Evidence‡
Herbals	Hawthorn (80–300 mg b.i.d., tincture 4–5 mL t.i.d.)		Cinnamon (2–3 mg/d, tincture 2–3 mL t.i.d.)
Diet and Nutrition/ Lifestyle	Coenzyme Q10 (30–100 mg t.i.d.) Magnesium (300 mg/d) Thiamine (20–100 mg/d)	Carnitine (500 mg b.i.d.–t.i.d.) Taurine (3–6 g/d)	L-Arginine (1500 mg–12 g/d)
Mind-Body Interventions	Relaxation and stress management Screen and treat for depression Guided imagery	Cognitive-behavioral therapy Social support Anger/hostility management Meditation Tai chi Yoga	

*Therapies with the highest degree of scientific support for efficacy and safety
†Therapies that are often helpful but that do not have the highest degree of supporting evidence for efficacy and safety
‡Therapies that may be useful but that have limited scientific evidence for efficacy and safety

Case Summary

Although Monica's prognosis remains guarded, the supplements, close monitoring of her weight and diet, and some regular exercise are simple measures that have improved her life. Because of the high adrenergic tone of patients in CHF, some mind-body and relaxation techniques could be suggested to help her cope more effectively so that stress is less likely to cause further decompensation. Social support, such as spending time with her family, has also been shown to improve metabolic reserve (Greenwood et al 1996, Brezinka et al 1996). Maintaining a view of the "big picture" is the best that can be done to help her manage her long-term condition. Other important measures include boosting immunizations to prevent respiratory infections that can tip her into an exacerbation of CHF, controlling the diabetes mellitus and cholesterol, evaluating her mood state to rule out and treat depression, and working closely with her cardiologist. An integrative approach to CHF is summarized in Table 21–2.

Chapter

22

Diabetes

Up to 90% of cases of diabetes mellitus (DM) result from consuming too many calories. Although type 1 diabetes mellitus (formerly called juvenile-onset or insulin-dependent diabetes) is thought to result from immune or infectious causes, the major risk factor for the much more common type 2 diabetes (formerly known as adult-onset or non–insulin-dependent diabetes mellitus) is obesity. There is some association with genetic factors, but the pattern is clear: diabetes, hypercholesterolemia, coronary artery disease (CAD), hypertension (HTN)—all are related to **too many calories**.

Once a patient is diagnosed with diabetes, how do alternative and integrative therapies fit in? Type 1 DM, which relentlessly led to ketoacidosis, coma, and death before the discovery of insulin, now is commonly survived for many years. One study that needs to be replicated with a larger number of cases showed that this type of diabetes may be completely reversed if treated early with niacinamide supplementation (Vague et al 1987). Without a doubt, dietary modification is essential to both types 1 and 2 diabetes, as are a number of other lifestyle and supplemental measures. Those with type 2 diabetes have a slower progression of their disease than those with type 1 but still are at high risk for a shortened lifespan, despite numerous excellent oral hypoglycemic medications.

As we think about alternative approaches to DM, we need to keep in mind the severe consequences of the

disease in the untreated state: retinopathy, CAD, renal failure, peripheral neuropathy, and vasculopathy resulting in chronic ulceration,
gangrene, and amputation. As with other life-threatening conditions,
the standard of care requires that we adhere to proven treatments as we
integrate alternative therapies. The best applications of alternative
therapies for diabetes are in certain types of patients:

1. The patient with impaired glucose tolerance, formerly known as
   "borderline" or "chemical" adult-onset diabetes
2. The patient who does not respond to oral hypoglycemic agents
   and resists switching to insulin injections or whose clinician resists such a switch
3. The patient with type 2 diabetes that is relatively easily controlled with standard therapy and for whom nonpharmacologi-
   cal treatment is preferred
4. The patient with newly diagnosed diabetes without ketoacidosis
   who prefers to try a lifestyle or natural approach before starting
   medications. Let us look at an illustrative case of this last type:

Case Study: Type 2 (Adult-Onset) Diabetes Mellitus

Maria G. is a 47-year-old obese Latin American woman who comes to
your office for a well-woman exam. During the history, you note her
complaints of fatigue, blurring vision, a recurrent vaginal yeast infection,
and episodic numbness of the legs. Her history shows that she is a
G3P3Ab0, has had a tubal ligation, and has occasional urinary tract
infections, but it is otherwise unremarkable. She is taking no medications and does not take any over-the-counter products except a daily
multivitamin. She is married, works as an administrative assistant in the
local community college, and has three grown children living outside the
home. Her husband works as a marketing director for a local software
firm. She neither smokes nor drinks alcohol. She smoked marijuana as a
college student but has used no drugs since her early 20s. Her family
history is positive for type 2 diabetes in both her parents and several
aunts and uncles. Her paternal grandparents have had heart problems,
and her maternal grandmother has had a stroke. Review of systems
reveals several complaints: She has gained 20 pounds in the last
2 years. She has had problems with blurred vision though she has never
worn glasses. She has increasing fatigue, frequent diarrhea, and vaginal
yeast infections with itching and discharge at this time, and has nocturia
2 times nightly. Her feet tingle and feel numb on occasion. She also says
that she needs to drink a lot of water because her mouth often feels dry.
   Physical exam shows a pleasant woman who is 5' 1" and weighs

156 pounds. Her BP is 125/80, P 72, RR 14, T 37°C. HEENT shows normal tympanic membranes and benign funduscopic, nasal, and pharyngeal exams, with no adenopathy or thyromegaly. Heart and lung exams are normal, as is the abdominal exam except for the finding of moderate obesity. A pelvic exam, done because of the complaint of vaginal symptoms, reveals a discharge resembling cottage cheese, erythema of the introitus and vagina, and normal bimanual and rectal exams. Extremity exam reveals normal sensation, reflexes, and vibratory sense. You order lab work, which includes a CBC, thyroid test, urinalysis, wet prep and KOH, renal profile, blood glucose levels, electrolyte levels, and cholesterol level. When these come back, the CBC, thyroid, renal profile, and electrolytes are normal; but the urinalysis shows 500 mg of glucose but no protein, the KOH prep and Pap both reveal yeast forms, her blood glucose is 285, and her cholesterol is 223.

What Is Your Next Step?

You ask Maria to come in for a fasting blood glucose test, explaining that you strongly suspect she has diabetes. You order a lipid profile as well, and tell her to go to the local pharmacy to pick up an antifungal vaginal cream. The results arrive in a couple of days: her fasting blood glucose is 187, cholesterol is 240, and triglycerides are 445. Her HDL-C ratio is high at 5.9.

Now What?

In discussing the new diagnosis of diabetes with patients, it is essential to relieve fears about the disease and help them become aware of what they can do to control their condition. In Maria's case, you provide some education and literature about the condition, the variety of treatments available besides insulin, and the importance of a dietary and exercise plan. Because this is all new to her, you schedule a follow-up visit with a diabetic counselor to reinforce what you have taught her.

The best dietary approach for diabetics is a high-fiber, low-fat diet that is rich in complex carbohydrates. You recommend such a diet and encourage her to start a regular exercise program at least 3 times a week, with a goal of losing at least 20 pounds over the next year. Maria has spoken to a Hispanic curandera about some traditional herbal agents used in that culture for diabetes. She asks you if she should try them.

What Do You Say?

Because she is symptomatic, you must reduce her blood sugar levels soon and reliably. You recommend that she buy a blood glucose monitoring system for home use and that she start monitoring her blood sugar levels regularly. You explain that you would like to see the effects of a change in diet and exercise on her blood sugar levels and would be willing to observe for a short while for the effects of the curandera's herbs. You tell her that she may be able to control this condition without medication, even at this stage. Maria is pleased by your openness to her cultural approach and asks if you have any other recommendations.

Are There Other Herbs or Supplements That May Be Helpful?

To try to reduce the oxidative stress on the tissues, you may recommend supplementation with vitamin C, 500 to 1000 mg 2 to 3 times/day, and vitamin E, 400 IU 2 to 3 times/day (Sinclair et al 1994, Paolisso et al 1993). You also recommend additional vitamin B_6, 50 mg/day, because it is protective against diabetic neuropathy, which is suggested by her complaints of numbness and tingling (Levin et al 1981). In addition, supplemental chromium (200 μg/day) and magnesium citrate or aspartate (300 to 500 mg/day) can be helpful to diabetic patients in stabilizing blood sugar levels, because both minerals are involved in glucose metabolism (Ravina et al 1995, Paolisso et al 1992). Vitamin B_6 helps in the transport of magnesium into the cells. Zinc at 30 mg/day can be helpful for its effects on insulin metabolism plus its benefits in wound healing (Engel et al 1981). A high-potency multiple vitamin and mineral supplement may contain much of what you have recommended, although Maria will need to add some separate supplements. You also order a glycohemoglobin level for a baseline reading.

Follow-Up

Maria agrees with this plan and returns to see you in 3 weeks. She has met with the diabetic counselor, has begun exercising almost daily at a local aerobics class, and is adjusting her diet. She has also started the supplements you recommended as well as a *yerba* (herb) from the curandera, cheerfully assuring you that several members of her family have taken it over the years for their diabetes. Your fears about this unknown herb are allayed somewhat when she shows you her blood glucose record. The range of sugar readings is 120 to 160. The glycohemoglobin result drawn at the last visit was 8.5, so this looks like progress. (**Pearl:** To get an estimate of the average blood sugar level, simply multiply the glycohemoglobin reading by 25—in this case 8.5 × 25 = 212, her pre-treatment average blood glucose.) Some of her symptoms, such as the tingling in her feet, have gone away; her vision and energy have improved; and the yeast infection is cleared up. She has lost about 4 pounds and is feeling a good deal better overall.

You continue to monitor her over the next year and are pleased that her blood sugar readings continue to decline to near normal with the combination of diet, exercise, supplements, and herbs she is taking. You check her glycohemoglobin level every 3 months and are pleased to

Table 22–1 ALTERNATIVE THERAPIES FOR DIABETES

Therapy	Best Evidence*	Probably Useful†	Least Evidence‡
Herbals		Bilberry *(Vaccinium myrtillus)* (retinopathy 80–160 mg t.i.d.) Bitter melon *(Momordica charantia)* (30–60 mL of juice/d) Coccinia indica *Gymnema sylvestre* (200 mg b.i.d.) Ginkgo biloba (retinopathy, neuropathy, and vascular complications: 40 mg t.i.d.) Garlic Green tea *(Camellia sinensis)* (2 c/d) *Trigonelle foenum-graecum*	Dandelion leaves Eleutherococcus Fenugreek *(Trigonella foenum-graecum)* (50 g/d defatted seed powder) Ginseng (100 mg t.i.d.) Glucomannan Guar gum Horehound Juniper Lavender Myrrh Neem Primrose oil (neuropathy) Salt bush *(Atriplex halimus)* Silymarin (cirrhosis in diabetes) Spanish needles *(Bidens pilosa)* Tragacanth Yellow bells *(Tecoma stans)*
Diet and Nutrition/ Lifestyle	Regular exercise Weight loss Diet high in fiber, low in simple sugars and fats Pritikin diet Ornish diet	Alpha-lipoic acid Biotin (type 1 and type 2 DM: 9–16 mg/d) Chromium (200 µg/d) Essential fatty acids (cold-water fish, 480 mg/d; gamma linoleic acid, 1 T/d flaxseed oil) Magnesium (300–500 mg/d) Onions Potassium (dietary) Vitamin C (>2 g/d in divided doses) Vitamin B_3 (prevention of new-onset type 1: 25 mg/kg/d) Inositol hexaniacinate (hyperlipidemia: 500–1000 mg/d)	Flavonoids (dietary, 1–2/d) Manganese (30 mg/d)

Table 22–1   ALTERNATIVE THERAPIES FOR DIABETES *(Continued)*

Therapy	Best Evidence*	Probably Useful†	Least Evidence‡
Diet and Nutrition/ Lifestyle *(Continued)*		Vitamin B_6 (neuropathy: 50–100 mg/d) Vitamin B_{12} (neuropathy: 1000–3000 μg/d.p.o.) or 1000 μg/wk IM Vitamin E (800–900 IU/d) Zinc (30 mg/d)	
Mind-body Interventions	Self-care, personal locus of control and responsibility	Biofeedback Reduction of threat of DM (adolescents) Relaxation therapy Social support Spiritual approaches Yoga	Treatment of depression Qi Gong
Bioelectromagnetic Therapies		Therapeutic touch	Electrical stimulation
Alternative Systems of Care		Acupuncture (neuropathy) Traditional Chinese medicine	Ayurveda Curanderismo herbalism
Hands-on Healing Techniques			Massage

*Therapies with the highest degree of scientific support for efficacy and safety
†Therapies that are often helpful but that do not have the highest degree of supporting evidence for efficacy and safety
‡Therapies that may be useful but that have limited scientific evidence for efficacy and safety

see it dropping gradually to 5.3. Her lipids have also normalized, as they often do, with control of the diabetes. Although there are other supplements, drugs, and herbs that can be useful, she is doing well enough that you make no additional changes. At one point you consider adding a sulfonylurea when her blood sugars climb over 160, but you hold off on the prescription because the loss of control was because of dietary indiscretion and decreased exercise over the Christmas holiday. By mid-January, the blood sugars are again running around 120.

CONCLUSION

Although many diabetics will require medication to keep their blood sugar levels well controlled, motivated patients like Maria can keep their diabetes in check with lifestyle changes. Even when a patient with diabetes requires medication, I continue to stress the importance of diet, exercise, weight control, and nutritional supplements. Some patients ignore these simple measures and depend only on their medications to manage their condition, a less effective approach to whole-person health and well-being. Table 22–1 summarizes alternative measures for the management of diabetes mellitus.

Chapter

23

Gastrointestinal Problems

Chronic problems of the digestive system are another common complaint in the primary care setting. Some abdominal complaints—acute obstruction, vomiting and diarrhea with dehydration, appendicitis, bleeding ulcers, cancer, acute pancreatitis or cholecystitis, and others—are emergencies that may require hospitalization or surgery. On the other hand, many are managed chronically. Chronic conditions that can be treated using alternative therapies may include gastroesophageal reflux disease (GERD), peptic ulcers or dyspepsia, irritable bowel syndrome (IBS), cholecystitis, inflammatory bowel disease (IBD), constipation or diarrhea, and hepatitis (Table 23–1). This chapter will illustrate the integrative approach to the treatment of three of these common problems: GERD, hepatitis, and IBS.

Case Study: Gastroesophageal Reflux Disease

John M. is a moderately obese 52-year-old who comes to your office complaining of recurrent chest pains. John tells you that the pain is provoked by eating a big meal, lying down, bending over, and drinking coffee. It has been relieved by Tums or other antacids, but these have not worked as well lately. The pain is a burning, cramping sensation located in the middle of his chest and the back of his throat. He says he has had some symptoms for several years, but the pains now are lasting

Table 23–1 ALTERNATIVE THERAPIES FOR MISCELLANEOUS GASTROINTESTINAL COMPLAINTS

Therapy	Best Evidence*	Probably Useful†	Least Evidence‡
Herbals	Aloe (constipation) (30 mL t.i.d.) Cascara (constipation) (tea from 1 tsp. bark b.i.d.; 1 mL tincture b.i.d.) Deglycyrrhizinated licorice (DGL) (PUD) (380–760 mg t.i.d./ac) Peppermint (indigestion: 0.2 mL–0.4 mL enteric-coated oil b.i.d.–t.i.d./ac) Senna (constipation)	Aloe (heartburn: 30 mL t.i.d.) Bilberry (diarrhea) Boldo (cholagogue, indigestion) Caraway Chamomile (antispasmodic, colic, PUD: 2–3 g/d; 3–5 mL tincture t.i.d.; as tea t.i.d.–q.i.d.) Ginger (nausea: 500mg t.i.d.) Goldenseal (diarrhea: 500 mg t.i.d.; use with caution) Fennel (colic, antispasmodic: tea 1 cup t.i.d.; 600 mg caps t.i.d.; for infants, 2 tsp seeds t.i.d.) (as tea) Garlic (antispasmodic: up to 3 g b.i.d.) Lemon balm Marijuana (nausea) Raspberry tea (antispasmodic) Sage (antispasmodic) White wine (increases gastric emptying)	Bitters (indigestion: barberry, dandelion) Oregon grape, yellow dock, wormwood Butcher's broom (hemorrhoids) Horse chestnut (hemorrhoids)
Diet and Nutrition/ Lifestyle	Lactase (for those with lactose intolerance) Lipase (pancreatic insufficiency)	Bismuth (PUD: 240 mg subcitrate b.i.d./ac, subsalicylate 500 mg q.i.d./ac) Cabbage (PUD: 1 L juice daily, effects possibly due to glutamine content) Charcoal (excess gas) Lactobacillus acidophilus (diarrhea, antibiotic-induced diarrhea)	Betaine HCL (low stomach acidity) Flavonoids (PUD: 500 mg t.i.d.) Proteolytic enzymes Yogurt (antibiotic-induced diarrhea) Vitamin A (up to 25,000 IU/d) Vitamin C (500 mg t.i.d.) Vitamin E (100 IU t.i.d.) Zinc 20 mg/d

**Table 23–1   ALTERNATIVE THERAPIES FOR MISCELLANEOUS
GASTROINTESTINAL COMPLAINTS** *(Continued)*

Therapy	Best Evidence*	Probably Useful†	Least Evidence‡
Mind-Body Interventions	Depression (functional bowel complaints), detect and treat Exercise (constipation) Psychotherapy Stress management (PUD)		
Alternative Systems of Care		Acupuncture (nausea) Acupressure (nausea) Ayurveda	**Homeopathy:** *Colic:* Cuprum metallicum (6C t.i.d.–q.i.d.) Chamomile (6C t.i.d. for 3–4 d) Colocynthis (30C t.i.d.) Nux vomica (6C q 15 min until vomiting ceases) Belladonna (6C q 1 hr for up to 6 doses) Bryonia (6C q 1 hr for up to 6 doses) *Constipation:* Nux vomica (6C t.i.d. for 10 d) Sepia (30C: 3 doses in 24 hr once a month) Sulfur (6C t.i.d. up to 10 d) *Diarrhea:* Arsenicum album (6C q 30 min for up to 6 doses, then t.i.d.) Argentum nitricum (6C q 1 hr up to 6 doses) Podophyllum (30C t.i.d.–q.i.d. for 2 d) Pulsatilla (6C q 2 hr for up to 6 doses) Sulfur (6C q 1 hr up to 6 doses, then t.i.d.) *Hemorrhoids:* Hamamelis (6C t.i.d. for 3 d) Calcarea fluorica (6C t.i.d.–q.i.d. for 3–4 d)

(Continued)

Table 23–1   ALTERNATIVE THERAPIES FOR MISCELLANEOUS GASTROINTESTINAL COMPLAINTS *(Continued)*

Therapy	Best Evidence*	Probably Useful†	Least Evidence‡
Alternative Systems of Care *(Continued)*			Arnica (30C q.i.d. for 2–3 d) Aesculus hippo-castanum (30C t.i.d. for 3 d) *Heartburn, Indigestion, and Gas:* Nux vomica (6C q 30 min for 2 hr) Carbo vegetabilis (6C q 30 min for 2 hr) Lycopodium (6C 2–3 times after meals) Natrum phosphoricum (6C q 30 min for 2 hr) Arsenicum album (6C q 1 hr up to 6 doses, then t.i.d.)

*Therapies with the highest degree of scientific support for efficacy and safety
†Therapies that are often helpful but that do not have the highest degree of supporting evidence for efficacy and safety
‡Therapies that may be useful but that have limited scientific evidence for efficacy and safety
PUD = Peptic ulcer disease

an hour or more and getting bad enough to take his breath away. He had an upper GI series when they first started, which showed a hiatal hernia, but now he is concerned that he might be having heart problems because of his recent weight gain and his family history of heart disease.

At this point, you are reasonably sure that John is suffering from reflux esophagitis, chronic in nature owing to a hiatal hernia. It has probably been aggravated lately by the weight gain, which increases intra-abdominal pressure and the tendency to reflux. Your exam findings of his lungs, heart, and chest wall are normal. He has some tenderness when you press deeply in the epigastric area. An EKG done in your office is normal. Although you are fairly confident that these chest pains are gastrointestinal in origin, you are cautious not to jump to this conclusion and miss a life-threatening problem, so you order an exercise stress test and chest x-ray.

Because he has had a good response to antacids in the past, you decide to use ranitidine, an H_2 antagonist, holding the more powerful proton pump inhibitor, omperazole, in reserve. Additionally, you tell John your impression, that he has GERD, and print a handout on lifestyle measures that will support the treatment of his condition. You recommend that he lose weight; avoid lying down within 2 hours of a meal; eat smaller meals; avoid tobacco, alcohol, and any spicy foods that seem to aggravate the condition; and elevate the head of his bed about 6 inches to reduce reflux in the recumbent position. You also tell him to avoid high-fat foods, which delay gastric emptying, and peppermint, which may increase reflux by reducing gastroesophageal sphincter tone.

John returns in a couple of weeks, feeling much better. The cardiologist pronounced his treadmill test normal even though John didn't stay on it as long as he would have liked. The chest x-ray was clear, but a small hiatal hernia could be seen in the lateral view.

John doesn't really want to take medication every day and wants to consider other options (Table 23–2). You tell him that GERD is often a chronic condition; sometimes it responds to surgery, but more often it is treated by the lifestyle measures and medication you have already advised. You mention that deglycyrrhizinated licorice (DGL) may be useful as an antacid, at a dosage of 250 to 500 mg t.i.d. of the dry powdered extract in capsules (Kassir 1985). Other approaches, such as acupuncture or osteopathic manipulation, could likewise be tried. You also suggest that relaxation therapies may help by reducing excess acid production due to stress. If he continues with chronic H_2-blocker therapy, it might be helpful to check later for deficiency of B_{12}, calcium, and iron, because the absence of acidity in the stomach affects their absorption.

Case Study: Chronic Hepatitis C

Bill T. is a 34-year-old paramedic who is known to have hepatitis C. He thinks he probably got it during his paramedic training when a jaundiced patient with a massive upper GI bleed came to the ER. While starting the IV, Bill had a needlestick accident and was exposed to the patient's blood. Subsequent testing revealed a positive hepatitis C antibody, and although he had been immunized against hepatitis B, there is no vaccine for C. He feels well but wants to get his liver enzymes checked. You feel his abdomen to determine the size of his liver. (**Pearl:** Placing your stethoscope over the midline about midway between the xiphoid and the umbilicus, you gently scratch over the area of the liver with your finger, starting inferiorly and working upward toward the costal margin, a technique call a *scratch percussion test*, which is particularly useful with obese patients, if tenderness prevents palpation, or in those with ascites. You can hear precisely where the liver edge is; the tone of the scratching changes to a higher frequency.) Bill's liver is not enlarged.

Table 23–2 ALTERNATIVE THERAPIES FOR GASTROESOPHAGEAL REFLUX DISEASE (GERD)

Therapy	Best Evidence*	Probably Useful†	Least Evidence‡
Herbals	Deglycyrrhizinated licorice (DGL) (380–760 mg t.i.d./ac)	Caraway Lemon balm Raspberry tea White wine (increases gastric emptying)	Oregon grape, yellow dock, wormwood
Diet and Nutrition/ Lifestyle	Lactase (for those with lactose intolerance) Lipase (pancreatic insufficiency) Weight loss Small meals Don't lie down for 2 hr after a meal Elevate head of bed 6'' Avoid foods that promote reflux, such as alcohol, tobacco, caffeine, onions, spicy foods, peppermint		Proteolytic enzymes Vitamin A (up to 25,000 IU/d) Vitamin C (500 mg t.i.d.) Vitamin E (100 IU t.i.d.) Zinc 20 mg/d
Alternative Systems of Care		Acupuncture Ayurveda	*Homeopathy:* Bryonia (6C q 30 min for 2 hr) Carbo vegetabilis (6C q 30 min for 2 hr) Lycopodium (6C 2–3 times after meals) Natrum phosphoricum (6C q 30 min for 2 hr) Nux vomica (6C q 30 min for 2 hr)

*Therapies with the highest degree of scientific support for efficacy and safety
†Therapies that are often helpful but that do not have the highest degree of supporting evidence for efficacy and safety
‡Therapies that may be useful but that have limited scientific evidence for efficacy and safety

His enzymes are slightly increased, but not alarmingly so. Because you are aware that hepatitis C is a "stealth virus" that can cause significant liver damage and cirrhosis with minimal evidence on testing liver enzymes, you refer him to a gastroenterologist who specializes in diseases of the liver. The specialist performs a viral load study and liver biopsy, and after reviewing the results, starts Bill on interferon and retroviral therapy. He feels weak, achy, and flu-like throughout the treatment course but finishes with the protocol. When he comes to see you next, he asks if you can make any suggestions besides the medications.

You advise him to avoid drugs or other substances that can further damage the liver, such as alcohol, nonsteroidal anti-inflammatory drugs (NSAIDs) or acetaminophen, antifungal drugs, or some of the lipid-lowering agents. He admits to an occasional beer when out with friends and acetaminophen for headache, but these are not usual in his life. You recommend switching to a tasty nonalcoholic beer. You also advise that he consider a different headache therapy, such as acupressure or an herb like willow bark.

You recommend that Bill start taking milk thistle (*Silybum marianum*) at doses of 140 mg 2 to 3 times a day. When his paramedic curiosity prompts him to ask how it works, you explain that it protects against fibrosis by stabilizing membranes through increased production of ribosomal RNA for cellular repair, and it also acts as a free-radical scavenger and antioxidant.

"Why didn't the liver specialist recommend it if it is so good?" Bill asks.

You reply, "Some hepatologists routinely recommend milk thistle for this condition but perhaps Dr. Jones hasn't been convinced yet of its safety and effectiveness. On the basis of all my experience and reading, I recommend it." You make a mental note to talk with Dr. Jones and to give him some articles on the use of milk thistle in hepatitis (Blumenthal 2000, Robbers 1999, Blumenthal 1998).

A few months later, Bill returns for a repeat liver test and you both happily note that his liver functions have returned to a normal range. He has eliminated beer and acetaminophen. Dr. Jones is now enthusiastically prescribing milk thistle for similar patients and is considering a study to measure the decrease in abnormal liver enzymes he has observed.

Bill's case is one more example of the limits of conventional therapy in curing conditions such as chronic hepatitis. Though silymarin does not cure it either, the safety and efficacy studies, including the recommendations of the German Commission E (Blumenthal 1998), suggest that it should be a regular part of your prescription for this condition (Table 23–3).

Case Study: Irritable Bowel Syndrome (IBS)

Heather A. comes in for her annual well-woman exam. She is an attractive 28-year-old securities broker who feels healthy except for

Table 23–3 ALTERNATIVE THERAPIES FOR HEPATITIS

Therapy	Best Evidence*	Probably Useful†	Least Evidence‡
Herbals	Milk thistle (hepatitis, cirrhosis: 70–140 mg t.i.d.)	Artichoke (Astragalus membranaceus) Caraway Glycyrrhizin, licorice root (<100 mg/d, 1g root t.i.d.; higher doses affect electrolytes, BP) Goldenseal (500 mg t.i.d.; use with caution) Lemon balm Raspberry tea Turmeric (250–500 mg b.i.d.)	Oregon grape, yellow dock, wormwood Evening primrose oil (alcoholic liver disease) Sho-saiko-to (TJ-9) Coumpound 861 Phyllanthus amarus
Diet and Nutrition/ Lifestyle			Proteolytic enzymes Vitamin A (up to 25,000 IU/d) Vitamin C (500 mg t.i.d.) Vitamin E (100 IU t.i.d.) Zinc (20 mg/d)
Mind-Body Interventions	Psychotherapy		
Alternative Systems of Care		Ayurveda	

*Therapies with the highest degree of scientific support for efficacy and safety
†Therapies that are often helpful but that do not have the highest degree of supporting evidence for efficacy and safety
‡Therapies that may be useful but that have limited scientific evidence for efficacy and safety

recurrent feelings of abdominal bloating, gas, episodic diarrhea, and colicky abdominal pain. She tells you that as a child she often stayed home from school because of abdominal pain, and her mother has told her that even as an newborn infant, she had a lot of colic.

As a teenager and again in her early 20s, Heather had a series of tests, including endoscopy and radiographic studies of the abdomen, which failed to find any tumors, stones, malrotations of the gut, obstruction, IBD, or other serious problem. She was told there was nothing wrong and that she should try to live with the condition.

You perform her regular yearly exam. Except for some mild general-ized abdominal pain with an increase in bowel sounds, she appears to be a healthy young woman. After she dresses, she asks, "What can I do about this abdominal pain? It is really affecting my life. I've missed days off work, I have to run to the bathroom a lot, and I have embarrassing stomach rumblings and gas."

You review her chart and note that she has tried an antispasmodic in the past with some relief. "When you took metoclopramide, how did that work?" you ask.

"It helped some, but it made my mouth dry and made me drowsy," Heather responds.

When you ask what seems to make her GI problems worse, she mentions dairy products (especially ice cream), caffeine, most sweets, alcohol, and some grains. And especially stress—such as her recent discovery that her boyfriend, Corey, whom she was considering marrying after dating for 4 years, has been seen out with a cocktail waitress. Her GI complaints also have been worsened by another layer of stress at work: since the stock market has been rising so fast, her firm's mutual funds are selling like hotcakes. She is making lots of money but has been having trouble keeping up with all her clients' trades and is not getting much sleep.

You consider the situation in its entirety: a chronic problem recently exacerbated by work and relationship stress, in a patient who is also sensitive to dietary factors and intolerant of pharmaco-therapy. You believe that Heather has IBS and recall reading that the four major treatments from a natural perspective are (1) increas-ing dietary fiber, (2) eliminating allergenic foods, (3) using enteric-coated volatile oil preparations, and (4) controlling psychological factors through stress reduction and exercise (Murray & Pizzorno 1998).

Although you know how difficult it is to ask a patient to make too many lifestyle changes at once, you feel Heather is ready for a serious and intense approach to this problem. You tell her, "Here's a plan, Heather. We will work on this together over the next few weeks to make sure it is working, but it will require some effort on your part."

"I'm ready to try anything. This is no way to live," Heather replies eagerly.

"First, we have to increase your dietary fiber. Since IBS is thought to be a motility disorder, it seems that increasing the bulk of the stool slows the passage of intestinal contents and also reduces the spasm of the walls of the large intestine. I want you to increase your intake of fruits and vegetables to at least 7 servings a day. And let's start you on a psyllium-seed powder (Hotz et al 1994) and gradually increase the amount in the next few weeks. If you take too much at first, it will cause excess flatus.''

"I sure don't need that!" she replies, "That's already a bad problem.''

"Right, that's why we are starting slowly, with 1 teaspoon twice a day and working up to a higher dose if we need to. This can also help to prevent colon cancer, by the way. Next, I'd like you to eliminate dairy products, at least for a while. I'd like you to cut out milk, cheese, and ice cream, but you can have yogurt a couple of times a week, because it contains helpful bacteria for your gut. Also, since caffeine and sweets seem to aggravate your problem, let's switch to herbal teas or decaffeinated beverages and cut out soft drinks, refined sugars, and desserts.''

"Now you are starting to get to me," Heather says. "Giving up milk is one thing, but coffee and ice cream . . . that may be hard.''

"As I said, this will require some effort on your part. We'll be patient with the process and approach it gradually. Next, I would like you to start taking a 300-mg capsule of enteric-coated peppermint oil 3 times a day before meals. That should relax the painful spasms in your gut" (Blumenthal 2000, Dew et al 1984, Liu et al 1997, Rees et al 1979).

"I'll be happy for that," she says. "Is that it?''

You continue, "People with IBS often find that it's aggravated by stress. What do you do to relax? Are you interested in learning some new techniques?''

"Like what?''

"I have a number of options in mind. One is increasing your regular exercise, say going to the gym and working out 3 or 4 times a week.''

"With my schedule? You must be kidding!''

"Do you want to feel better or not?''

"Well, sure. I know you're right. When I work out, my stress level goes way down.''

"Heather, another option is to get some short-term counseling about the anger and pain you are expressing about ending your relationship. Here is the name of a psychologist I trust. In addition to supportive counseling, he teaches relaxation and biofeedback. Both of these are very useful in IBS and stress management in general.''

"I'll think about it," she says warily.

About a month later, Heather returns to your office. She is wearing a frown.

"How has it been going?" you ask.

"Well it was going just fine until that jerk, Corey, called me to see if I would see him again. Apparently his new girl dumped him, just like he did me. Serves him right, I say! No chance I'll see him again. Anyway, after he called, my stomach started hurting again. I had been doing quite a bit better, though not perfect, with the changes in diet, the peppermint oil, and getting regular exercise.''

''Fine,'' you respond. ''It sounds as if we're making some progress.''

''We were!'' she retorts. ''I'm so mad at him I could just scream.'' She bends over and grabs her abdomen as a painful cramp hits her.

''What do you think you would like to do? How can you handle this better?'' you inquire.

''Maybe that shrink wasn't such a bad idea. If I don't do something, I might kill the %$@&*.''

''OK, it doesn't have to get to that. In the meantime, your emotions are just making you feel worse. Go see Dr. Borstein as I recommended and see if he can help you with the anger and the effect it's having on your abdominal symptoms. I'll call and talk with him. Would you like me to make the appointment?''

''Sure, anytime this week after 4 would be good,'' Heather responds, still grimacing from her pain.

Before you discharge her, you re-examine her abdomen to make sure nothing else is going on. Even patients with IBS can develop something acute or even life-threatening, such as appendicitis or an ectopic pregnancy. The background complaints may lull a clinician into dismissing a new presentation of pain as the same old condition when it is something more serious.

At her next visit, a month later, Heather comes in smiling. ''Doc Borstein was great. He just listened while I blew up about Corey and then suggested some ways to handle it. He also taught me some deep-breathing exercises and showed me some relaxation exercises that have really helped.''

''How have your bowel complaints been doing?'' you ask.

''That's what I mean,'' Heather replies. ''I have felt a lot better since I stopped being so mad about Corey. I'm also learning to handle stress better at work. Except for when I slipped and ate a pint of ice cream, my stomach really is doing better.''

You reinforce the dietary changes and regular exercise, and suggest a little chamomile tea at bedtime and as a substitute for coffee because it also has an antispasmodic effect (Robbers 1998). Heather suggests that she make her next appointment in 2 months rather than 1. You agree, and find that over the ensuing months she continues to have episodes of discomfort from time to time but nothing that she can't handle. They are less intense than before and do not last as long.

Table 23–4 ALTERNATIVE THERAPIES FOR IRRITABLE BOWEL SYNDROME (IBS)

Therapy	Best Evidence*	Probably Useful†	Least Evidence‡
Herbals	Peppermint (0.2 mL–0.4 mL enteric-coated oil b.i.d.–t.i.d./ac)	Caraway Chamomile (2–3 g/d; 3–5 mL tincture t.i.d.; as tea t.i.d.–q.i.d.) Fennel (colic, antispasmodic): tea 1 cup t.i.d., 600 mg caps t.i.d.; for infants, 2 tsp seeds t.i.d. (as tea) Garlic (antispasmodic: up to 3 g b.i.d.) Lemon balm Raspberry tea Sage (antispasmodic)	Oregon grape, yellow dock, wormwood
Diet and Nutrition/ Lifestyle	Lactase (for those with lactose intolerance) Lipase (pancreatic insufficiency) Fiber Food allergy: identify and eliminate if present; dairy and grain most common factors	Charcoal (excess gas) Lactobacillus acidophilus Refined sugar: reduce amount in diet	Proteolytic enzymes Vitamin A (up to 25,000 IU/d) Vitamin C (500 mg t.i.d.) Vitamin E (100 IU t.i.d.) Zinc (20 mg/d)
Mind-Body Interventions	Cognitive behavioral therapy Depression (functional bowel complaints), detect and treat Exercise Hypnotherapy Biofeedback Progressive muscle relaxation Psychotherapy Stress management		

Table 23–4   ALTERNATIVE THERAPIES FOR IRRITABLE BOWEL SYNDROME (IBS) *(Continued)*

Therapy	Best Evidence*	Probably Useful†	Least Evidence‡
Alternative Systems of Care		Traditional Chinese medicine herbals Acupuncture Ayurveda	*Homeopathy:* (follow label dosages) Argentum nitricum Asafoetida Colocynthis Lillium tigrinum Lycopodium Natrum carbonicum Nux vomica Podophyllum Sulphur

*Therapies with the highest degree of scientific support for efficacy and safety
†Therapies that are often helpful but that do not have the highest degree of supporting evidence for efficacy and safety
‡Therapies that may be useful but that have limited scientific evidence for efficacy and safety

Case Summary

Heather illustrates the benefit of a natural and holistic approach to a chronic problem. Many lifestyle factors often play a role in a chronic condition like IBS, and until they are all addressed, only part of the problem can be solved (Table 23–4).

Chapter

24   *Headache*

CURBSIDE CONSULT

Migraine Headache

■ Avoidance of precipitating causes, including food allergens (particularly chocolate, some cheeses, beer, and red wine), inhaled allergens, smoke, and air pollution

■ Management of stress, pain, and muscle tension with biofeedback, relaxation therapies, imagery, meditation, yoga, tai chi

■ Herbal therapies such as feverfew, ginger, and ginkgo

■ Other supplements such as vitamins B_2 and D, magnesium, and calcium

■ Acupuncture, acupressure, and other methods from traditional Chinese medicine (TCM) or Ayurvedic traditions

Chronic headaches are a very common affliction, often resistant to standard therapy. Though acute-onset headaches and certain kinds of headaches resulting in neurologic impairment may be associated with serious infectious, neoplastic, or inflammatory conditions, chronic headaches are generally benign, though bothersome. Each patient with headache needs to be assessed fully with standard diagnostic techniques including thorough history and physical. Some need specialized radiological imaging and otolaryngologic, neurologic, and psychiatric evaluations. Changes in the patterns and intensity of headaches may signal the change of a chronic headache to a more serious problem such as a ruptured aneurysm, a subdural hematoma, meningitis, or a neoplasm. Systemic conditions such as connective tissue disease, arthritis, allergy, hypertension, or the abuse of drugs or alcohol also can be contributing factors. Chronic daily headaches in patients who use analgesic medications such as acetaminophen and butalbital (Fioricet, Esgic) on a regular basis increasingly are being recognized as the result of analgesic withdrawal.

For the purpose of this book, I will limit my discussion to the two most common types of chronic headaches: vascular headaches, such as migraine, and tension headache. Each requires a different approach, although the types of alternative therapies that can be useful overlap somewhat.

MIGRAINE

Migraine headache is characterized by a pounding, unilateral headache often preceded by an "aura," or sensation of premonitory symptoms, such as visual and psychological disturbance, numbness, or tingling. The headache itself is often accompanied by not only severe, sharp, and throbbing pain but also photophobia, temporary loss of part of the vision, paresthesias, nausea and vomiting, and dizziness. It is followed by a period of fatigue and drowsiness. It may last from several hours to several days. In the acute phase, this is a "sick headache," very severe, all-encompassing, and a serious disruption to the life of the patient. Some chronic, less intense but persistent headaches are called "transformed migraines."

The exact etiology of migraine is unclear but it seems to be polyfactorial. Several lines of evidence suggest that it is related to an interaction among serotonin and other neurotransmitters such as substance P (a pain-related peptide), platelets, and vascular instability. It is much more common among women than men and runs in some families, suggesting a genetic influence. Certain factors such as stress, some foods, alcohol, and even changes in weather can precipitate a migraine. Fatigue, muscle tension, drug withdrawal, changes during the menstrual cycle, some chemicals, sinus problems, and eyestrain all can contribute to or trigger a migraine. With so many imputed causes and such a variety of precipitating factors, the migraine headache probably represents a spectrum of disorders with various presentations in different people.

Conventional treatment involves prophylactic therapy to prevent headache, abortive therapy to stop it at its onset, and ablative therapy to treat it in its full-blown manifestation. Prophylaxis is accomplished by the use of beta blockers or calcium channel blockers given regularly to prevent the onset of headaches and to decrease their frequency. Examples of abortive agents are caffeine, ergotamine derivatives, and serotonin agonists such as sumatriptan. Ablative agents include opioids such as meperidine, given to suppress or eliminate the full-blown attack once it occurs. In many cases, these medical approaches solve the patient's problem. For others, however, standard therapy does not sufficiently control the frequency of the headaches, their intensity, and their effect on the person's life. Let us look at a case of migraine that benefits from an integrative approach (Table 24–1).

Case Study: Migraine

Joan B. is a 28-year-old who has suffered with migraine headaches since adolescence. They are unilateral, almost always over the right side

Table 24–1 ALTERNATIVE THERAPIES FOR MIGRAINE HEADACHE

Therapy	Best Evidence*	Probably Useful†	Least Evidence‡
Herbals	Feverfew (0.25–0.5 mg parthenolide b.i.d.)	Ginger (4–6 g/d, 1.5–3 mL tincture t.i.d., 500 mg q.i.d. dried ginger; also treats nausea) Ginkgo biloba (40–60 mg t.i.d.)	Capsaicin intranasal Yucca
Diet and Nutrition/ Lifestyle	Vitamin B_2 (riboflavin) (400 mg/d for at least 3–4 mo)	Magnesium (250–400 mg t.i.d., especially for premenstrual migraine and those with low Mg levels) Calcium 800 mg/d Vitamin D 400 IU/d Avoid dietary amines, which provoke migraine: chocolate, cheese, beer, red wine Food allergy: detect and eliminate most common allergenic foods: dairy, wheat, chocolate, eggs Use elimination diet Vitamin B_6 (25 mg t.i.d.)	Fish oil, EPA/DHA S-adenosyl-L-methionine (SAMe) (400 mg q.i.d.; gradually increase dose from 200 mg b.i.d. to 400 mg q.i.d. over 3 wk) 5-Hydroxytryptophan (5-HTP) (100–200 mg t.i.d.)
Mind-Body Interventions	Relaxation therapy Biofeedback	Guided imagery Meditation Stress management Tai chi Therapeutic Touch Yoga	
Bioelectro-magnetic Therapies			Energy healing Magnets Transcutaneous electrical nerve stimulation (TENS)

Table 24–1   ALTERNATIVE THERAPIES FOR
MIGRAINE HEADACHE (Continued)

Therapy	Best Evidence*	Probably Useful†	Least Evidence‡

Alternative Systems of Care		Acupuncture
		TCM
		Ayurveda
			Homeopathy:
			Belladonna (6C q
			   30 min for 1½ hrs)
			Bryonia (6C q 30 min
			   for 1½ hrs)
			Gelsemium (30C q
			   30 min for 1½ hr)
			Kali bichromicum
			   (6C q 1 hr up to
			   6 doses, then t.i.d.)

Hands-on Healing Techniques			Chiropractic

*Therapies with the highest degree of scientific support for efficacy and safety
†Therapies that are often helpful but that do not have the highest degree of supporting evidence for efficacy and safety
‡Therapies that may be useful but that have limited scientific evidence for efficacy and safety

of her head and behind the right eye. She describes them as pounding, throbbing, and sharp, and they are accompanied by nausea and vomiting. She rarely if ever has a prodromal aura. Her mother and both sisters also suffer from migraine. She has found that her menstrual cycle, stress, and cigarette smoke aggravate her headaches, but the headaches often come at unpredictable times without clear-cut precipitating factors. She is a Southern Baptist and doesn't use alcohol, but she has found that some foods, particularly certain cheeses, chocolate, and dairy products, can sometimes trigger an attack. When she gets a headache, she takes a combination of butalbital and acetaminophen, along with promethazine for the nausea. These medications sometimes control her pain, but most times she just goes to bed in a darkened room and waits for it to pass, which can take from 12 hours to 3 days. Her husband, a physician assistant, encouraged her to start taking a beta blocker a couple of years ago for prophylaxis, but she quit taking it after a few months, claiming that it made her feel tired and didn't seem to help much. She has taken sumatriptan at the onset of a migraine on occasion with relief.

Joan comes in today, not for her headache, but because she has missed her period. A home pregnancy test was positive, and she has come for confirmation of pregnancy. Your exam and urine pregnancy test confirm the diagnosis of intrauterine pregnancy of 8 weeks' duration.

Then Joan asks about her migraines. "I don't want to take medication if I am pregnant. If I get a headache, what shall I do?"

Though you assure her that the medications she is taking are generally safe during pregnancy, you share her concern and want to minimize drugs during pregnancy, especially the sumatriptan, which is a relatively new agent. "Some types of migraine go away during pregnancy. Let's hope this will be the case for you, Joan," you tell her.

The next week, during her prenatal exam and counseling, she reports that she had a really bad headache during the week. She took some acetaminophen, which didn't help much, and went to bed. Because of the nausea, she wasn't able to eat or drink much for a couple of days. You see from her chart that she has lost a couple of pounds. You give her prenatal vitamins and a pregnancy information packet and set up a visit for a month later.

Before that visit, she calls to report that her headaches seem to be getting worse. She is missing work several days a week, can't tolerate the prenatal vitamins, and is not eating regularly. You advise her to come in for an evaluation.

You examine her to make sure that she has not developed a new problem besides the migraine, and you find that she has lost 2 more pounds. You confer with Joan and her husband Mark.

"What can I do?" Joan asks. "I don't think I can go through my whole pregnancy like this."

You express your concern as well. "Joan, I am concerned about the weight loss, inability to keep down the vitamins, and the progressive nature of the headaches. Though the usual medications you take can help, they never really broke up your headaches before."

"We really don't want her to take anything stronger while she's pregnant," Mark says. "Are there any herbs or anything that can help?"

"Feverfew, an herb used widely for preventing migraines, has not been proven safe in pregnancy [Robbers & Tyler 1999]. Several vitamins can reduce the nausea of pregnancy and we could try those when you get a headache with nausea. Vitamin B_6 [Vutyananich et al 1995] and over-the-counter antihistamine may help. But I have another idea," you tell them. "I have had good results with acupuncture in several patients with migraine. It can both break an attack and lessen the frequency and intensity" (NIH 1998).

"Is it safe during pregnancy?" Joan asks.

"Yes, though there are some points that we need to avoid because they can stimulate uterine contractions. We would treat you weekly at first, using points on your hands and lower legs, then space out the treatments as you improve."

Joan agrees, and over the next several weeks you administer

acupuncture using about a dozen needles at each session, including one for nausea, along with a low-frequency electrical stimulation of the needles. At one of the visits, Joan has a headache, but it is nearly gone at the end of the treatment. Gradually, she notes that the headaches are not coming as often or lasting as long. By the sixth acupuncture session, you have spaced her sessions out to every 2 weeks and she is headache-free between sessions. You continue to see her monthly for prenatal visits and do acupuncture prophylactically at each one, keeping the headaches at bay for most of the pregnancy.

She delivers a healthy 9-lb baby. At her postpartum check, 6 weeks later, Joan notes that her headaches are starting to return. Despite the benefit of the acupuncture, she prefers not to continue this approach now that the baby is born.

"I just don't want to take the time to come in with the baby and all, and besides, we found out Mark's insurance doesn't cover acupuncture. What else can we do?" Joan asks.

You suggest that she abstain from chocolate, milk, and cheese (dairy products provoke a high incidence of food allergy) (Pizzorno & Murray 1999), but remind her to get plenty of protein from other sources and to take a calcium supplement while breast-feeding. You also refer her to a local biofeedback expert, who teaches some simple techniques that seem to help her relax. You also prescribe supplemental magnesium and vitamin B_6.

"Once you are done breast-feeding," you say to her, "we can start you on feverfew to prevent migraines. It is widely used in Europe and Canada for this problem and is probably safe during breast-feeding, but we can wait until you're done nursing to start it."

Joan comes in with the baby at the 6-month checkup. Both mother and baby are fine, and she has been getting by with very few headaches.

"The relaxation and biofeedback really help, especially if the baby is keeping me up at night," she tells you (Shellenberger et al 1994). "Fatigue used to trigger headaches all the time. I was a little worried when my periods came back too, but so far, so good. Maybe it is the feverfew." She reports starting the herb about 2 months earlier, when she went back to work and tapered off nursing.

Case Summary

The special problems involved in pregnancy and nursing make this migraine case a bit more difficult to manage than most. The approach used is another example of a drugless approach to a chronic problem. Safe, effective, alternative therapies can be used for migraine, though often the best result comes from a combination of conventional and alternative therapies.

▬▬ TENSION HEADACHE

CURBSIDE CONSULT

Tension Headache
• •

- ■ Relaxation therapies and stress management: the relaxation response, progressive muscle relaxation, biofeedback, and imagery; also cognitive-behavioral therapy
- ■ Yoga, tai chi, and regular physical exercise
- ■ Massage, therapeutic touch, or osteopathic or chiropractic manipulation
- ■ Acupuncture, acupressure, and other methods from traditional Chinese medicine (TCM) or Ayurvedic traditions
- ■ Transcutaneous electrical nerve stimulation (TENS), magnets

Tension headaches, though not as severe as migraines, are much more common. They are characterized by a steady, dull or aching sensation, often arising from the back of the head or involving the forehead and temples. They may be described as squeezing or like a band or vise around the head. They are considered a result of chronic muscle contraction, which puts traction on nerves and connective tissue and impairs blood flow. Stress, poor posture, prolonged typing or other upper body activity in a fixed position, jaw clenching, temporomandibular joint (TMJ) dysfunction, and arthritis of the neck all may contribute to muscle contraction and tension headaches. Analgesic rebound also can play a role in tension headaches. As with migraine, tension headache must be differentiated from more serious causes of headache, but it is clinically less alarming and less likely to mask a serious condition. Excluding hypertension or other medical conditions as a cause of headache is essential to a good clinical evaluation.

Once the diagnosis of tension headache is made, treatment should be directed at relieving the underlying muscle contraction, structural abnormality, or stressful condition underlying the headache. Physical or hands-on therapies such as massage or chiropractic or osteopathic manipulation are useful, as are acupuncture and acupressure (Table 24–2). Relaxation therapies and stress management play a significant role in treatment. Some supplements, such as magnesium, also can be useful. Let's look at a case.

Case Study: Tension Headache

Peggy S. is a 31-year-old transcriptionist at a law firm. She spends her days typing at a computer workstation, usually for 6 to 8 hours at a time. Her workspace was evaluated by a specialist in occupational therapy, who looked at ergonomic factors such as lighting, screen size, height of

Table 24–2   ALTERNATIVE THERAPIES FOR TENSION HEADACHE

Therapy	Best Evidence*	Probably Useful†	Least Evidence‡
Diet and Nutrition/ Lifestyle		Magnesium (250 mg b.i.d.–t.i.d.)	
Mind-Body Interventions	Relaxation therapy Biofeedback Cognitive therapy	Guided imagery Meditation Progressive muscle relaxation Stress management Tai chi Therapeutic Touch Yoga	
Bioelectro- magnetic Therapies			Energy healing Magnets TENS
Alternative Systems of Care		Acupuncture TCM Ayurveda	*Homeopathy:* Belladonna (6C q 30 min for 1½ hrs) Bryonia (6C q 30 min for 1½ hrs) Gelsemium (30C q 30 min for 1½ hrs) Kali bichromicum (6C q 1 hr up to 6 doses, then t.i.d.)
Hands-on Healing Techniques			Chiropractic

*Therapies with the highest degree of scientific support for efficacy and safety
†Therapies that are often helpful but that do not have the highest degree of supporting evidence for efficacy and safety
‡Therapies that may be useful but that have limited scientific evidence for efficacy and safety

the keyboard, and chair position, because often simple adjustments in such factors can reduce workplace overuse injuries, but Peggy continues to have chronic headaches in her neck and the back of her head, which develop through the day. In the morning she has a minimal headache, but it starts up again in a repeat cycle each day. She takes naproxen or acetaminophen regularly, but when they wear off, her headache seems to come back worse than before. Muscle relaxants have helped temporarily, but she doesn't like them because they affect her thinking and her work requires accuracy and close attention to detail.

Your exam shows some localized tenderness at the base of her occiput and temples, and in the paracervical muscles. She has full range of motion of the neck and her neurologic exam is normal.

What Are Your Initial Recommendations?

Given Peggy's history, the nature of her headaches, and her normal neurologic exam, laboratory tests and x-rays are unlikely to be helpful. Her symptoms and findings are consistent with tension headaches.

One thing that might be helpful initially is to decrease her chronic analgesic use. The rebound nature of the headaches when her medication wears off is typical of analgesic withdrawal headaches. Thus, you suspect that Peggy is actually suffering from two types of headaches—tension and analgesic withdrawal. She is reluctant to stop her medications, however.

''If I don't take something, the pain is really bad and it is hard to get through work. I am afraid if I stop the medications, the headache will just be worse,'' she says.

You offer her a schedule of gradually decreasing the medications. She is willing to try. You also suggest a massage therapist who has worked with some of your patients (Field et al 1997). Peggy says she will try to make an appointment.

A few weeks later, she reports that decreasing the medication has actually helped her headaches. Although the massage felt really good and relieved her discomfort, she is still getting headaches at the end of each day of transcription.

What Else Can You Suggest?

Though acupuncture might be useful, you decide to try a referral to an osteopathic physician of your acquaintance. She starts doing weekly manipulation treatments on Peggy (Murray & Pizzorno 1998). You recommend magnesium (250 mg 3 times/day) for muscle relaxation (Mazzotta 1996) and some general stress-management techniques. You suggest that she get up from her chair at work several times a day to do neck rolls, stretching, and other measures to release tension in her neck (Benson & Stuart 1992).

A few weeks later, Peggy comes in for her annual well-woman exam and reports that her headache pain is reduced by 90%. Now and then she takes an aspirin or acetaminophen, but many days she takes nothing. Besides doing some neck manipulation on Peggy, your osteopathic colleague has recommended that she adjust the angle of her computer screen about 15 degrees. These measures seem to have made her more comfortable. She has gone through several days without pain and has been promoted to transcription pool supervisor.

Case Summary

Peggy's case illustrates several aspects of the management of tension headaches. In addition to addressing structural problems, drug rebound headaches, and ergonomic considerations, you were able to reduce this patient's chronic headaches by relaxation and muscle stretching, and perhaps magnesium and stress management. Although each case must be assessed individually to determine which component may be most significant, an integrative approach that addresses the problem from several sides often will help the patient when other methods have failed.

Chapter

25

Hypercholesterol-
emia

Heart disease, stroke, atherosclerosis, and vascular disease are all increased in the presence of elevated cholesterol in the bloodstream. Total cholesterol levels above 200 are considered abnormal. This is further subdivided into the relative amounts of HDL (high-density lipoprotein), LDL (low-density lipoprotein), and triglycerides (VLDL or very–low-density lipoproteins), and the ratios of total cholesterol to HDL and of LDL to HDL. Desirable levels for most lipids should not exceed the levels listed in the accompanying box. The level of HDL, however, the "good cholesterol" that returns fats back to the liver, ought be *over* 35 mg/dL. Some people have a familial tendency to a lower HDL and are at higher risk for the complications of cholesterol than are those with higher levels. Another lipoprotein, Lp(a), is related to LDL and causes adherence of LDL to the intimal wall of blood vessels and subsequent damage to the vessels. Levels of Lp(a) higher than 30 mg/dL increase the risk of heart disease.

Since the recognition in the 1980s of the contribution of cholesterol to vascular problems, many useful and potent pharmacological agents have been developed to reduce total cholesterol and triglyceride levels and to improve the cardiac risk ratios. These drugs are often helpful and effective, but I have seen significant controversy in the medical literature about their safety. Although I certainly prescribe lipid-lowering drugs regularly, concerns about liver toxicity, carcinogenicity, depletion of coenzyme Q10 levels, and a possible increase in all-cause mortality make me think twice before writing a prescription. An integrative approach offers alternatives for patients who prefer to avoid drug therapy, who have side effects while using it, or whose lipid levels are not adequately controlled by it.

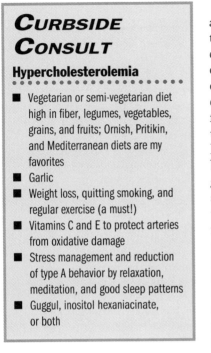

CURBSIDE CONSULT

Hypercholesterolemia

- Vegetarian or semi-vegetarian diet high in fiber, legumes, vegetables, grains, and fruits; Ornish, Pritikin, and Mediterranean diets are my favorites
- Garlic
- Weight loss, quitting smoking, and regular exercise (a must!)
- Vitamins C and E to protect arteries from oxidative damage
- Stress management and reduction of type A behavior by relaxation, meditation, and good sleep patterns
- Guggul, inositol hexaniacinate, or both

I have found the naturopathic approach to be most useful in treating the very common problem of hypercholesterolemia. These interventions overlap conventional therapies in recommending a number of lifestyle changes, such as reducing fat, fried foods, animal products, and cholesterol in the diet; increasing exercise; losing weight; consuming more fiber by eating fruits, vegetables, nuts, legumes, and whole grains; avoiding smoking; and reducing caffeine intake. Interestingly, nutritionists have noted that in the absence of an excess of calories, even fats in the diet are converted to acetone in the liver and then to harmless carbon dioxide and water. When too many calories are consumed, however, these same fats are reconstructed into cholesterol and other lipid moieties. These go on to wreak their negative effects on the vascular system by the accumulation of obstructing LDL-rich plaques within the arteries. Dietary changes thus are critical to lowering cholesterol (see "How to Lower Cholesterol with Diet").

Some people have conditions that make treatment of hypercholesterolemia more challenging. Among these are certain familial or genetic forms of dyslipidemias and untreated diabetes or thyroid disease. Those with untreated diabetes or untreated or undiagnosed hypothyroidism often have very high triglycerides, for instance. Management of the underlying problem will normalize the lipid levels. Recognition of special problems can lead to more appropriate treatment and expectations for outcomes. I have been working with one unhappy lady who has a severe form of familial dyslipidemia. Maximal pharmacological and lifestyle management has failed to reduce her total cholesterol below 350 mg/dL. Another woman in my practice has had nine angiograms, several angioplasties, and bypass surgery. At 48 years old, she, too, clearly has a resistant form of lipid disorder that has caused a persistent cholesterol level of more than 270 and premature atherosclerosis. Unfortunately, both women smoke, which further accelerates their vascular problems. Though these patients are unusual, such cases need to be identified and managed as well as possible, using both conventional and alternative therapies. Let us now proceed with a more typical case.

HOW TO LOWER CHOLESTEROL WITH DIET

INSTEAD OF THESE . . .	EAT THESE
High-fat dairy products, eggs, butter, lard	Skim or low-fat milk, yogurt, and cottage cheese; Egg Beaters, other egg substitutes, or tofu; vegetable-oil spreads, unsaturated vegetable oils (such as olive oil)
High-fat meats, hamburgers, sausage, bacon, lunch meats, hot dogs	Fish, chicken, turkey, lean cuts of beef or pork in small quantities
High-calorie and high-fat desserts, ice cream, and other rich sweets	Fruits
Refined and simple carbohydrates, cereals, white bread	Whole grains, granola (low-fat, unsweetened, or unprocessed), whole wheat breads, and other unprocessed cereals such as oatmeal
Fried or fatty "fast food" and snacks	High-fiber snacks like carrots, celery, other vegetables, salad
Salted foods and snacks	"Lite" salt, herbal seasoning, low-sodium products
Coffee, caffeinated, high-sugar soft drinks	Herbal teas, green tea, fruit or vegetable juice

Case Study: Hypercholesterolemia

John W. is a 44-year-old construction worker. He is from an Italian family with a high incidence of heart disease, peripheral vascular disease, and stroke. They prefer rich sauces and fried foods, and John's wife has cooked this way for him since they were married 20 years ago. A look into her shopping cart would find sausage, prepared cold cuts, potato chips, eggs, bacon, pork chops, steaks, hot dogs, and cheese, but few fresh fruits or vegetables except for salad preparations; John loves salad. When John visits your office, he has no current complaints but wants a checkup because his father, who is 63, has just suffered a myocardial infarction and was released from the hospital last week. John doesn't smoke but enjoys a glass or two of red wine, particularly with his wife's excellent pasta dishes. He doesn't do any regular fitness type of exercise, but his job is fairly active. "I'm just too tired to exercise after work," he says.

Your exam shows John to be about 20 lbs overweight, with normal blood pressure and pulse. He has a normal funduscopic exam without vessel changes, and no xanthelasma or carotid bruits. His heart and lung exams are normal. His abdomen is slightly obese, but you find no organomegaly or bruits. The peripheral pulses and EKG are normal, but on the blood testing you find that he has a cholesterol of 252 with an LDL of 190, HDL of 45, and triglycerides of 292 [Chol/HDL = 5.6 (N < 4.0), LDL/HDL = 4.2 (N = <2.5)]. The blood tests for renal, liver, and thyroid function and blood glucose are normal. John's urine shows trace protein but is otherwise normal.

What Are Your Initial Recommendations?

John's case is fairly typical. He is an overweight man with a strong family history of vascular disease and probably lipid problems, due to either lifestyle or genetics. His diet, though traditional for him and his family, is quite high in animal fats and low in essential fruits, vegetables, whole grains, and other antioxidants. Though his work is active, he needs to lose some weight and is unlikely to do so without some conditioning type of exercise. He inquires about taking a cholesterol-lowering drug, but you recommend starting with some lifestyle modifications instead.

Given John's normal exam, we can afford to initiate changes slowly and gradually rather than making too many at once, despite his family history and his abnormal lipid panel. The goal of lifestyle modification is enduring change, not just temporary risk reduction. You recommend that he lose a few pounds and take a daily walk. John readily agrees, wishing to avoid the problems his father has had with his heart.

To facilitate the weight loss, you recommend that he keep track of his diet, eating what he usually does for the next 2 weeks. You encourage him to bring in his wife at the next visit to review the diet diary.

In 2 weeks John and Anne come in together. She is a bit worried about his health, but not unduly so. John reports that he has been walking with Anne about 3 times a week and is happy to note that he has lost a couple of pounds. The diet diary you asked him to keep is incomplete but enough has been recorded to give you a general idea of his eating habits. They are about what you'd expect from the snapshot of his wife's shopping cart above. A typical day's diet:

Breakfast—coffee, two eggs, three slices of bacon, white toast with butter, fried potatoes, and orange juice

Morning snack—coffee and a sweet roll or donuts

Lunch (usually purchased from the lunch wagon that comes out to his construction site)—a couple of beef and bean burritos or a hamburger and chips, a soft drink, and a pastry

Dinner—salad, fried pork chops, mashed potatoes and gravy, corn on the cob with butter, a couple of glasses of Chianti, and a slice of pie. Some nights Anne makes spaghetti with meatballs or makes meat sauce from boiled pork neckbones. They usually have garlic toast with pasta, along with a salad, and maybe a vegetable.

"What do you think of this diet, John and Anne, now that we have found the high cholesterol levels?" you ask.

"Not so great, huh?" John admits.

Anne bristles a bit and says, "It's all he will eat! I've tried to make him eat more vegetables but he just won't touch them. If I cook differently, he just complains about it."

At this point, you have a number of challenges on the dietary side. First you must convince John of the importance of changing his diet and give him the information he needs to select a better mix of foods with lower cholesterol content. Another challenge is to recruit his wife, cook, and life companion to join you in helping John's lifestyle change. After all, if she doesn't bring home the bacon, fry the eggs, and boil the pork necks, he is unlikely to prepare them on his own. The very reason that you invited her to this visit was to partner with her in helping John make necessary lifestyle changes.

Though you punch up a couple of patient information sheets on low-cholesterol diets from the database in your office computer, you realize that an individualized approach is more likely to be effective. You recommend increasing John's regular intake of garlic to a clove or two daily (Warshafsky 1993, Jain 1993) and increasing the fruits and vegetables in his diet to include at least 7 portions each day. You make some practical suggestions, like having Anne pack a lunch with a salad and some fruit to replace the high-fat foods John had been buying at the construction site. You name a couple of books with tasty and healthful recipes, including excellent Italian dishes and pasta meals that use fish or chicken instead of higher fat meats (Brody & Flaste 1994, Moosewood Collective 1996, Schlesinger & Earnest 1990).

"How about my wine with dinner?" John asks as you rise to leave the room.

"A glass or two with dinner is fine," you reassure him. "In fact, it has been shown to increase your HDL, the good cholesterol, when taken in moderation [Hein 1996, Hendricks 1994, Rimm 1996]. And keep up the exercise. Let's see you in a couple of months."

When he returns his weight is down 5 more pounds, he is walking almost daily, and he has made a number of dietary modifications. You check his cholesterol and find that the total is down to 220 and triglycerides are down to 160.

What Do You Advise Next?

At this stage, I would encourage continued lifestyle measures with the diet and exercise plans previously outlined and encourage further weight loss; but John is still concerned about his cholesterol reading—although it's better—because of his family history and because his brother just had an abnormal stress test.

You have already worked with John and his wife to adopt a lower-fat diet. John has significantly reduced his fat intake. He eats fruit and whole-grain cereal for breakfast and has a low-fat yogurt, granola bar, or piece of fruit for mid-morning snack. He now carries his lunch, which may include a sandwich made with low-fat tuna, ham, or turkey; a salad; some fruit; and juice. Or he may have some raw vegetables, like baby carrots or celery, with a thermos full of homemade minestrone soup and some whole-grain bread from the new breadmaker he and his wife bought. Though he got a bit of a ribbing from the other construction workers for awhile, several of them have now started bringing their lunches and including healthier foods. The lunch wagon driver (30 lbs overweight himself and a heavy smoker) is not entirely pleased with this turn of events but has started to bring oranges, apples, bananas, yogurt, granola bars, noodles, and other healthier offerings on his truck. For dinner, John and Anne are eating fewer fried foods and animal products in general and more vegetables, pasta, salads, and soups. Their two teenagers grumbled for awhile, but after taking a health class in school, they realized that their family was eating in a healthier fashion, and they have been more enthusiastic about the new menu.

Despite these changes, John's lipid profile still puts him at risk, though he is doing better than before. Because of his concern and your experience that diet and exercise often will not reduce the cholesterol much further, you tell him to start taking niacin as inositol hexaniacinate (Head 1996, Murray 1995). You prescribe 500 mg 3 times/day to start. Another possible recommendation is an herbal product from the Indian mukul myrrh tree (*Commiphora mukul*), gugulipid 500 mg 3 times daily (Pizzorno 1999, pp. 680–681), but you keep this in reserve in case he cannot tolerate the inositol hexaniacinate or it doesn't work for him. You also tell him to take 500 mg of vitamin C and 400 IU of vitamin E twice daily for their antioxidant effects and protective benefit to his arteries (Rimm 1993, Frei 1991). Some nutritionally oriented practitioners also add flaxseed oil. You suggest 1 T daily drizzled over salad or cooked into other menu items to provide the cardiovascular benefits of its omega-3 and omega-6 fatty acids.

When you see John in another 3 months, his weight is down another 8 lbs, for a loss of almost 20 lbs in less than a year. He feels good and

Table 25–1 ALTERNATIVE THERAPIES FOR HYPERCHOLESTEROLEMIA

Therapy	Best Evidence*	Probably Useful†	Least Evidence‡
Herbals	Garlic (1–4 cloves/d, tabs 300 mg t.i.d. [4000–5000 µg of allicin], tincture 2–4 mL t.i.d.) Guggul (500 mg tab t.i.d. [5–10% gugulsterones or total of 25 mg t.i.d.]) Psyllium (5–10 g/d) Chinese red yeast rice (Cholestin) (*Monascus purpureus*) (2 600-mg capsules b.i.d.)	Artichoke (320 mg of std extract t.i.d.) Avocado Barley Evening primrose oil Flax seeds (20 g/d, 1 T flaxseed oil daily) Glucomann Pectin Plantain	Fenugreek (5–30 g with meals t.i.d. or 15–90 g once daily with a meal) Fo-ti (3–5 g/d as tea t.i.d., 500 mg tabs, up to 5 tabs t.i.d.) Ginseng Proanthocyanidins (grape seed extract, pine bark) Wild yam (2–3 mL tincture t.i.d., 1–2 tabs t.i.d.) Yogurt
Diet and Nutrition/ Lifestyle	Exercise 5–7 servings/d fruits and vegetables (source of bioflavonoids and beta carotene) Fiber Mediterranean diet Quit smoking Soy protein (30 g/d) Vegetarian diet Very low-fat diet (Ornish) Vitamin B_3 (niacin) (up to 3 g/d [potential hepatotoxicity]) Weight loss	Calcium (800–1000 mg/d) Coenzyme Q10 (100–200 mg/d) Fish intake (EPA/DHA omega-3 oils) Inositol hexaniacinate (500–1000 mg t.i.d.) Olive and canola oil Pritikin program Reduce intake of refined sugars Reduce caffeine intake Red wine or other form of alcohol (1–2 drinks/d) Selenium (200 µg /d) Vitamins B_5 (pantethine) (300 mg b.i.d.–q.i.d. esp. for diabetics, hypertriglyceridemia) Vitamin C (100–1000 mg/d) Vitamin E (100–800 IU/d)	Beta–sitosterol Brewer's yeast (2 T/d) Carnitine (1–4 g/d) Chitosan (3–6 g/d) Chromium (200 µg /d) Green tea (3 c/d) Lecithin Magnesium (400 mg/d) Mushrooms: shiitake, maitake Oats Octacosanol Vitamins B_6 (pyridoxine) (50 mg/d); B_9 (folic acid) (400 µg / d); B_{12} (cyanocobalamin) (1000 µg/d) (May lower homocysteine levels, alone or together) Quercetin (>35 mg/d) (apples, onion, black tea) Safflower oil

Table 25–1   ALTERNATIVE THERAPIES FOR HYPERCHOLESTEROLEMIA *(Continued)*

Therapy	Best Evidence*	Probably Useful†	Least Evidence‡
Mind-Body Interventions		Modifying Type A behavior, stress reduction, reducing hostility, time urgency, competitiveness Reducing chronic emotional arousal Improving sleep pattern Relaxation therapy	Meditation Qi Gong
Pharmacological and Biological Treatments			Chelation therapy
Alternative Systems of Care		Ayurveda Traditional Chinese medicine	

*Therapies with the highest degree of scientific support for efficacy and safety
†Therapies that are often helpful but that do not have the highest degree of supporting evidence for efficacy and safety
‡Therapies that may be useful but that have limited scientific evidence for efficacy and safety

has recently been promoted to foreman. His total cholesterol is 172, LDL 120, HDL 55 (Total/HDL = 3.1; LDL/HDL = 2.2).

The following year, you see him for a general physical. His lipid profile remains excellent and he is feeling well. He hands you a gift certificate for a meal for two at Anne's "Healthy Paisano" Italian restaurant.

Table 25–1 lists the alternative approaches to hypercholesterolemia.

Chapter 26

Hypertension

Hypertension is estimated to be present in up to 20% of the adult population in developed countries. Because it is much less frequent in underdeveloped countries, we can infer that it arises from some element of our lifestyles. The factors most commonly cited as contributing to hypertension are excess sodium and fat in the diet, obesity (there we go again . . . *too many calories!*), inactivity, stress, too much alcohol and coffee, and smoking.

Treatment of elevated blood pressure demonstrably reduces the risk of heart attack, stroke, and heart and renal failure. (The double insult to the kidneys of hypertension and diabetes is a leading cause of renal failure and the need for dialysis.)

Interestingly, about 20% of those with elevated blood pressure readings in the medical office have normal readings at home and elsewhere. This condition has been called "white coat hypertension." It is an important reason to obtain outside readings whenever possible, from a home BP cuff, a reading at the drugstore or a health fair, or from another health care provider such as a school or work nurse. I suspect that many of these "white coat hypertensives" are in a state of increased adrenergic tone and eventually may develop true hypertension. This idea recently was confirmed by a study in which these folks wore 24-hour ambulatory blood pressure monitoring devices. They showed a heightened response of blood pressure elevation during their day-to-day activities (Stassen et al 1997, Hornsby et al 1991).

I clearly recall the high numbers of stroke patients in our teaching hospitals when I was a medical student and resident. At that time, there were few drugs for hypertension, and its association with stroke and heart attacks was not so well known. We have become more and more sophisticated in our pharmacological approaches to hypertension, and there are now dozens of agents and several new, major classes of drugs used for this widespread condition. As we have learned to manage hypertension better, we have by no means eliminated strokes but our caseload has been reduced dramatically.

With the wide array of effective drugs available to treat hypertension, what is the role of alternative therapies in this condition? Why

Levels of Hypertension*
••••••••••••••••••••••

BORDERLINE ("HIGH NORMAL")
130–139 systolic
or 85–89 diastolic

MILD (STAGE 1)
140–159 systolic
or 90–99 diastolic

MODERATE (STAGE 2)
160–179 systolic
or 100–109 diastolic

SEVERE (STAGE 3)
≥180 systolic
or ≥110 diastolic

*In adults ≥18 yr

CURBSIDE CONSULT

Hypertension
•••••••••••••••••••••••

■ Low-sodium, high-potassium diet high in fruits (e.g., the DASH diet)
■ Less caffeine and fewer than 3 drinks of alcohol per day
■ No smoking
■ Weight loss
■ Aerobic exercise
■ Mind-body measures such as stress and anger management, deep-breathing exercises and meditation, religious attendance, social support
■ CoQ10, garlic, magnesium, calcium, hawthorn
■ Tai chi, yoga

should we use them at all? Isn't treatment just a simple matter of telling the patient to pop a pill?

You may be surprised to know that the standard of care for hypertension in the borderline to moderate range (see box) is not to initiate medication right away. Instead, nondrug therapies and lifestyle modification are considered first-line treatment. How do we manage a newly diagnosed hypertensive, a patient with borderline hypertension? Let's look at a case to illustrate an integrative approach.

Case Study: Hypertension

Tyrone W. is a 39-year-old African-American male who presents to your office for a work physical. He is on the local police department, where he has attained the position of sergeant. He feels well, but he does admit to some work-related stress since his promotion last year. His past medical history is notable only for the arthroscopic repair of a meniscus that was injured when he played college football. He is not taking any medications but does take a B-complex vitamin pill daily. He is married with three children. He smokes a cigar on occasion but not regularly, drinks 4 to 6 cups of coffee daily, and has 2 or 3 beers every night and more on the weekend. His diet is often composed of fast foods, and he often salts his food before tasting it. He used to exercise regularly, including lifting weights, playing racquetball, and running 3 miles a day, but he has quit working out in the past few months because of time pressures at work. His family history is positive for hypertension, stroke, heart failure, and lung cancer. Review of systems is entirely normal except for a 12-lb weight gain in the last year. When his cholesterol was checked last year, the total was 192.

He appears to be healthy and looks younger than his stated age. Vitals are weight 197 lbs, height 5′ 11″, pulse 74, BP 144/94, respirations 12, temperature normal. A funduscopic exam is normal, as are his ears, nose, and throat. He has no carotid bruit, jugular venous distention, or thyromegaly. His lungs are clear. His heart feels slightly hyperdynamic on the precordium, the apical pulse is in the mid-clavicular line, and the heart sounds are normal, with no murmur or extra sounds. His abdomen is soft, without organomegaly or renal bruits. The rest of the exam is normal.

What Do You Recommend?

First of all, a diagnosis of hypertension cannot be made by a single reading. To verify the diagnosis requires at least three separate elevated readings at least 2 weeks apart. In addition to ordering a cholesterol level and possibly a urinalysis, the proper step at this point would be to repeat Tyrone's blood pressure readings. You repeated the nurse's reading while doing his exam and found essentially the same value. You ask him to come in a couple of times over the next month to have your nurse take his readings. He replies that the doctor who comes to see prisoners at the jail will take his pressure if he asks him to do so. You agree with that plan and ask him to bring in the readings in a month or two.

"But with my family history and all, do you think I should do something about my blood pressure *now*?" Tyrone asks.

"We haven't made a diagnosis of high blood pressure, Tyrone, but several factors in your lifestyle concern me and may be putting you at higher risk for that diagnosis," you tell him. "Salting your food before tasting it can result in consuming as much as 10 g of sodium a day, more than 3 times the recommended amount, and can contribute to elevated blood pressure. The facts that you have quit running, have gained 12 lbs, and are under increased stress at work are all possible contributors to this elevated reading. In addition, the amount of coffee and beer you mention may bear some adjustment."

"Whew, that sounds like a lot of changes! Can't you just give me a pill or something?" Tyrone asks.

"I am not convinced yet that you have hypertension. Even if we make that diagnosis, the standard approach is to gradually modify lifestyle factors like those I have mentioned over at least a 6-month period and observe the effect. Many times, some simple changes will normalize readings and avoid the need for medication."

"That sounds OK. I just don't think I can do all those things at once," Tyrone tells you.

"Let's talk about it more at your next visit. In the meantime, why don't you slack off on the salt shaker and consider getting some exercise?" you advise.

"I can do that. I've been meaning to get back to running anyway. I have heard that exercise is one of the best things for stress," says Tyrone as you and he walk to the receptionist's desk together.

When he comes back in a couple of months, he brings with him several BP readings obtained at work. They are in the range of 128–140 over 82–89. Though these are not diagnostic of hypertension, they are definitely in the borderline area and call for further evaluation and treatment through lifestyle changes.

You tell Tyrone that his blood pressure is borderline and that no other intervention is needed right now besides exercising regularly; reducing his intake of salt, caffeine, and alcohol; and losing that extra 12 lbs. You give him a copy of the DASH diet (see Chap. 11), which emphasizes fruits, vegetables, and low-fat dairy foods, because its low levels of saturated fat and total fat have been shown to substantially lower blood pressure (Appel 1997). Tyrone seems less than satisfied with this approach and inquires about other options.

So far, the recommendations you have given Tyrone are standard therapy for managing his blood pressure. What are some of the nondrug alternative methods that can be integrated with the lifestyle prescriptions you have given him so far?

Relaxation and stress management have long been advised for lowering blood pressure. Although this makes intuitive sense, the scientific literature doesn't really show a dramatic benefit except in blacks (Johnston et al 1993, Schneider et al 1995, Jacob et al 1991). Because of his job-related stress and his ethnicity, you recommend to Tyrone that he learn and practice some form of relaxation therapy such as deep breathing and meditation. He readily agrees and acknowledges that it might help him control his temper, which has created problems at work and at home lately. You tell him to include plenty of garlic and onions in his diet, as both have shown a slight benefit for lowering blood pressure. Taking foods high in potassium—such as citrus, melons, berries, and bananas—and substituting potassium-containing "lite" salt for regular table salt will also help.

You also tell Tyrone about a number of supplements that may be helpful.

"Depending on how much you want to do, I would recommend supplementing with 500 to 1000 mg of vitamin C up to 3 times/day [Ness et al 1997], vitamin E 400 IU twice a day, magnesium 800 to 1200 mg/day [Kawano et al 1998], and 1500 mg of calcium daily, in the

Table 26–1 ALTERNATIVE THERAPIES FOR HYPERTENSION

Therapy	Best Evidence*	Probably Useful†	Least Evidence‡
Herbals		Garlic Hawthorn	Ginseng (1 g dried root/d) Guar gum (5 g t.i.d.) Yellow root Yucca
Diet and Nutrition/ Lifestyle	DASH diet Fiber Aerobic exercise Potassium in diet Quit smoking Reduce caffeine Low sodium Weight loss	Vegetarian diet CoQ10 (50 mg b.i.d.) Alcohol intake <3 drinks/d Calcium (800–1500 mg/d) Magnesium (350–500 mg/d [esp. if taking diuretics]) Fish oil, EPA/DHA, omega-3 fatty acids >3 g/d	Check for heavy metals, such as lead Reduce sugar intake Vitamin C Chitosan Arginine (2 g t.i.d.)
Mind-Body Interventions		Anger prevention or management Anxiety reduction (men) Guided imagery Meditation Music therapy Religious attendance Social support Stress management Tai chi Yoga	
Pharmacological and Biological Treatments			Chelation therapy
Alternative Systems of Care		Ayurveda Traditional Chinese medicine	Homeopathy

*Therapies with the highest degree of scientific support for efficacy and safety
†Therapies that are often helpful but that do not have the highest degree of supporting evidence for efficacy and safety
‡Therapies that may be useful but that have limited scientific evidence for efficacy and safety

citrate form. The calcium has been shown to be particularly helpful for someone like you, a black person whose blood pressure seems to be salt-sensitive [Resnick 1999]. You could also take a number of herbs and other supplements, such as hawthorn and coenzyme Q10 [Langsjoen et al 1994, Digiesi et al 1990], but I don't think your borderline pressure warrants this now," you advise.

"That sounds like a good plan. My wife has been after me to take more vitamins and eat less salt," Tyrone replies.

You encourage him to monitor his blood pressure at work a couple of times a month, which he does. He returns a year later for his checkup and his BP in your office is 130/80, with similar readings at work. He has lost about 10 lbs and continues to restrict his sodium and fat intake and exercise regularly. His total cholesterol is 168. He is managing stress much better and is handling his anger more productively. In fact, a larger neighboring town offered him a position on their police force with a substantial increase in responsibility and salary. He is considering it, although it means the children will need to change schools.

"I feel my health overall has improved a lot," he tells you, "not just my blood pressure. Thanks for the suggestions. I'll see you in a year, unless I need a new physical for my new position!"

◼◼◼◼ CONCLUSION

As with diabetes, cancer, and heart disease, alternative therapies for hypertension are best used as adjuncts to standard therapy. Those with moderately or severely elevated blood pressure will generally require medication, though adjunctive measures can be helpful in minimizing dosages. A problem with giving medication for borderline to mild hypertension is that people often won't make the necessary lifestyle changes. They often ask if they will need to take the medication forever, once it is started. I tell them that unless they modify their lifestyles, most likely they will need to take it indefinitely. I point out that, although taking prescription medication is vastly superior to leaving hypertension untreated, these medications have potential side effects such as impotence, fatigue, edema, constipation, cough, and electrolyte disturbances, not to mention their cost. These potential problems make a nondrug approach (Table 26–1) a wise first step.

As with any chronic condition, regular monitoring of hypertension and follow-up are essential. Such monitoring has been made easier by the availability of simple-to-use home blood pressure monitors.

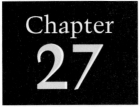

Chapter

27

Musculoskeletal Problems

Among the most common problems seen in any health care setting are musculoskeletal complaints. Every day, minor injuries from falls, overuse, sports, and work cause patients to come to the office seeking (1) reassurance that nothing is broken, (2) relief from pain, and (3) recovery of function. On top of this are the chronic, painful conditions such as backache, fibromyalgia, and muscle spasm that set up housekeeping in some of our patients.

Rather than try to cover all the kinds of musculoskeletal problems and alternative approaches in this chapter, I will give examples of both acute and chronic problems. These examples will give a flavor of the integrative approach to musculoskeletal complaints and offer some practical techniques you can start using right away with your patients.

Case Study: Acute Ankle Sprain

Bret W. is an active physician assistant student who plays on his school's intramural softball team. During a recent play-off game, he was stealing second base. As he slid into the base, his shoe caught on the ground and he twisted his ankle. He felt pain instantly but he was able to get up and walk around. Though he was happy to have stolen the base successfully, he asked the coach to put in a substitute runner, and he sat out the rest of game with his ankle elevated and packed in ice. The next day he hobbles into your office on crutches.

You obtain the history, asking about any prior injury to this ankle (there was none), and learn that he was able to bear weight on it after the injury. On examination, the ankle is swollen and tender, with a purplish discoloration on the lateral aspect. Your exam is limited by Bret's pain, but it shows point tenderness over the anterior talofibular ligament. Tests for joint laxity are negative.

"Do you think it is broken?" Bret asks worriedly. "We are in the middle of the play-offs and they want me to pitch in the next game."

"No, I don't," you respond. You order an x-ray anyway, mainly because of his anxiety and eagerness to get back to softball. The x-ray is negative for fracture.

What Do You Recommend?

The standard approach to an acute injury is the **RICE** method:

- **R**est
- **I**ce/**I**mmobilization
- **C**ompression
- **E**levation

You tell him to rest the injured ankle by avoiding weight bearing for a few days until he is more comfortable. The crutches are fine for this purpose, but you add an Aircast walking brace (Aircast, Inc., Summit, NJ), a molded plastic splint with interior inflatable segments that both immobilize and compress the area, preventing further injury and swelling. You also advise Bret to continue icing the area intermittently for another day and to elevate the ankle as much as possible.

Because of the upcoming play-offs, Bret asks if there is anything you can do to help him heal faster. Other patients are waiting, but you understand Bret's eagerness to get back to softball and his youthful impatience to be done with this annoying and inconvenient sprain. When you advise him that this kind of tissue injury will take up to 6 weeks to heal completely, he moans. He tries to negotiate with you about pitching next weekend, promising to have someone else run for him if he gets on base.

"I'm not the coach, Bret, but there are some things you can do to help yourself heal. When you go back to playing, how much you can do will depend a lot on how you feel. I'll be glad to re-evaluate you, of course, and help make a decision."

"Tell me what I can do," he pleads.

"I recommend *Arnica montana,* a homeopathic remedy for reducing the swelling and pain. Comfrey poultices or arnica ointment can also help, but don't take either arnica or comfrey internally, except for the highly diluted homeopathic version [Lininger et al 1999]. Something you can take by mouth is bromelain, a pineapple-derived enzyme, which will help reduce swelling [Lininger et al 1999]. Take one capsule 4 times/day until the swelling and pain are improved."

"That sounds good. Anything else?"

"As soon as the soreness subsides, start doing some gentle mobilization exercises to stretch the tissue. And you may want to take extra vitamin C to help with tissue healing [Kanter 1998]. I also know a local osteopathic physician who enjoys sports medicine, and she uses a technique called 'strain-counterstrain' to relieve acute pain and spasm quickly following a sprain. You may want to call her."

"I'm on it," he says. "I've got to get ready for the game this weekend."

You have your doubts about his pitching this weekend, but you figure that the injury was only a grade-1 sprain without any ligamentous damage, so it should heal relatively quickly. Bret's motivation to get back to his softball tournament and the absence of prior injury predict a good outcome.

The following week he comes in smiling.

"We won the game! I pitched six innings, and with our great fielders, they only scored two runs to our six. Next week we play the Family Medicine team. They're tough, I hear. By the way, that osteopath was on vacation but my buddy recommended a local acupuncturist. He stuck some needles in my ankle and toe, and even one in my face. I felt a lot better by the next day. I also took the homeopathic remedy and the bromelain like you said, and they seemed to help, too."

You examine the ankle and note with satisfaction that the swelling and tenderness are almost gone. Bret has stopped using his crutches, but he is still wearing the Aircast brace. You give him a patient education handout explaining some mobilization and weight-bearing exercises. A couple of weeks later you see a report in the campus newspaper saying that the physician assistant team won the play-offs and that Bret pitched the last three innings of the final game.

Case Summary

Though many minor sprains and strains resolve with little intervention, athletes are often eager, as in this case, to return quickly to their regular activities. Limiting their sports activities too much is a mistake, but this must be balanced with the potential mistake of returning them too early and risking re-injury or more serious injury. In this case, the ankle was protected and the modified activity of pitching without running allowed him to participate. (He missed fielding a bunt because of his ankle, but his pitching was so good, his teammates forgave him.) At times, we have to prescribe a different sport to maintain fitness, such as a regimen of weight training, cycling, or swimming for a runner with a grade-2 ankle sprain. This is always more acceptable to an athlete than just sitting around waiting for things to heal. And as illustrated by this case, alternative therapies may be useful even for an acute injury, both psychologically and structurally (Table 27–1).

Case Study: Chronic Low Back Pain

Manuel L., a 43-year-old man previously seen by you only for an annual physical, comes in because of back pain. A couple of months ago he suffered a back injury at his work as a longshoreman. He was helping to unload a ship when a load of bananas shifted and caught him off balance. He was thrown back with a twisting injury and felt immediate pain in his lower back, radiating to his left leg. A herniated disc was suspected, and he was taken off duty for 6 weeks while his symptoms gradually improved. At the end of this period, about 2 weeks ago, he had minimal residual pain and no neurologic signs, so he was returned to limited duty. He continued to take ibuprofen regularly, as prescribed by the company doctor who saw him initially.

Now he comes in to see you, complaining of increasing back pain and protesting that "where I work, there is no such thing as light duty."

You order an aggressive program of back-strengthening exercises, stretching, range-of-motion exercises, and physical therapy. He remains off work. A month later he comes in for a recheck, still complaining of pain despite the therapy. You refer him to an orthopaedic surgeon, who orders an MRI. It confirms your initial impression of a herniated disc, though it shows only minimal impingement on the spinal cord and left L4 nerve root. The surgeon recommends continued physical therapy and further rest from work. He also prescribes a transcutanous electrical nerve stimulator (TENS) unit for Manuel and gives him a prescription for hydrocodone and acetaminophen.

Manuel sees you a month later, now almost 4 months since his injury. The TENS unit helped a bit initially but doesn't seem to be doing much now. He is taking 4 to 6 hydrocodone tablets a day and goes to physical therapy 3 times/week, but he feels he is still in too much pain to go back to his heavy work as a longshoreman. He has no other job skills and barely finished high school after he emigrated to the United States from Mexico 30 years ago.

Table 27–1 ALTERNATIVE THERAPIES FOR MUSCULOSKELETAL PROBLEMS

Therapy	Best Evidence*	Probably Useful†	Least Evidence‡
Herbals	Arnica ointment/gel (topical) Tiger balm White willow (salicylate)	*Topical agents for wound and tissue healing, pain:* Aescin (horse chestnut) Aloe gel Angelica Calendula Comfrey Echinacea St. John's wort oil Tea tree Witch hazel Wintergreen oil Curcumin (anti-inflammatory)	*Tissue and wound healing:* Cat's claw Gotu Kola Aromatherapy Lavender, camphor, eucalyptus, chamomile, rosemary *Athletic performance enhancement:* Asian ginseng, eleuthero Guarana
Diet and Nutrition/ Lifestyle	Stretching, conditioning, warm-up to prevent injuries Bioflavonoids: citrus (900–1800 mg/d [improves healing time of injuries]) Enzymes: bromelain (500 MCU q.i.d. [proteolytic, anti-inflammatory])	Calcium (800–1000 mg/d [bone, muscle injury]) Magnesium (300 mg t.i.d. [muscle spasm, injury]) Vitamin C (400–3000 mg/d [connective tissue support, muscle damage]) Vitamin E (400–1200 IU/d [muscle damage]), topically for scars Eliminate food allergy (may worsen inflammation)	*Tissue/wound healing:* Vitamin A Copper, managanese, silicon, zinc Chondroitin sulfate Glucosamine sulfate Arginine, glutamine, l-carnitine *Bursitis:* Vitamin B$_{12}$ (1000 µg q.d. for 2–4 wk IM or subcutaneously) *Fibromyalgia:* Vitamin B$_1$ (10–100 mg/d) Magnesium (300–600 mg/d) Vitamin E (100–300 IU/d) D,L-Phenylalanine (500–750 mg t.i.d. [for pain]) *Enhancing athletic performance:* Antioxidants, B-complex vitamins, chromium, zinc, iron, magnesium, branched-chain amino acids, carnitine, pyruvate whey protein, leucine, inosine, ornithine, ornithinine alpha-ketoglutarate, glutamine, creatine, gamma oryzanol, medium-chain triglycerides

Table 27–1   ALTERNATIVE THERAPIES FOR MUSCULOSKELETAL PROBLEMS (Continued)

Therapy	Best Evidence*	Probably Useful†	Least Evidence‡
Mind-Body Interventions	Regular exercise, stretching Tai chi Yoga	Biofeedback Guided imagery Hypnosis Music therapy Qi Gong Relaxation therapy Spiritual interventions	
Pharmacological and Biological Treatments			Hydrotherapy (add essential oils, Epsom salts) Spa therapy DMSO topically
Bioelectromagnetic Therapies	TENS unit	Energy medicine Healing touch Reiki Therapeutic Touch	Hyperbaric oxygen Light therapy Magnet therapy
Alternative Systems of Care		Acupuncture Acupressure Traditional Chinese medicine: cupping Ayurveda: massage, oil, herbal techniques	Homeopathy: *Broken bone support:* Arnica (30C q 15–30 min for 2 hr, then t.i.d. for 2 d) Ruta graveolens (6C t.i.d. for 2–3 d) *Sprains and injuries:* Arnica (30C t.i.d.–q.i.d. for 2–3 d) Ruta graveolens (6C t.i.d. for 2–3 d) Ledum (30C t.i.d. for 2–3 d) *Bursitis:* Rhus toxicodendron (6C t.i.d.–q.i.d. for 3–4 d) Ruta graveolens (6C t.i.d. for 3–4 d) Belladonna (6C t.i.d.–q.i.d. for 1–2 d)
Hands-on Healing Techniques		Craniosacral Feldenkrais Rolfing Trager	Chiropractic Massage Osteopathy

*Therapies with the highest degree of scientific support for efficacy and safety
†Therapies that are often helpful but that do not have the highest degree of supporting evidence for efficacy and safety
‡Therapies that may be useful but that have limited scientific evidence for efficacy and safety
MCU = Milk clotting units.

What Other Treatment Options Do You Have?

At this stage, Manuel is approaching a critical point with his back pain. The acute problem has become chronic. Those who fail to return to work within 6 months of a back injury rarely ever do so, most often becoming disabled permanently. The scenario is all too familiar: an increasingly poor quality of life with a cycle of pain, habit-forming analgesic drugs, sometimes unsuccessful back surgery, depression, disability insurance payments reducing the motivation to return to work, and high use of the medical system.

You decide to continue his physical therapy, send him to a pain clinic, get a second opinion from another back surgeon or neurosurgeon, repeat his MRI, add amitryptiline to his medications to try to reduce his narcotic use, and start a work-hardening program. All of these are reasonable options and have some degree of success.

While these referrals are in the works, however, you decide to move ahead with a parallel plan of integrative care. After getting approval from his workmen's compensation plan, you refer him to a local acupuncturist. You also set him up with a psychologist who uses biofeedback to reduce pain, spasm, and anxiety (Schneider 1987). A local class in yoga is just getting started, and you recommend that he enroll to improve his flexibility, strength, pain control, and ability to move more normally after months of discomfort (Telles et al 1997, Nespor 1989). You prescribe calcium and magnesium supplements to reduce his back spasms and vitamin C to improve tissue healing.

At this point, Manuel has a new full-time job—getting his back well. Despite his disability payments, he tells you that he really wants to get back to work; at 50% of his previous income, the payments do not meet his family's financial needs. His wife has had to start work to help make up for the lost income. You decide to follow him closely and see him in 2 weeks. The acupuncture relieved some of his pain, even after one treatment. He tells you that the yoga stretches feel more helpful than the standard physical therapy exercises, which he has been doing for months. He hasn't met yet with the biofeedback specialist, but the neurosurgeon has reassured him that the disc in his back, though still bulging, does not require surgery. Manuel has reduced his hydrocodone to a bedtime dose only but continues taking the ibuprofen during the day. He tells you that a friend's daughter is a massage therapist and has offered to give him massage treatments, but he wanted to check with you first.

Where Are We Now in His Treatment?

Though he is still having pain, the encouraging thing is that Manuel has reduced his narcotic use. The second opinion from the surgeon is also a relief; you have seen many chronic back pain patients who still have pain after one or more surgeries. Work-hardening will help him condition his back and improve his lifting habits so that he will be in optimal condition when (and if) he goes back to work. The early response to acupuncture is also heartening, but it is too early to draw any conclusions.

At this point, while you are using many different modalities to try to turn this problem around, frequent visits are useful. You tell him to come back in 2 weeks and that, yes, a massage from a licensed massage therapist can often be helpful for back pain (Pope et al 1994, Weintraub 1992). You write a prescription for it so it will be covered by his accident policy. You tell him to continue with the yoga and acupuncture. He has an appointment for biofeedback that afternoon, and you encourage him to keep it.

At the next visit, he continues to express his satisfaction with the results of the acupuncture and yoga and says the massages have been really helpful as well. He didn't like the biofeedback approach, and after two sessions decided it wasn't for him. His pain is better, so he has stopped his hydrocodone but still takes an ibuprofen most nights.

You check him every couple of weeks for another month or so. After the 8-week work-hardening program is over, workmen's compensation sends you a form inquiring if he is at MMI (maximum medical improvement). You re-examine him and find him to be free of limitations in terms of pain, range of motion, or strength, and recommend that he return to work. He reminds you about the absence of limited duty at the docks, so you call his foreman to discuss it.

The foreman likes Manuel, who was a very good worker before his injury. He is willing to use him to check inventory, do some cleanup around the warehouse, and move some lighter things. You advise that, until you see how he responds to a return to the workplace, Manuel should not lift anything over 25 lbs and should not do repetitive lifting for longer than 1 hour, as the work-hardening program recommended.

At his next visit, Manuel reports a little stiffness at the end of the workday, but says he is doing well. He feels that it is helpful to continue to see the acupuncturist and masseuse weekly. He also does yoga and back stretching every day. You decide to release him to full duty and see him again in a month. He is apprehensive about his future; this incident has made him realize how dependent his family is on him and his physical health.

Three months later, he not only feels fine, but he has enrolled in an evening program in electronics at a technical school. He is continuing his yoga exercise but no longer has regular acupuncture or massage, though he still goes in for an acupuncture treatment or massage "tune-up" if his back starts to act up.

Case Summary

This case shows how severely a chronic back problem can affect a person's life, not only physically but also financially, psychologically, and socially. A prolonged back problem can reach a critical point at which long-term pain and disability will result if the problem is not resolved soon. The many modalities that may be used at this point are reminiscent of the way a team of professionals may join in various activities to get a patient through an acute emergency room event.

This case also shows that not every modality is equally preferred or acceptable to each patient. Manuel enjoyed and benefited from the massage but not the biofeedback. He was willing to go to an acupuncturist but was not interested in surgery. The key to successful treatment is for the primary care provider to recognize the slippery slope toward chronicity and respond with a plan acceptable to the patient.

If Manuel had come to you as a new patient who had been off work for nearly a year, had already had back surgery, and was taking narcotics daily, the problem would have been more difficult to treat. But you might have addressed it in a similar way, offering him multiple modalities such as massage, physiotherapy, acupuncture, and perhaps osteopathic or chiropractic treatment. At that point, the disability lifestyle would have been more firmly established, and psychological intervention, retraining, detoxification, and graded work-hardening may all have played a role in the rehabilitation process.

In the acute phase of Manuel's injury, it might have been helpful to introduce some of the therapies earlier, such as chiropractic (Shekelle et al 1997, Carey et al 1995), acupuncture (MacDonald et al 1983, Thomas et al 1994), and massage (Field et al 1997). Clinical outcome studies are now in progress to verify their early benefit, so it is too soon to know whether this will be become the standard of care in the future. Some argue that watchful waiting is more cost-effective than such an intense intervention program, because as many as 90% of back injuries, even the more serious ones involving a ruptured disc, resolve within 6 months. The difficulty lies in knowing which 10% of back pain patients will go on to chronic pain and disability. In the meantime, safe and helpful alternative therapies should be offered to patients whose pain is not resolving through conventional methods.

Chapter 28

Upper Respiratory Infection

The common cold is a benign but bothersome affliction that affects many children and adults up to several times a year. Caused by a variety of viruses, this condition is usually self-limited within a week or so but occasions huge numbers of visits to health-care settings. Many times, the suffering adult or anxious parent of an sick child falsely believes that an antibiotic can speed the resolution of the infection and its familiar symptoms of runny nose, cough, fever, fatigue, body aches, and general malaise.

One of the challenges of clinical training is to properly diagnose secondary bacterial infections such as otitis media, sinusitis, bacterial tonsillitis, meningitis, or pneumonia, which may initially present similarly. These do require treatment with antibiotics and are outside our focus.

Allergic rhinitis is another common problem masquerading as a cold. It may be distinguished by its chronic nature, clear nasal discharge, itching of the eyes, absence of high fever, and blue to white, boggy nasal passages versus the red, inflamed mucosa found in infections.

Most often a tincture of time, rest, fluids, and chicken soup are as effective as any over-the-counter or prescription agent. Nonetheless, many alternative therapies have been proposed and used for the common cold (Table 28–1). This chapter will discuss the most common of these and present a rational approach to the treatment of upper respiratory infections.

Table 28–1   ALTERNATIVE THERAPIES FOR UPPER RESPIRATORY INFECTIONS

Therapy	Best Evidence*	Probably Useful†	Least Evidence‡
Herbals	*Echinacea:* 3–5 mL tincture or juice t.i.d. 300-600 mg caps t.i.d. Dried root or as tea 0.5–1.0 g t.i.d.	Garlic (300 mg [4000–5000 µg allicin] t.i.d., 1–4 cloves/d) Goldenseal (4–6 g t.i.d.)	*Immune support:* Asian ginseng, astragalus, eleuthero, schisandra *Antiviral/antibiotic:* Elderberry, horseradish, myrrh, usnea *Symptomatic relief:* Slippery elm, marshmallow, red raspberry, blackberry, blueberry, sage, yarrow, eucalyptus oil, meadowsweet *Aromatherapy*
Diet and Nutrition/ Lifestyle	Avoid exhausting exercise Bedrest Drink large amounts of fluids	Vitamin C (1–3 g/d) Avoid dietary allergens *Gargle:* Salt water and vinegar Hot water with lemon juice and honey	Zinc gluconate or gluconate-glycine lozenges (10/d until better) L-Lysine (4–5 g/d initially, then 500 mg t.i.d. for cold sores; L-lysine cream) Vitamin A (15,000–25,000 IU/d [unless pregnant]) Beta carotene (50,000–100,000 IU/d)
Mind-Body Interventions	Social support Stress management and awareness		
Pharmacological and Biological Treatments	Control respiratory allergies with antihistamines, nasal steroids, avoidance of allergens	Hyperthermia	
Bioelectromagnetic Therapies			Energy medicine Hydrotherapy Magnet therapy

Table 28–1   ALTERNATIVE THERAPIES FOR UPPER RESPIRATORY INFECTIONS (Continued)

Therapy	Best Evidence*	Probably Useful†	Least Evidence‡
Alternative Systems of Care		Ayurveda Traditional Chinese medicine Acupuncture Cupping	*Homeopathy:* Aconite (30C q 2 h for 3 doses only) Kali bichromicum (6C t.i.d.–q.i.d. for 2–3 d) Rhus toxicodendron (6C t.i.d. for 1–2 d) Natrum muriaticum (6C q 2 hrs up to 6 doses) Euphrasia (6C q.i.d.)
Hands-on Healing Techniques		Percussion	

*Therapies with the highest degree of scientific support for efficacy and safety
†Therapies that are often helpful but that do not have the highest degree of supporting evidence for efficacy and safety
‡Therapies that may be useful but that have limited scientific evidence for efficacy and safety

THE INFLUENCE OF STRESS

It is important for you to realize the connection between the occurrence of colds and life stressors. Because we are all exposed to viral agents regularly, especially in the colder months, why doesn't everyone catch a cold? Why does a person come down with an infection at a particular time? The immune system is the key to resisting any infection. When immunity is depressed for any reason, a person is more prone to getting a cold or secondary bacterial infection (McEwan et al 1993, Cohen et al 1991).

Stressors such as lack of sleep, poor diet, work or relational difficulties, or a recent loss may be obvious to patients. Sometimes colds and other illnesses can occur in the wake of long-standing stress, because an initial heightened immune reaction provoked by stress is followed by depleted immunity (Klein 1993). Scales that attempt to quantify stress show that the accumulation of a certain number of stress "points" in a year is highly associated with the occurrence of acute illness (Holmes et al 1967). We should help our patients understand the connection of stress to upper respiratory infections for several reasons:

■ Recognizing a cold as a marker of stress encourages patients to take measures to recover from the stress and prevents them from adding new tasks and responsibilities that could compound it.

■ Ignoring stress that is announced by the arrival of a cold may make patients more prone to a variety of other, more serious illnesses, perhaps even cancer or heart disease, because stress accumulates over time.

■ Realizing that their lifestyle choices affect their health in even such a simple condition as an upper respiratory infection keeps patients from feeling like victims of illness and helps them realize that they can make healthier choices.

▨▨▨▨ OTHER FACTORS

Other factors besides stress contribute to colds, of course. A diet high in sugar can suppress the uptake of vitamin C into white blood cells (Sanchez et al 1973). Allergy to foods such as dairy products, especially in children, can produce more mucus and make a cold more likely or more difficult to treat. Exposure to extremes of temperature and drafts can certainly deplete immune reserves. (Chinese practitioners refer to this as an invasion of "cold and wind.") In cold climates, people cluster indoors during the winter months, increasing the concentration of viruses excreted and aerosolized through coughs and sneezing. Thus more people may be exposed.

Influenza immunization can definitely prevent or reduce the severity of the respiratory "flu," which is a certain kind of upper respiratory infection that can be severe, especially in the elderly and immunocompromised. Therefore, flu shots are recommended every fall for those who are older than 65, who have a cardiac or respiratory condition, or whose immunity is impaired by other illnesses such as diabetes or HIV disease.

Case Study: Upper Respiratory Infection

Mona K. is a 27-year-old waitress who comes into your office with signs and symptoms of a cold, including cough, nasal congestion, headache, low-grade fever, and "just feeling miserable" for the past 2 days. She has been working long hours at the diner because one of the other waitresses has been off for surgery. She reports that a lot of her customers seem to be coughing, and their cigarette smoke bothers her, even though she smokes half a pack a day herself. Her two children, ages 3 and 6, have also had colds. In the past month, Mona has finalized a divorce; she retains custody of her children. Her mother helps her take care of the two children and has moved into their small apartment. Mona's general health has been good, though at her well-woman exam 3 months ago she reported feeling fatigued.

"Can you give me an antibiotic or something to get over this?" Mona asks you.

What Are This Patient's Risk Factors?

As with any illness, many factors may contribute to a cold. In Mona's case, she not only has been working long hours but also has been exposed at home and at work to lots of people with colds. She smokes, which dries out her mucus membranes and depresses her local and systemic immunity. Her recent divorce is a major stressor as well.

After examining her ears, nose, throat, and lungs, you tell her that she just seems to have a cold, and although it is making her feel miserable, antibiotics really won't help.

What Do You Recommend?

You recommend rest; drinking plenty of fluids like chicken soup and juices; and taking echinacea (Dorn et al 1997, Blumenthal 1998 pp. 121–123), big doses of vitamin C, at least 3 to 4 g/day (Murray & Pizzorno 1998 p. 373, Hemila et al 1995, Hemila 1992), and perhaps zinc lozenges, but only the kind sweetened with glycine, not mannitol, sorbitol, or citric acid because they do not deliver adequate levels of ionized zinc (Pizzorno & Murray 1999 p. 1588, Mossad et al 1996, Zarembo et al 1992). You tell her that inhalation of fragrant oils like eucalyptus, peppermint, or tea tree also can bring relief in colds and flu, and though no firm evidence exists, many people prefer the safe homeopathic remedies. Even acupuncture and acupressure can help resolve symptoms.

"I need a rest but can't take time off work just now," Mona replies. "I really need the job since the divorce."

"How has that been for you, Mona?" you ask kindly.

A tear comes to her eye as she responds, "Pretty rough. If it weren't for Mom moving in to help with the kids, I don't know what I'd do. Still, the kids are cranky and haven't adjusted well, and the apartment is just too small. Some days I don't know how I'm going to make it."

"Often, Mona, a lot of stress like you've been having really builds up and makes you more prone to colds, flu, and other illness," you advise.

"Really?" she asks, "I thought colds just get passed around from other people that have them."

You explain briefly that her immune system has been under assault from the stressors in her life, making a cold almost inevitable for her. You also use this moment to encourage her to quit smoking. You urge her to make a follow-up appointment to address these issues after she is feeling better.

She agrees that this is a good idea and asks, "What is echinacea and how do I take it?"

"It is an herb that helps your white blood cells fight infection. It is available in most pharmacies, grocery stores, and health food stores. Look on the bottle for the dose. I recommend 300 mg 3 times/day of the capsules, or 2 to 3 mL of the juice. The tea form is also helpful and relaxing."

A couple of weeks later, Mona brings one of the children with asthma in for treatment. After examining the child and recommending some home remedies (Lewith et al 1996, see Chapter 19), you talk with her about her personal stress level and that of the whole family. You recommend a single-parent support group at a local church, which provides child care during the sessions. You also recommend a couple of self-help books and make some recommendations on quitting smoking. Mona says she appreciates your concern and is glad to know that there are things she can do to help herself.

Case Summary

You may think that I have gone on too long about Mona's stress rather than discussing the viral causes of upper respiratory infections. I believe a holistic approach includes more than zinc lozenges, vitamins, and echinacea. Helping patients identify the underlying insults to their immunity that precede a cold is potentially more effective as a long-term solution than simply addressing the cold symptoms. The symptoms of a cold might just be a cold, or they might be symptoms of another life dysfunction, as in Mona's case (Cohen et al 1997 pp. 59–72, Cohen et al 1997 pp. 1940–1949, Klein 1993).

Some patients really are not ready for this kind of discussion about the parallel between a common cold and other factors in their lives. They may just want you to give them a prescription. But an illness often presents a "teachable moment." The discomfort of an acute illness is an irrefutable event and can be the stimulus for your patients to quit smoking, get more rest, or handle stress better if you can draw a clear-cut association for them. This may be your best opportunity to influence the future lifestyle choices of your patients. Don't simply hand out a prescription for a decongestant and let it pass by.

Chapter 29

Urinary Tract Infections

CURBSIDE CONSULT

Urinary Tract Infections
● ●

■ High fluid intake, urination after intercourse
■ Cranberry or blueberry juice
■ Uva-ursi
■ Homeopathic remedies

Although bladder infections are hardly a leading cause of mortality in our society, they can be a source of recurrent discomfort and can lead to more potentially serious problems such as pyelonephritis, renal damage, and urosepsis, a life-threatening infection of the blood. Infections in childhood require evaluation for obstruction and other anatomic causes. The vast majority of cases occur in healthy women in the years between adolescence and menopause. These infections also occur in elderly patients, who are prone to obstruction from problems such as prostatism, incontinence, and indwelling catheters. The infections are often more serious in this age group.

I wish to focus this chapter on the very common problem of urinary tract infections (UTIs) in the otherwise healthy woman patient. The symptoms of cystitis are burning on urination; increased frequency; foul-smelling, cloudy, or bloody urine; and pain in the lower abdomen. Bladder infections are increasingly common after the commencement of sexual intercourse; the diagnosis of "honeymoon cystitis" is well-known to health care practitioners. Many women suffer from several infections a year. The standard of care is to prescribe an antibiotic, which is generally quickly effective. Over-the-counter products containing pyridine derivatives can relieve symptoms by providing a local anesthetic effect, but they do not eliminate the bacteria, usually *Escherichia coli*, that cause the infection. On the other hand, antibiotics may cause problems for the patient, commonly an antibiotic-induced vaginal yeast infection. Drug allergy is another potential problem. Taking a good history of medication allergy can reduce the likelihood of problems, but there is always the risk of newly developing allergy, particularly with repeated use of an antibiotic. Keep in mind that women experienced bladder infections for centuries before the discovery of antibiotics. Most cases have been self-limited, although the risk of complications of upper tract infections has always been present.

A naturalistic approach is well-known to patients: increase fluids and drink cranberry juice. The increased fluid flow through the bladder serves to dilute the urine and bacterial concentrations. A half-gallon of

Table 29–1 ALTERNATIVE THERAPIES FOR URINARY TRACT INFECTIONS

Therapy	Best Evidence*	Probably Useful†	Least Evidence‡
Herbals		Cranberry juice (0.5 L/d, 400 mg/ b.i.d. of extract) Blueberry juice (0.25 L/d)	Uva-ursi (3–5 mL tincture, 100–250 mg t.i.d. [as arbutin in herbal extract]) (requires alkaline urine—potassium or sodium citrate, ½ tsp sodium bicarbonate, Alka Seltzer) Garlic (300 mg t.i.d., 1–4 cloves/d) Goldenseal (250–300 mg t.i.d. std extract, 3–4 g/d root caps, tabs, tincture) Sandalwood oil (1–2 drops t.i.d.) *Herbal diuretic teas:* Asparagus, birch, couch grass, horsetail, Java tea, juniper lovage, spiny restharrow, nettle, parsley (1–3 tsp [5–15 g] steeped for 15 min and taken t.i.d.)
Diet and Nutrition/ Lifestyle	Drink large amounts of low-sugar juices, water, other fluids (>2 L/d) Urinate after intercourse (women) Eliminate obstruction		Identify and eliminate food allergies in recurrent infections Vitamin C (5 g/d) Vitamin A (25,000 IU/d) Beta-carotene (200,000 IU/d) Zinc 30 mg/d Bromelain Multivitamins

Table 29–1   ALTERNATIVE THERAPIES FOR URINARY TRACT INFECTIONS *(Continued)*

Therapy	Best Evidence*	Probably Useful†	Least Evidence‡

Alternative Systems of Care		Ayurveda
		Traditional Chinese
		  medicine
			Homeopathy:
			Cantharis (30C t.i.d.
			  for 2 d)
			Sepia (30C t.i.d.
			  for 2 d)
			Belladonna (6C q 2 hr
			  up to 6 doses)
			Staphysagria (12C
			  t.i.d. for 2 d)
			Nux vomica (q 2 hr up
			  to 6 doses)

*Therapies with the highest degree of scientific support for efficacy and safety
†Therapies that are often helpful but that do not have the highest degree of supporting evidence for efficacy and safety
‡Therapies that may be useful but that have limited scientific evidence for efficacy and safety

fluids daily, made up of pure water, fruit and vegetable juices, or herbal tea, is generally recommended. I suggest abstaining from liquids containing alcohol, caffeine, or high concentrations of sugar (for example, soft drinks). Some experts recommend diluting the fruit juices with water because the sugar content of juices may be high and their acidity may irritate the bladder further. Better yet, taking fresh cranberry juice (blueberry juice is also effective), perhaps sweetened with apple or grape juice, is the preferable method (Sobota 1984, Ofek et al 1991). Those who do not like the taste may use cranberry extracts available in pill form. Voiding after intercourse can also help by flushing out bacteria that may have been introduced (Table 29–1).

Case Study: Cystitis

A 39-year-old woman presents to your office with repeated UTIs. She has been evaluated by a urologist, and x-rays of the urinary tract showed no structural abnormality. You have recommended that she drink plenty of fluids daily, that she void after intercourse, and that she start drinking cranberry juice at the onset of symptoms. You explain that cranberry juice has been found to decrease the adherence of bacteria to the wall of the bladder (Robbers 1999 pp. 96–100). She reports that she had used this approach when she was younger but was dissuaded from it by her former physician.

Additionally, you recommend that when she is symptomatic and not getting relief with fluids and cranberry juice, she should try an herb called Uva-ursi or bearberry, which has an active antiseptic component called arbutin. Another herbal option is goldenseal, which also has antibiotic properties. According to Murray and Pizzorno's *Encyclopedia of Natural Medicine* (1998 p. 288), both of these herbal products work better when the urine has been alkalinized (rather than acidified) with potassium, sodium citrate (4 g 3 times/day), or both. You also make some general dietary recommendations such as reducing simple sugars, refined carbohydrates, and undiluted fruit juices, and identifying and eliminating any food allergens.

Appendix

Tools and Resources

BOOKS

ACA Chiropractic: State of the Art. 1994–1995. Printed by American Chiropractic Association.

Achterberg J, et al. 1994. *Rituals of Healing: Using Imagery for Health and Wellness.* New York: Bantam.

Ardell D. 1999. *14 Days to Wellness—The Easy, Effective, and Fun Way to Optimum Health.* Novato, CA: New World Library.

Ballentine R. 1999. *Radical Healing—Integrating the World's Great Therapeutic Traditions to Create a New Transformative Medicine.* New York: Harmony Books.

Benson H. 1975. *The Relaxation Response.* New York: William Morrow.

Benson H. 1984. *Beyond the Relaxation Response.* New York: Times Books.

Benson H. 1996. *Timeless Healing: The Power and Biology of Belief.* New York: Simon & Schuster.

Benson H, and Stuart E. 1992. *The Wellness Book: The Comprehensive Guide to Maintaining Health and Treating Stress-Related Illness.* New York: Simon & Schuster.

Blumenthal M (ed). 1998. *The Complete German Commission E Monographs—Therapeutic Guide to Herbal Medicines.* Boston, MA: Integrative Medicine Communications.

Blumenthal M, et al. 2000. *Herbal Medicine—Expanded Commission E Monographs.* Boston, MA: Integrative Medicine Communications.

Burton Goldberg Group. 1995. *Alternative Medicine—The Definitive Guide.* Fife, WA: Future Medicine Publishing.

Chapman-Smith D. 1997. *The Chiropractic Report* II(2), March.

Chopra D. 1990. *Quantum Healing: Exploring the Frontiers of Mind/Body Medicine.* New York: Bantam.

Chopra D. 1993. *Ageless Body, Timeless Mind.* New York: Harmony Books.

D'Adamo P. 1996. *Eat Right for Your Type: The Individualized Diet Solution to Staying Healthy, Living Longer and Achieving Your Ideal Weight.* New York: Putnam.

Dillard J, and Ziporyn T. 1998. *Alternative Medicine for Dummies.* Foster City, CA: IDG Books.

Dossey B, et al. 1999. *Holistic Nursing—A Handbook for Practice.* Gaithersburg, MD: Aspen.

Dossey L. 1993. *Healing Words: The Power of Prayer and the Practice of Medicine.* San Francisco: HarperCollins.

Dossey L. 1999. *Reinventing Medicine—Beyond Mind-Body to a New Era of Healing.* San Francisco: HarperCollins.

Duke JA. 1997. *The Green Pharmacy.* Emmaus, PA: Rodale Press.

Eisenberg D. 1987. *Encounters with Qi: Exploring Chinese Medicine.* New York: Penguin Books.

Ferguson T (ed). 1980. *Medical Self-Care: Access to Health Tools.* New York: Summit Books.

Filshie J, and White A (eds). 1998. *Medical Acupuncture—A Western Scientific Approach.* Edinburgh: Churchill Livingstone.

Frankl V. 1984. *Man's Search for Meaning.* New York: Simon & Schuster.

Gatterman M. 1995. *Foundations of Chiropractic: Subluxation.* St. Louis: Mosby.

Gordon J. 1996. *Manifesto for a New Medicine—Your Guide to Healing Partnerships and the Wise Use of Alternative Therapies.* Reading, MA: Addison Wesley.

Helms J. 1995. *Acupuncture Energetics.* Berkeley, CA: Medical Acupuncture Publishers.

Jonas W, and Levin J (eds). 1999. *Essentials of Complementary and Alternative Medicine.* Philadelphia: Lippincott/Williams & Wilkins.

Kabat-Zinn J. 1990. *Full Catastrophe Living: Using the Wisdom of Your Body and Mind to Face Stress, Pain and Illness.* New York: Delacorte Press.

Kaptchuk T. 1983. *The Web That Has No Weaver: Understanding Chinese Medicine.* New York: Congdon & Weed.

Kemper K. 1996. *The Holistic Pediatrician.* New York: HarperCollins.

Krieger D. 1993. *Accepting Your Power to Heal.* Santa Fe, NM: Bear & Co.

Kritek PB (ed). 1997. *Reflections on Healing: A Central Nursing Construct.* New York: NLN Press.

Kushi M, with Jack A. 1983. *The Cancer Prevention Diet: Michio Kushi's Nutritional Blueprint for the Relief and Prevention of Disease.* New York: St. Martin's Press.

Larson D. 1993. *The Faith Factor, Volume II: An Annotated Bibliography of Systematic Reviews and Clinical Research on Spiritual Subjects.* NIHR.

Lerner M. 1994. *Choices in Healing—Integrating the Best of Conventional and Complementary Approaches to Cancer.* Cambridge, MA: MIT Press.

Lininger S (ed), Wright J, Austin S, Brown D, Gaby A. 1998. *The Natural Pharmacy*, ed 2. Rocklin, CA: Prima Health, revised and expanded, 1999.

Lininger S, et al. 1999. *A–Z Guide to Drug-Herb-Vitamin Interactions.* Rocklin, CA: Prima Publishing.

Matthews D et al. 1993. *The Faith Factor: Volume I: An Annotated Bibliography of Clinical Research on Spiritual Subjects.* NIHR.

Matthews D, and Larson D. 1995. *The Faith Factor, Volume III: An Annotated Bibliography of Clinical Research on Spiritual Subjects.* NIHR.

Matthews D. 1997. *The Faith Factor, Volume IV: An annotated bibliography of clinical research on spiritual subjects: Prevention and treatment of illness, addictions, and delinquency.* NIHR.

Matthews D. 1998. *The Faith Factor—Proof of the Healing Power of Prayer.* New York: Viking.

Micozzi M (ed). 1996. *Fundamentals of Complementary and Alternative Medicine*. New York: Churchill Livingstone.

Milton D, and Benjamin S. 1999. *Complementary & Alternative Therapies—An Implementation Guide to Integrative Health Care*. Chicago: American Hospital Association Press.

Monte T (ed). 1997. *The Complete Guide to Natural Healing*. New York: Perigree.

Moore J. 1993. *Chiropractic in America: The History of a Medical Alternative*. Baltimore: Johns Hopkins University Press.

Moyers B. 1993. *Healing and the Mind*. New York: Doubleday. (also a PBS series)

Murray M, and Pizzorno J. 1998. *Encyclopedia of Natural Medicine*. Rocklin, CA: Prima Publishing.

Northrup C. 1994. *Women's Bodies, Women's Wisdom—Creating Physical and Emotional Health and Healing*. New York: Bantam.

Novey D. 2000. *Clinician's Complete Reference to Complementary/Alternative Medicine*. St. Louis: Mosby.

Ornish D. 1992. *Dr. Dean Ornish's Program for Reversing Heart Disease without Drugs or Surgery*. New York: Ballantine.

Ornish D. 1998. *Love & Survival—The Scientific Basis for the Healing Power of Intimacy*. New York: HarperCollins.

Ornstein R, and Sobel D. 1989. *Healthy Pleasures*. Reading, MA: Addison-Wesley.

Ottarian S. 1999. *Medicinal Herbal Therapy—A Pharmacist's Viewpoint*. Portsmouth, NH: Nicolin Fields.

PDR for Herbal Medicines. 2000. Montvale, NJ: Medical Economics.

Pelletier K. 1977. *Mind as Healer, Mind as Slayer: A Holistic Approach to Preventing Stress Disorders*. New York: Delta.

Pizzorno J, and Murray M. 1999. *Textbook of Natural Medicine*. Edinburgh: Churchill Livingstone.

Pressman A, and Buff S. 1997. *The Complete Idiot's Guide to Vitamins and Minerals*. New York: Macmillan.

Pressman A, and Buff S. 1999. *The Complete Idiot's Guide to Alternative Medicine*. New York: Alpha Books.

Robbers J, and Tyler V. 1999. *Tyler's Herbs of Choice—The Therapeutic Use of Phytomedicinals*. New York: Haworth Press.

Rosenfeld I. 1996. *Dr. Rosenfeld's Guide to Alternative Medicine—What Works, What Doesn't—And What's Right For You*. New York: Random House.

Rossman M. 1987. *Healing Yourself: A Step-by-Step Program for Better Health through Imagery*. New York: Walker.

Siegel B. 1986. *Love, Medicine, and Miracles: Lessons Learned about Self-Healing from a Surgeon's Experience with Exceptional Patients*. New York: Harper & Row.

Siegel B. 1993. *How to Live between Office Visits: A Guide to Life, Love, and Health*. New York: Harper & Row.

Sears B. 1995. *The Zone: A Dietary Road Map*. New York: Regan Books.

Simonton O, et al. 1978. *Getting Well Again: A Step-by-Step Guide to Overcoming Cancer for Patients and Their Families*. New York: Bantam.

Sobel D, and Ornstein R. 1996. *The Healthy Mind, Healthy Body Handbook.* Los Altos, CA: DR Press.

Spencer J, and Jacobs J. 1999. *Complementary/Alternative Medicine—An Evidence-Based Approach.* St. Louis: Mosby.

Steward J, et al. 1998. *Sugar Busters! Cut Sugar to Trim Fat.* New York: Ballantine.

Watkins A. 1997. *Mind-Body Medicine—A Clinician's Guide to Psychoneuroimmunology.* New York: Churchill Livingstone.

Weil A. 1995. *Spontaneous Healing.* New York: Knopf.

Weil A. 1997. *8 Weeks to Health.* New York: Knopf.

Weil A. 2000. *Eating Well for Optimum Health: The Essential Guide to Food, Diet, and Nutrition.* New York: Knopf.

Wirth S (ed). 1999. *Integrative Medicine—A Balanced Account of the Data.* Ukiah, CA: Boitumelo Publishing.

Workshop on Alternative Medicine, Chantilly, VA. 1992. *Alternative Medicine: Expanding Medical Horizons.* A report to the National Institutes of Health on Alternative Medical Systems and Practices in the United States. Washington, DC: U. S. Government Printing Office.

COMPLEMENTARY AND ALTERNATIVE MEDICINE RESEARCH CENTERS

National Institutes of Health (NIH) NCCAM Clearinghouse
P.O. Box 8218
Silver Spring, MD 20907-8218
http://nccam.nih.gov/
Toll Free Hotline: (888) NIH-OCAM (644-6226)
TTY/TDY: (888) 644-6226
FAX: (301) 495-4957

Addictions

Center for Addiction and Alternative Medicine Research (CAAMR)
Minneapolis Medical Research Foundation
914 South Eighth St., Suite D917
Minneapolis, MN 55404
Phone: (612) 347-7670
Fax: (612) 337-7367
http://www.mmrfweb.org/caamrpages/caamrcover.html
Principal Investigator: Thomas J. Kiresuk, PhD
Contact: Jennifer Shinn, caamr@winternet.com

Aging

Complementary and Alternative Medicine Program at Stanford University (CAMPS)
http://scrdp.stanford.edu/camps.html
730 Welch Rd.
Palo Alto, CA 94304-1583
Principal Investigator: William L. Haskell, PhD
Contact: Ellen M. DiNucci, MA, edinucci@scrdp.stanford.edu

Asthma, Allergy, and Immunology

Center for Complementary and Alternative Medicine Research in Asthma
Department of Nutrition
3150 Meyer Hall
University of California, Davis
One Shields Ave.
Davis, CA 95616-8669
Phone: (530) 752-6575
Fax: (530) 752-1297
http://www.camra.ucdavis.edu/
Principal Investigator: M.E. Gershwin, MD
Contact: Paul A. Davis, Ph.D, camra@ucdavis.edu

Chiropractic

The Palmer Center for Chiropractic Research
Palmer College
741 Brady St.
Davenport, IA 52803

The Palmer Center for Chiropractic Research
Palmer College West
90 East Tasman Drive
San Jose, CA 95134
Principal Investigator: William Meeker, DC, MPH, Meeker_b@palmer.edu

General Medical Conditions

Center for Alternative Medicine Research
Beth Israel Hospital Deaconess Medical Center
Harvard Medical School
330 Brookline Ave.
Boston, MA 02215
Principal Investigator: David M. Eisenberg, MD

HIV/AIDS

Bastyr University AIDS Research Center
http://www.bastyr.edu/research/buarc/
14500 Juanita Drive NE
Bothell, WA 98011
Phone: (425) 823-1300
Fax: (425) 823-6222
Principal Investigator: Leanna J. Standish, ND, PhD
Contact: Cherie Reeves, MS, cherie@bastyr.edu

Pain

University of Maryland School of Medicine
Division of Complementary Medicine
2200 North Forest Park, 3rd Floor
Baltimore, MD 21207-6693
Principal Investigator: Brian M. Berman, MD
Contact: E. Victor Leino, PhD, vleino@kernan2.ummc.ab.umd.edu

University of Virginia Center for the Study of Complementary and Alternative Therapies (CSCAT)
McLeod Hall, Suite 5006
15th and Lane St.
Charlottesville VA 22903-3395
http://www.nursing.virginia.edu/centers/alt-ther.html
Principal Investigator: Ann Gill Taylor, EdD

Pediatrics

Program in Integrative Medicine
College of Medicine
The University of Arizona
P.O. Box 245153
Tucson, AZ 85724-5153
Phone: (520) 626-7222
Fax: (520) 626-6484

Stroke and Neurological Conditions

Kessler-UMDNJ Center for Research in Complementary and Alternative Medicine
Kessler Medical Rehabilitation Research and Education Corporation (KMMREC) Research Department
Center for Research in Complementary and Alternative Medicine
1199 Pleasant Valley Way
West Orange, NJ 07052
Phone: (973) 243-6972
Fax: (973) 243-6984
Principal Investigator: Samuel C. Shiflett, PhD, shiflesc@umdnj.edu
Contact: Nancy Schoenberger, PhD, schoenbe@umdnj.edu

Women's Health

Center for CAM Research in Women's Health
Columbia University
630 West 168th St.
New York, NY 10032
Principal Investigator: Fredi Kronenberg, PhD
Contact: Christine Wade, wade@columbia.edu

JOURNALS AND NEWSLETTERS

Alternative Medicine Alert. Published by American Health Consultants. Phone: (800) 688-2421*

Alternative Therapies in Health and Medicine. Published by the Innovision Communications, a division of American Association of Critical Care Nurses, 101 Columbia, Aliso Viejo, CA 92656. Phone: (800) 899-1712*

Alternative Therapies in Women's Health. Published by American Health Consultants. Phone: (800) 688-2421*

The Ardell Wellness Report Newsletter. 345 Bayshore Blvd., #414, Tampa, FL 33606. Phone: (813) 251-4567*

Clinical Pearls Newsletter. 3301 Alta Arden, #2, Sacramento, CA 95285. Phone: (916) 483-1085. http://www.prescription2000.com/

Herbalgram. American Botanical Council. Phone: (800) 373-7105*

Integrative Medicine. Edited by Dr. Andrew Weil. Phone: (520) 626-7222

Integrative Medicine Consult. Integrative Medicine Communications, 1029 Chestnut St., Newton, MA. 02464. Phone: (800) 217-1938.

Journal of Complementary and Alternative Therapy. Published by Mary Ann Liebert, Inc., New York, NY 10128. Phone: (212) 289-2300.

Journal of Holistic Nursing. Sage Publications, Inc. 2455 Teller Rd. Thousand Oaks, CA. 91320. Phone: (520) 526-2196.

Natural Health. Phone: (800) 526-8440.

New Age Journal. New Age Publishing, 42 Pleasant St, Watertown MA 02472. Phone: (800) 782-7006 or (617) 926-0200; Fax: (617) 926-5021.

Prevention. Rodale Press, Emmaus, PA. Phone: (800) 666-1920 or (610) 967-8038; Fax: (610) 967-7654. http://www.prevention.com.

Dr. Andrew Weil's Self Healing: Creating Natural Health for Your Body and Mind. Edited by Dr. Andrew Weil, Thorne Communications. Phone: (800) 523-3296.

Spirituality and Health: The Soul/Body Connection. 74 Trinity Pl., New York, NY 10006. Phone: (212) 602-0705.

Yoga Journal. P.O. Box 469088, Escondido, CA 92046-9088. Phone: (800) 600-YOGA.

ORGANIZATIONS

Academy for Guided Imagery
P.O. Box 2070
Mill Valley, CA 94942
Phone: (800) 726-2070

Acupressure Institute
1533 Shattuck Ave.
Berkeley, CA 94709
Phone: (800) 442-2232

Alexander Technique International Inc.
1692 Massachusetts Ave.
Cambridge, MA 02138
Phone: (617) 497-2242

*Check under **Websites** for a URL for this publication.

American Academy of Medical Acupuncture*
5820 Wilshire Blvd., Suite 500
Los Angeles, CA 90036
Phone: (323) 937-5514

American Association of Naturopathic Physicians*
601 Valley St., Suite 105
Seattle, WA 98109
Phone: (206) 298-0126

American Association of Oriental Medicine*
433 Front St.
Catasauqua, PA 18032
Phone: (610) 266-1433

American Association for Therapeutic Humor
222 Meramec, Suite 303
St. Louis, MO 63105
Phone: (314) 863-6232

American Board of Chelation Therapy
1407-B N. Wells
Chicago, IL 60610
Phone: (800) 356-2228

American Botanical Council*
P.O. Box 201660
Austin, TX 78720
Phone: (512) 331-8868

American Chiropractic Association*
1701 Clarendon Blvd.
Arlington, VA 22209
Phone: (703) 276-8800

American Holistic Medical Association*
4101 Lake Boone Trail, Suite 201
Raleigh, NC 27607
Phone: (919) 787-5181

American Holistic Nurses' Association*
P.O. Box 2130
Flagstaff, AZ 86003
Phone: (800) 278-2462

American Massage Therapy Association*
820 Davis St., Suite 100
Evanston, IL 60201
Phone: (708) 864-0123

American Osteopathic Association*
142 East Ontario St.
Chicago, IL 60611
Phone: (312) 280-5882 or (800) 621-1773

---

*Check under **Websites** for a URL for this organization.

American Society for Clinical Hypnosis
2200 E. Devon Ave., Suite 291
Des Plaines, IL 60018
Phone: (847) 297-3317

American Yoga Association
513 Orange Ave.
Sarasota, FL 34236
Phone: (941) 953-5859

Association for Applied Psychophysiology and Biofeedback*
10200 W. 44th Ave., Suite 304
Wheat Ridge, CO 80033
Phone: (800) 477-8892

Ayurvedic Institute
11311 Menaul NE, Suite A
Albuquerque, NM 87112
Phone: (506) 291-9698

Bastyr University of Natural Health Sciences
College of Naturopathic Medicine*
144 NE 54th
Seattle, WA 98105
Phone: (206) 523-9585

Bio-Electro-Magnetics Institute
2490 Moana Lane
Reno, NV 89509
Phone: (702) 827-9099

Center for Mind-Body Medicine
5225 Connecticut Ave. NW, Suite 414
Washington, DC 20015
Phone: (202) 966-7338

Feldenkrais Guild of North America
524 Ellsworth St. SW
Albany, OR 97321
Phone: (800) 775-2118

Fetzer Institute*
9292 West KL Ave.
Kalamazoo, MI 49009
Phone: (616) 375-2000

Herb Research Foundation*
1007 Pearl St., Suite 200
Boulder, CO 80302
Phone: (800) 748-2617

Himalayan Institute of Canada
371 Berkeley St.
Toronto, Ontario, Canada M5A 2X8
Phone: (416) 960-5062

---

*Check under **Websites** for a URL for this organization.

International Center for Reiki Training
21421 Hilltop, #28
Southfield, MI 48034
center@reiki.org

International Chiropractors Association
1120 North Glebe Rd., Suite 1000
Arlington, VA 22201
Phone: (800) 423-4690

International Society for the Study of Subtle Energies and Energy Medicine
356 Goldco Circle
Golden, CO 80401
Phone: (303) 425-4625

Linus Pauling Institute of Science and Medicine
440 Page Mill Rd.
Palo Alto, CA 94306
Phone: (650) 327-4064

Maharishi International University
1000 N 4th St.
Fairfield, IA 52557
Phone: (515) 472-7000 or (515) 472-1166

Mind-Body Medical Institute
110 Francis St., Suite 1A
Boston, MA 02215
Phone: (617) 632-9525

National Association for Holistic Aromatherapy
P.O. Box 17622
Boulder, CO 80308
Phone: (800) 566-6735

National Association for Music Therapy
8455 Colesville Rd., Suite 1000
Silver Spring, MD 20910
Phone: (301) 589-3300

National Center for Homeopathy
801 N. Fairfax St., Suite 306
Alexandria, VA 22314
Phone: (703) 548-7790

National Center for Complementary and Alternative Medicine (NCCAM)*
P.O. Box 8218
Silver Spring, MD 20907
Phone: (888) 644-6226 (888-NIH-OCAM)

National Certification Commission for Acupuncture and Oriental Medicine (NCCAOM)
11 Canal Center Plaza, Suite 300
Alexandria, VA 22314
Phone: (703) 548-9004

---

*Check under **Websites** for a URL for this organization.

Nurse Healers and Professional Associates*
1211 Locust St.
Philadelphia, PA 19107
Phone: (215) 545-8079

Office of Alternative Medicine (OAM) Information Clearinghouse
Qi Gong Institute/East-West Academy of Healing Arts
450 Sutter St., Suite 2104
San Francisco, CA 94108
Phone: (415) 788-2227

Professional Registry: International Association of Reiki Professionals (IARP)
P.O. Box 481
Winchester, MA 01890
Phone: (781) 729-3530

WEBSITES

The University of Texas Medical Branch Alternative and Integrative Health-care Program
http://atc.utmb.edu/altmed

Acupuncture
http://www.acupuncture.com

Alternative Link, LLC (information on billing codes)
http:// www.alternativelink.com

Alternative Medicine Health Care Information Resources
http://hsl.mcmaster.ca/tomflem/altmed.html

Alternative Medicine Homepage—University of Pittsburgh
http://www.pitt.edu/~cbw/altm.html

American Academy of Medical Acupuncture
http://www.medicalacupuncture.org

American College for the Advancement in Medicine (chelation therapy)
http://www.acam.org

American Association of Naturopathic Physicians
http://www.naturopathic.org

American Botanical Council
http://www.herbalgram.org

American Chiropractic Association
http://www.americhiro.org

American Health Consultants
http://www.ahcpub.com

American Holistic Medical Association
http:// www.holisticmedicine.org

American Massage Therapy Association
http://www.AMTAMASSAGE.org

American Osteopathic Association
http://www.am-osteo-assn.org/

---

*Check under **Websites** for a URL for this organization.

The Ardell Wellness Report
http:// www.yourhealth.com

Ask Dr. Weil
http://www.drweil.com

Association for Applied Psychophysiology and Biofeedback
http:// www.aapb.org

Bastyr University—AIDS
http://www.bastyr.edu/research/research/html

Biotecnoquimica (Venezuela—Spanish language)
http://www.biotecnoquimica.com

Children's Hospital, Boston: Center for Holistic Pediatric Education and Research (CHPER)
http://www.childrenshospital.org/holistic/index.html

Choices for Health
http://www.choicesforhealth.com

Columbia University Rosenthal Center for Complementary and Alternative Medicine—Women's Health
http://cpmcnet.columbia.edu/dept/rosenthal

Consortorial Center for Chiropractic Research (CCCR)—Palmer Center for Chiropractic Research
http://www.palmer.edu/pccr/pccrhome.htm

Duke's Phytochemical and Ethnobotanical Database
http://www.ars-grin.gov/duke/

Fetzer Institute (a nonprofit organization promoting the study of the spiritual elements of life)
http://www.fetzer.org

Global Health 2000 (10 languages)
http://www.globalhealth2000.com

Guided Imagery Resource Center
http://www.healthjourneys.com

Harvard Medical School—General Medical Conditions
http://www.bidmc.harvard.edu/medicine/camr

Healing Touch International
http://www.healingtouch.net

Healthfinder
http://healthfinder.com

HealthNotes Online
http://www.healthnotes.online

HealthWWWeb—Paracelsus—Clinical Practice in the Healing Arts
http://www.healthwwweb.com/paracelsus.html

Herb Research Foundation
http://www.herbs.org

Hippocrates—The Clinical Practice of Integrative Medicine
http://www.healthweb.com/hippocrates.html

Holistic Medicine Interest Group
http://www.ohsu.edu/ohmig

International Center for Reiki Training
http://www.reiki.org

Kessler-UMDNJ Center for Research in Complementary and Alternative
Medicine
http://www.umdnj.edu/altmdweb

Longwood Herbal Task Force
http://www.mcp.edu/herbal/Default.htm

Medical College of Wisconsin: Alternative Medicine Resources
http://www.intmed.mcw.edu/gimcme/altmed.html

National Association of Nurse Massage Therapists
http://members.aol.com/nanmt1/about.html

National Center for Complementary and Alternative Medicine
http://altmed.od.nih.gov/nccam

National Center for Homeopathy
http://www.healthy.net/pan/pa/homeopathic

National Council for Reliable Health Information (NCRHI)
http://www.ncahf.org

National Health Information Center (NHIC)—Alternative Medicine Database
Search Returns
http://nhic-nt.health.org/Scripts/
Hitlist.cfm?Keyword=ALTERNATIVE%20MEDICINE

National Institute of Ayurvedic Medicine
http://niam.com

Natural Healthline
http://www.naturalhealthvillage.com

Nurse Healers – Professional Associates International
http://www.therapeutic-touch.org

Office of Dietary Supplements (National Institutes of Health): The International Bibliographic Information on Dietary Supplements (IBIDS)
http://odp.od.nih.gov/ods/databases/ibids.html

Orthomolecular Medicine Online
http://www.orthomed.org

Professional Registry: International Association of Reiki Professionals (IARP)
http://www.iarp.org

Qi Gong Association of America
http://www.qi.org

Quackwatch
http://www.quackwatch.com

Stanford University Complementary and Alternative Program—Aging
http://scrdp.stanford.edu/camps.html

Tufts University Nutrition Navigator
http://www.navigator.tufts.edu

University of Arizona Program in Integrative Medicine—Pediatrics
http://integrativemedicine.arizona.edu

University of California, Davis—Allergy, Asthma, Immunology
http://www-camra.ucdavis.edu

University of Maryland—Pain
http:// www.compmed.ummc.ab.umd.edu

The University of Texas Center for Alternative Medicine Research—Cancer
http://www.sph.uth.tmc.edu/utcam

University of Virginia—CAM and Nursing
http://www.med.virginia.edu/nursing/centers/alt-ther.html

References

CHAPTER 1—WHAT IS INTEGRATIVE HEALTH CARE?

Astin JA. 1998. Why patients use alternative medicine: results of a national study. *JAMA* 279:1548–1553.

Eisenberg D, et al. 1993. Unconventional medicine in the United States. Prevalence, costs, and patterns of use. *N Engl J Med* 328:246–252.

Eisenberg D, et al. 1998. Trends in alternative medicine use in the United States, 1990–1997: results of a follow-up national survey. *JAMA* 280:1569–1575.

Lazarou J, et al. 1998. Incidence of adverse drug reactions in hospitalized patients. *JAMA* 279:1200–1205.

Workshop on Alternative Medicine, Chantilly, VA.1992. *Alternative Medicine: Expanding Medical Horizons. A report to the National Institutes of Health on Alternative Medical Systems and Practices in the United States.* Washington, DC: U. S. Government Printing Office.

CHAPTER 2—HOW TO TALK TO PATIENTS ABOUT INTEGRATIVE HEALTH CARE

Coppes MJ, et al. 1998. Alternative therapies for the treatment of childhood cancer. Letter to the Editor. *N Engl J Med* 339:846.

Dossey L. 1999. *Reinventing Medicine—Beyond Mind-Body to a New Era of Healing.* San Francisco: HarperCollins.

Eisenberg D. 1997. Advising patients who seek alternative medical therapies. *Ann Intern Med* 127:61–69.

Lerner M. 1994. *Choices in Healing—Integrating the Best of Conventional and Complementary Approaches to Cancer.* Cambridge, MA: MIT Press.

CHAPTER 3—BEING WELL, BEING A ROLE MODEL

Ardell DB. 1979. *High Level Wellness: An Alternative to Doctors, Drugs and Disease.* New York: Bantam.

Ardell DB. 1982. *14 Days to a Wellness Lifestyle: The Easy, Effective, and Fun Way to Optimum Health.* Mill Valley, CA: Whatever Press.

Ardell DB. 1999. *14 Days to Wellness—The Easy, Effective, and Fun Way to Optimum Health.* Novato, CA: New World Library.

Ardell DB, and Tager MJ. 1982. *Planning for Wellness: A Guidebook for Achieving Optimal Health.* Dubuque, IA: Kendall/Hunt.

Benson H. 1975. *The Relaxation Response.* New York: William Morrow.

Benson H. 1984. *Beyond the Relaxation Response.* New York: Times Books.

Benson H, and Stuart E. 1992. *The Wellness Book, The Comprehensive Guide to*

Maintaining Health and Treating Stress-Related Illness. New York: Simon & Schuster.

Berkman LF, et al. 1979. Social networks, host resistance, and mortality: a nine-year follow-up study of Alameda County residents. *Am J Epidemiol* 109:186–204.

Dossey L. 1993. *Healing Words: The Power of Prayer and the Practice of Medicine.* San Francisco: HarperCollins.

Ferguson T. 1980. *Medical Self-Care: Access to Health Tools.* New York: Summit Books.

Levey J, and Levy M. 1998. *Living in Balance: A Dynamic Approach for Creating Harmony and Wholeness in a Chaotic World.* Berkeley, CA.: Conari Press. (Cited in *Noetic Sciences Review* April-July: 53.)

Schaeffer E, and Parkhurst L (eds). 1987. *The Art of Life.* Westchester, IL: Crossway Books.

Weil A. 1997. *Eight Weeks to Optimum Health: A Proven Program for Taking Full Advantage of Your Body's Natural Healing Power.* New York: Knopf.

CHAPTER 4—MIND, BODY AND NOW . . . SPIRIT

Arberry AJ (transl). 1955. *The Koran Interpreted.* New York: Collier Books.

Byrd R. 1988. Positive therapeutic effects of intercessory prayer in a coronary care unit population. *South Med J* 81(7): 826–829.

Dossey L. 1993. *Healing Words: The Power of Prayer and the Practice of Medicine.* San Francisco: HarperCollins.

Dossey L. 1999. *Reinventing Medicine—Beyond Mind-Body to a New Era of Healing.* San Francisco: HarperCollins.

Ellis MR, et al. 1999. Addressing spiritual concerns of patients—family physicians' attitudes and practices. *J Fam Pract* 48:105-109.

Foundation for Inner Peace. 1985. *A Course in Miracles.* Tiburon, CA: Foundation for Inner Peace.

Frankl VE. 1984. *Man's Search for Meaning.* New York: Simon & Schuster.

Holy Bible, multiple translations and editions.

King DE, et al. 1994. Faith healing and prayer among hospitalized patients. *J Fam Pract* 39(4):349–352.

Lao Tsu (Feng GF, et al., transl).1972. *Tao Te Ching.* New York: Vintage Books, Random House.

Lewis CS. 1944. *The Problem of Pain.* New York: Macmillan.

Matthews DA. 1998. *The Faith Factor—Proof of the Healing Power of Prayer.* New York: Viking.

Oxman TE, et al. 1995. Lack of social participation or religious strength and comfort as risk factors for death after cardiac surgery in the elderly. *Psychosom Med* 53:5–15.

Walsch ND. 1995. *Conversations with God: An Uncommon Dialog, Book 1.* New York: G.P. Putnam.

Walsch ND. 1997. *Conversations with God: An Uncommon Dialog, Book 2.* Charlottesville, VA: Hampton Roads Publishing Co.

Walsch ND. 1998. *Conversations with God: An Uncommon Dialog, Book 3.* Charlottesville, VA: Hampton Roads Publishing Co.

CHAPTER 5—PATIENT-CENTERED AND RELATIONSHIP-CENTERED CARE

Li JTC. 1999. Humility and the practice of medicine. *Mayo Clin Proc* 74:529–530.

Engel GL. 1977. The need for a new medical model: a challenge for biomedicine. *Science* 196(4286): 129–136.

Kabat-Zinn J.1990. *Full Catastrophe Living: Using the Wisdom of Your Body and Mind to Face Stress, Pain and Illness.* New York: Delacorte Press.

Tresolini CP, and the Pew–Fetzer Task Force. 1994. *Health Professions Education and Relationship-Centered Care.* San Francisco, CA: Pew Health Professions Commission.

CHAPTER 7—REIMBURSEMENT, LIABILITY, AND OTHER PRACTICE ISSUES

Berndtson K. 1998. Integrative medicine: business risks and opportunities. *The Physician Executive* Nov–Dec: 22–25.

Brown E. 1998. The daunting challenge. *The Physician Executive* Nov–Dec: 16–21.

Dalzell M. 1999. Health plans and alternative medicine: where do physicians fit in? *Manag Care* April: 14–23.

Kornblatt J. 1999. Legal and regulatory issues in integrative health care. In Milton D, and Benjamin S (eds.): *Complementary & Alternative Therapies—An Implementation Guide to Integrative Health Care.* Chicago: American Hospital Association Press. pp 123–138.

Pelletier KR, et al. 1997. Current trends in the integration and reimbursement of complementary and alternative medicine by managed care, insurance carriers, and hospital providers. *Am J Health Promot* 12(2):112–123.

Studdert DM, et al. 1998. Medical malpractice implications of alternative medicine. *JAMA* 280:1610–1615.

Weber D. 1998. Considering the alternatives. *The Physician Executive* Nov–Dec: 6–14.

CHAPTER 8—CONTINUING EDUCATION IN INTEGRATIVE HEALTH CARE

Gaudet TW. 1998. Integrative medicine: the evolution of a new approach to medicine and to medical education. *Int Med* 1(2):67–73.

Gordon J. 1996. Alternative medicine and the family physician. *Am Fam Physician* 54(7):2205–2212.

Kligler B, Gordon A, Stuart M, and Sierpina V. 2000. Suggested curriculum guidelines on complementary and alternative medicine: recommendations of the Society of Teachers of Family Medicine Group on Alternative Medicine, *Fam Med* 31(10):30–33.

Murray M, and Pizzorno J. 1998. *Encyclopedia of Natural Medicine.* Rocklin, CA: Prima Publishing.

Pizzorno J, and Murray M. 1999. *Textbook of Natural Medicine.* Edinburgh: Churchill Livingstone.

Sierpina V. 1999. The journal club: A forum for cultural change and the study of alternative and integrative medicine at a university health science center. *Intern Med* 2(1):31–34.

Sierpina V, et al. 1999. The changing face of medical education. Presentation at Alternative Therapies in Health and Medicine Annual Symposium, New York, March, 1999.

Wetzel MS, et al. 1999. Courses involving complementary and alternative medicine at US medical schools. *JAMA* 290:784–787.

CHAPTER 9—ALTERNATIVE SYSTEMS OF CARE

Ballentine R. 1999. *Radical Healing—Integrating the World's Great Therapeutic Traditions to Create a New Transformative Medicine.* New York: Harmony Books.

Chopra D. 1990. *Quantum Healing: Exploring the Frontiers of Mind/Body Medicine.* New York: Bantam.

Chopra D. 1993. *Ageless Body, Timeless Mind.* New York: Harmony Books.

Eisenberg D. 1987. *Encounters with Qi: Exploring Chinese Medicine.* New York: Penguin Books.

Filshie J, and White A (eds). 1998. *Medical Acupuncture—A Western Scientific Approach.* Edinburgh, UK: Churchill Livingstone.

Helms J. 1995. The five phases paradigm. In *Acupuncture Energetics.* Berkeley, CA: Medical Acupuncture Publishers. p 217.

Kaptchuk T. 1983. *The Web That Has No Weaver: Understanding Chinese Medicine.* New York: Congdon and Weed.

Jacobs J, et al. 1994. Treatment of acute diarrhea with homeopathic medicine: a randomized clinical trial in Nicaragua. *Pediatrics* 93(5):719–725.

Kleijnen J, et al. 1991. Clinical trials of homeopathy. *BMJ* 302:316–323.

Lazarou BH, et al. 1998. Incidence of adverse drug reactions in hospitalized patients. *JAMA* 279:1200–1205.

Linde K, et al. 1997. Are the clinical effects of homeopathy placebo effects? A meta-analysis of placebo controlled-trials. *Lancet* 350:834–843.

Mehl-Madrona LE. 1999. Native American medicine in the treatment of chronic illness: developing an integrated program and evaluating its effectiveness. *Altern Ther Health Med* 5(1):36–41.

Micozzi M (ed). 1996. *Fundamentals of Complementary and Alternative Medicine.* New York: Churchill Livingstone. p 71, pp 259–277.

Murray M, and Pizzorno J. 1998. *Encyclopedia of Natural Medicine.* Rocklin, CA: Prima Publishing.

Reilly D, et al. 1986. Is homeopathy a placebo effect? Controlled trial of homeopathy potency, with pollen in hay fever as a model. *Lancet* 2:881–885.

Reilly D. 1997. Data presented at Alternative Medicine Symposium. Harvard Medical School CME, March 9.

CHAPTER 10—HERBALS

Blumenthal M (ed). 1998. *The Complete German Commission E Monographs—Therapeutic Guide to Herbal Medicines.* Boston, MA: Integrative Medicine Communications.

Blumenthal M (ed), Goldberg A, and Brinckman J. 1999. *Herbal Medicine—Expanded Commission E Monographs.* Newton, MA: Integrative Medicine Communications.

Dincin Buchman D. 1979. *Herbal Medicine.* New York: David McKay. (Tables 10–1, 10–2). pp 189–269.

Duke JA. 1997. *The Green Pharmacy.* Emmaus, PA: Rodale Press.

Hoffman D. 1996. *The Complete Illustrated Holistic Herbal.* New York: Barnes & Noble Books. (Tables 10–1, 10–2). pp 22–31.

Lininger S (ed), Wright J, Austin S, Brown D, Gaby A. 1999. *The Natural Pharmacy,* ed 2. Rocklin, CA: Prima Publishing.

Lininger S (ed), Gaby AR, Austin S, Batz F, Yarnell E, Brown DJ, Constantine G. 1999. *A-Z Guide to Drug-Herb-Vitamin Interactions.* Rocklin, CA: Prima Publishing.

Liu JH. 1997. Enteric-coated peppermint oil capsules in the treatment of irritable bowel syndrome: a prospective, randomized trial. *Gastroenterology* 32:765–768.

Murray M, and Pizzorno J. 1998. *Encyclopedia of Natural Medicine.* Rocklin, CA: Prima Publishing.

Ottarian SG. 1999. *Medicinal Herbal Therapy—A Pharmacist's Viewpoint.* Portsmouth, NH: Nicolin Fields Pub.

PDR for Herbal Medicines. 1998. Montvale, NJ: Medical Economics.

Pizzorno JE, and Murray MT. 1999. *Textbook of Natural Medicine.* Edinburgh: Churchill Livingstone. (Tables 10–1, 10–2). pp 552–553.

Robbers J, and Tyler, V. 1999. *Tyler's Herbs of Choice—The Therapeutic Use of Phytomedicinals.* New York: Haworth Press p 70.

CHAPTER 11—DIET AND NUTRITION

Appel LJ, et al. 1997. A clinical trial of the effects of dietary patterns on blood pressure. DASH Collaborative Research Group. *N Engl J Med* 336:1117–1124.

Ardell D. 1999. *14 Days to Wellness—The Easy, Effective, and Fun Way to Optimum Health.* Novato, CA: New World Library.

Atkins R. 1999. *Dr. Atkins' New Diet Revolution.* New York: M. Evans.

D'Adamo P. 1996. *Eat Right for Your Type: The Individualized Diet Solution to Staying Healthy, Living Longer and Achieving Your Ideal Weight.* New York: Putnam.

DeLorgeril M, et al. 1994. Mediterranean alpha-linolenic acid rich diet, in secondary prevention of coronary heart disease. *Lancet* 343:1454.

DeLorgeril M, et al. 1998. Mediterranean dietary pattern in a randomized trial: prolonged survival and possible reduced cancer rate. *Arch Intern Med* 158:181–187.

Fraser G, et al. 1993. The application of results of some studies of California Seventh-Day Adventists to the general population. *Arch Intern Med* 153:533–534.

Janelle K, et al. 1995. Nutrient intakes and eating behavior scores of vegetarian and non-vegetarian women. *J Am Diet Assoc* 95(20):180–186, 189.

Jossa F, et al. 1996. The Mediterranean diet in the prevention of arteriosclerosis. *Recent Prog Med* 87(4):175–181.

Key T. 1999. Health benefits of a vegetarian diet. *Proc Nutr Soc* 58:271–275.

Kostreski F. 1999. Ornish program to get national test. *Family Practice News* 29(21):1, 5.

Kushi M, with Jack A. 1983. *The Cancer Prevention Diet: Michio Kushi's Nutritional Blueprint for the Relief and Prevention of Disease.* New York: St. Martin's Press.

Lerner M. 1994. *Choices in Healing, Integrating the Best of Conventional and Complementary Approaches to Cancer.* Cambridge, MA: MIT Press. pp 285–318, 335–351.

Merrell WC. 1999. How I became a low-carb believer. *Time* Nov 1: p 80.

National Research Council. 1989. *Diet and Health. Implications for Reducing Chronic Disease Risk.* Washington, DC: National Academy Press.

Ornish D, et al. 1983. Effects of stress management training and dietary changes in treating ischemic heart disease. *JAMA* 24:54–59.

Ornish D, et al. 1990. Can lifestyle changes reverse coronary atherosclerosis? The lifestyle heart trial. *Lancet* 336:129–133.

Ornish D. 1998. *Love & Survival—The Scientific Basis for the Healing Power of Intimacy.* New York: HarperCollins.

Ornstein R, and Sobel DS. 1989. *Healthy Pleasures.* Reading, MA: Addison-Wesley.

Sacks F, et al. 1974. Blood pressure in vegetarians. *Am J Epidemiol* 100 (5):390–398.

Sattilaro A. 1982. *Recalled by Life.* New York: Avon Books.

Sears B. 1995. *The Zone: A Dietary Road Map.* New York: Regan Books.

Stein J. 1999. The low-carb diet craze. *Time* Nov 1: pp 72–79.

Steward J, et al. 1998. *Sugar Busters! Cut Sugar to Trim Fat.* New York: Ballantine Books.

CHAPTER 12—NUTRICEUTICALS

Albanes D, et al. 1995. Effects of alpha-tocopherol and beta-carotene supplements on cancer incidence. *Am J Clin Nutr* 62(6 suppl):1427s.

The Alpha-Tocopherol, Beta Carotene Cancer Prevention Study Group. 1994. The effect of vitamin E and beta carotene on the incidence of lung cancer and other cancers in male smokers. *N Engl J Med* 330:1029–1035.

Baggio E, et al. 1994. Italian multicenter study on the safety and efficacy of coenzyme Q10 as adjunctive therapy in heart failure. CoQ10 Drug Surveillance Investigators. *Mol Aspects Med* 15:287–294.

Balz F. 1999. Antioxidant vitamins and heart disease. Presented at the 60th Annual Biology Colloquium. Oregon State University. February 25.

Gaby A, and Wright J. 1998. *Nutritional Therapy in Medical Practice* (syllabus). Nutrition Seminars. Kent, WA.

Goodwin JS, et al. 1998. Battling quackery: attitudes about micronutrient supplements in American academic medicine. *Arch Intern Med* 158:2187–2191.

The Heart Outcomes Prevention Evaluation Study Investigators. 2000. Vitamin E supplementation and cardiovascular events in high-risk patients. *N Engl J Med* 342:154–160.

Levine M, et al. 1996. Vitamin C pharmacokinetics in healthy volunteers: evidence for a recommended dietary allowance. *Proc Natl Acad Sci U S A* 93:3704–3709.

Levine M, et al. 1999. Criteria and recommendations for vitamin C intake. *JAMA* 281(15):1415–1423.

Morisco B, et al. 1993. Effect of coenzyme Q10 in patients with congestive heart failure: a long-term multi-center randomized study. *Clin Invest* 71:134–136.

Murray M, and Pizzorno J. 1998. *Encyclopedia of Natural Medicine.* Rocklin, CA: Prima Publishing.

Omenn GS, et al. 1996. Risk factors for lung cancer and for intervention effects in CARET, the Beta-Carotene and Retinol Efficacy Trial. *J Natl Cancer Inst* 88:1550–1559.

Reaven P, et al. 1993. Effect of dietary antioxidant combinations in humans. Protection of LDL by vitamin E but not by beta-carotene. *Arterioscler Thromb* 13:590–600.

Rimm E. 1993. Vitamin E consumption and the risk of coronary heart disease in men. *N Engl J Med* 328:1450–1455.

Stampfer J, et al. 1993. Vitamin E consumption and the risk of coronary disease in women. *N Engl J Med* 328:1444–1448.

Stephens N, et al. 1996. Randomized controlled trial of vitamin E in patients with coronary disease: Cambridge Heart Antioxidant Study (CHAOS). *Lancet* 347:781–786.

Walker W, et al. 1976. An investigation of the therapeutic value of the "copper bracelet": dermal assimilation of copper in arthritic/rheumatoid conditions. *Agents Actions* 6:454–459.

Weil A. 1999. My new vitamin C recommendation. *Self Healing*, August.

CHAPTER 13—PHARMACOLOGICAL AND BIOLOGICAL TREATMENTS

Drovanti A, et al. 1980. Therapeutic activity of oral glucosamine sulfate in osteoarthritis: a placebo-controlled, double-blind investigation. *Clin Ther* 3(4):260–272.

Ebeling P, and Koivisto VA, 1994. Physiological importance of dehydroepiandrosterone. *Lancet* 343:1479–1481.

Elihun N, et al. 1998. Chelation therapy in cardiovascular disease: ethylenediamine-tetraacetic acid, deferoxamine, and dexrazoxane. *J Clin Pharmacol* 38:101–105.

Ernst E. 1997. Chelation therapy for peripheral arterial occlusive disease: a systematic review. *Circulation* 96:1031–1033.

Gaby AR. 1996. Dehydroepiandrosterone: biological effects and clinical significance. *Altern Med Rev* 1:60–69.

Haimov I, et al.1994. Sleep disorders and melatonin rhythms in elderly people. *BMJ* 309:167.

Hilton E, et al. 1992. Ingestion of yogurt containing lactobacillus acidophilus as prophylaxis for candidal vaginitis. *Ann Intern Med* 116:353–357.

Katelaris PH, et al. 1995. Lactobacilli to prevent traveler's diarrhea? *N Engl J Med* 333:1360–1361.

Kelly GS. 1997. Sports nutrition: a review of selected nutritional supplements for bodybuilders and strength athletes. *Altern Med Rev* 2(3):184–201.

Kerzberg EM, et al. 1987. Combination of glycosaminoglycans and acetylsalicylic acid in knee osteoarthritis. *Scand J Rheumatol* 16:377.

Lee A, et al. 1983. Shark cartilage contains inhibitors of tumor angiogenesis. *Science* 221:1185–1187.

McAlindon TE, et al. 2000. Glucosamine and chondroitin for treatment of osteoarthritis: a systematic quality assessment and meta-analysis. *JAMA* 283(11):1483–1484.

Muller-Fassbender H, et al. 1994. Glucosamine sulfate compared to ibuprofen in osteoarthritis of the knee. *Osteoarthritis Cartilage* 2:61–69.

Petrie K, et al. 1993. A double-blind trial of melatonin as a treatment for jet lag in international cabin crew. *Biol Psychol* 33(7):526–30.

Pizzorno JE, and Murray MT. 1999. *Textbook of Natural Medicine.* Edinburgh: Churchill Livingstone.

Richardson MA. 1999. Texas Medical Association Seminar, Alternative Medicine. *Update on Alternative Treatments for Cancer.* University of Texas School of Public Health/MD Anderson Cancer Center. June.

Rovati LC, et al. 1994. A large, randomized, placebo controlled, double-blind study of glucosamine sulfate vs piroxicam and vs their association, on the kinetics of the symptomatic effect in knee osteoarthritis. *Osteoarthritis Cartilage* 2:56.

Scarpignato C, et al. 1995. Prevention and treatment of traveler's diarrhea: a clinical pharmacological approach. *Chemotherapy* 41:48–81.

Singer C, et al. 1996. Melatonin and sleep in the elderly. *J Am Geriatr Soc* 44:51[abstr #A1].

Vaz AL. 1982. Double-blind clinical evaluation of the relative efficacy of ibuprofen and glucosamine sulfate in the management of osteoarthritis of the knee in out-patients. *Curr Med Res Opin* 8:145–149.

Yen SSC, et al. 1995. Replacement of DHEA in aging men and women. *Ann NY Acad Sci* 774:128–142.

CHAPTER 14—BIOELECTROMAGNETIC THERAPIES

Algarin R. 1995. *Using Reiki as a harm reduction tool and as a stress management technique for participants and self.* Northeast Conference: Drugs, Sex, and Harm Reduction Conference syllabus. Harm Reduction Coalition and the Drug Policy Foundation, the ACLU AIDS Project and the City University of New York.

Ballock M. 1997. Reiki: A complementary therapy for life. *American Journal of Hospice and Palliative Care* 14(1):31–33.

Barnett L, et al. 1996. *Reiki Energy Medicine.* Rochester, VT: Healing Arts Press.

Bierman P, and Peters J (eds). 1991. *Proceedings of the Scientific Workshop on the Health Effects of Electric and Magnetic Fields on Workers.* Cincinnati,

OH, January 30–31. National Institute of Occupational Safety and Health (NIOSH) Report No. 91-111. NTIS Order No. PB-91-173-351/A13. Springfield, VA: National Technical Information Service.

Brewitt B, Vittetoe T, Hartwell. 1987. The efficacy of Reiki hands on healing: improvements in spleen and nervous system function as quantified by electrodermal screening. Alternative Therapies (3):4.

Frost M, et al. 1998. Nursing and alternative/complementary treatment modalities. Cited in Delaune SC, and Ladner PK: *Fundamentals of Nursing: Standards & Practice.* New York: Delmar Publishers.

Garrard CT. 1995. The effect of Therapeutic Touch on stress reduction and immune function in persons with AIDS. *Dissertation Abstracts International* 56(3692B).

Gordon A, et al. 1998. The effects of Therapeutic Touch on patients with osteoarthritis of the knee. *J Fam Pract* 47(4):271–277.

Heidt PR. 1991. Helping patients to rest: clinical studies in Therapeutic Touch. *Holist Nurs Pract* 5(4):57–66.

Hess B. 1999. Healing sailors with touch. *The Eagle* 17(77):1–2.

Hutchison CP. 1999. Healing touch: an energetic approach. *Am J Nurs* 99(4):43–48.

The International Association of Reiki Professionals (IARP) (Professional Registry). Winchester, MA URL address: http://www.iarp.org.

Ireland M. 1998. Therapeutic touch with HIV-infected children: a pilot study. *J Assoc Nurses AIDS Care* 9(4):68–77.

Krieger D. 1979. *Therapeutic Touch: How to Use Your Hands to Help or Heal.* Englewood Cliffs, NJ: Prentice Hall.

Macrae J. 1987. *Therapeutic Touch: A Practical Guide.* New York: Knopf.

Matthews DA, et al. 1993. *The Faith Factor: An Annotated Bibliography of Clinical Research on Spiritual Subjects.* Vols. I and II. NIHR.

Matthews DA, et al. 1995. *The Faith Factor: Volume III: An Annotated Bibliography of Clinical Research on Spiritual Subjects.* NIHR.

Matthews DA, and Saunders D. 1997. *The Faith Factor: Volume IV: An Annotated Bibliography of Clinical Research on Spiritual Subjects: Prevention and Treatment of Illness, Addictions, and Delinquency.* NIHR.

Meehan TC. 1998. Therapeutic Touch as a nursing intervention. *J Adv Nurs* 28(1):117–125.

Messenger, T et al. 1994. The terminally ill: Serenity nursing interventions for hospice clients. *J Gerontol Nurs* 20(11):17–22.

Olson M, et al. 1992. Therapeutic touch and post–Hurricane Hugo stress. *J Holist Nurs* 10:120–136.

Petter FA. 1997. *Reiki Fire: New Information about the Origins of the Reiki Power: A Complete Manual.* Twin Lakes, WI: Lotus Light Publications.

Petter FA. 1997. *Reiki Fire: New Information about the Origins of the Reiki Power—A Complete Manual.* Twin Lakes, WI, Lotus Light Publication.

Quinn JF. 1984. Therapeutic Touch as energy exchange: testing the theory. *ANS Adv Nurs Sci* 6(2):42–49.

Rand WL. 1998. *Reiki, The Healing Touch, First and Second Degree Manual.* Southfield, MI: Vision Publications, p B5.

The Reiki News. Vision Publications and The International Center for Reiki Training. 1997. Southfield, MI.

Rogers M. 1970. *Introduction to the Theoretical Basis of Nursing.* Philadelphia: FA Davis.

Rogers M. 1990. Nursing: science of unitary, irreducible human beings: update 1990. In Barrett EAM (ed): *Visions of Rogers' Science-Based Nursing.* New York: National League for Nursing.

Rogers M. 1994. Nursing science evolves. In Madrid M, and Barrett EAM (eds): *Rogers' Scientific Art of Nursing Practice.* New York: National League for Nursing.

Sell S. 1996. An ancient touch therapy, *RN* (59):57–59.

Turner JG. 1998. The effect of Therapeutic Touch on pain and anxiety in burn patients. *J Adv Nurs* 28(1):10–20.

Vallbona C. 1997. Response of pain to static magnetic fields in post-polio patients: a double-blind pilot study. *Arch Phys Med Rehabil* 78:1200–1203.

Wager S. 1996. *A Doctor's Guide to Therapeutic Touch.* New York: Berkley Publishing.

Winstead-Fry P, et al. 1999. An integrative review and meta-analysis of Therapeutic Touch research. *Altern Ther Health Med* 5(6):58–67.

Workshop on Alternative Medicine, Chantilly, VA.1992. *Alternative Medicine: Expanding Medical Horizons.* A report to the National Institutes of Health on Alternative Medical Systems and Practices in the United States. Washington, DC: U. S. Government Printing Office: 50–61, 134–146.

CHAPTER 15—MIND-BODY INTERVENTIONS

Bartrop RW, et al. 1977. Depressed lymphocyte function after bereavement. *Lancet* 1:834–836.

Benson H. 1972. The physiology of meditation. *Sci Am* 226:84–90.

Benson H. 1975. *The Relaxation Response.* New York: William Morrow.

Benson H, and Stuart E. 1992. *The Wellness Book, The Comprehensive Guide to Maintaining Health and Treating Stress-Related Illness.* New York: Simon & Schuster.

Benson H. 1998. Spirituality and Medicine (Lecture). Houston, TX.

Borysenko J. 1987. *Minding the Body, Mending the Mind.* Reading, MA: Addison Wesley.

Cannon W. 1939. *The Wisdom of the Body.* New York: WW Norton.

Cohen S, et al. 1991. Psychological stress and susceptibility to the common cold. *N Engl J Med* 325:606–612.

Cousins N. 1976. Anatomy of an illness (as perceived by the patient). *N Engl J Med* 295:1458–1463.

Cousins N. 1979. *Anatomy of an Illness.* New York: WW Norton.

Dossey L. 1999. *Reinventing Medicine: Beyond Mind-Body to a New Era of Healing.* San Francisco: HarperCollins.

Engel GL. 1977. The need for a new medical model: a challenge for biomedicine. *Science* 196:129–136.

Graham-Pole J. 2000. *Illness and the Art of Creative Self-Expression.* Oakland, CA: New Harbinger Publications.

Kabat-Zinn J.1990. *Full Catastrophe Living: Using the Wisdom of Your Body and Mind to Face Stress, Pain and Illness.* New York: Delacorte Press.

Kiecolt-Glaser JK, et al. 1986. Modulation of cellular immunity in medical students. *J Behav Med* 9:5–21.

Kiecolt-Glaser JK, et al. 1987. Marital quality, marital disruption, and immune function. *Psychosom Med* 49:13–34.

Kiecolt-Glaser JK, et al. 1988. Marital discord and immunity in males. *Psychosom Med* 50:213–229.

Kobasa S. 1990. Stress resistant personality. In Ornstein R (ed): *The Healing Brain: A Scientific Reader.* New York: Guilford. pp 219–239.

Rossman M. 1987. *Healing Yourself: A Step-by-Step Program for Better Health through Imagery.* New York: Walker.

Selye H. 1956. *The Stress of Life.* New York: McGraw-Hill.

Simonton OC, et al. 1978. *Getting Well Again: A Step-by-Step Guide to Overcoming Cancer for Patients and Their Families.* New York: Bantam.

Smyth J. 1999. Effects of writing about stressful experiences on symptom reduction in patients with asthma or rheumatoid arthritis. *JAMA* 281:1304–1309.

Speigel D. 1991. A psychosocial intervention and survival time of patients with metastatic breast cancer. *Advances* 7(3):10–19.

Stienstra K. 1998. *Psychoneuroimmunology or Mind Body Medicine.* Presentation at the Indiana Academy of Family Physicians, Indianapolis, IN. August.

Vaillant G, et al. 1970. Physicians' use of mood altering drugs. *N Engl J Med* 282:365–370.

Vaillant G, et al. 1977. *Adaptation to Life.* Boston: Little, Brown.

CHAPTER 16—HANDS-ON HEALING TECHNIQUES

Bigos S, et al. 1994. Acute low back pain problems in adults. *AHCPR Clinical Practice Guidelines.* No 14, AHCPR Pub No 9500642. Rockville, MD: U.S. Dept. of Health and Human Services.

Kaptchuk T, et al. 1998. Chiropractic—origins, controversies, and contributions. *Arch Intern Med* 158:2215–2223.

Manga P, et al. 1993. The effectiveness and cost effectiveness of chiropractic management of low back pain. Toronto: Ontario Ministry of Health.

Shekelle PG, et al. 1991. The appropriateness of spinal manipulation for low back pain: indications and ratings by an all-chiropractic expert panel. Santa Monica, CA: Rand.

Spitzer WO, et al. 1987. Scientific approach to the assessment and management of activity-related spinal disorders: a monograph for physicians. Report of the Quebec Task Force on Spinal Disorders. *Spine* 12(7).

Waddel G, et al. 1996. *Low Back Pain Evidence Review.* London: Royal College of General Practitioners.

Ward RC (ed). 1997. *Foundations for Osteopathic Medicine.* Baltimore: Williams & Wilkins.

CHAPTER 17—ANXIETY AND DEPRESSION

Benson H, and Stuart E. 1992. *The Wellness Book, The Comprehensive Guide to Maintaining Health and Treating Stress-Related Illness.* New York: Simon & Schuster.

Ernst E, et al. 1998. Complementary therapies for depression: an overview. *Arch Gen Psychiatry* 55:1026–1032.

Glenister D. 1996. Exercise and mental health: a review. *JR Soc Health* 116:7–13.

Hertsgaard D, et al. 1984. Anxiety, depression, and hostility in rural women. *Psychol Rep* 55:673–675.

Koenig H, et al. 1993. Religion and anxiety disorder. *J Anxiety Disord* 7: 321–342.

Koenig H, et al. 1994. Religious affiliation and psychiatric disorder among Protestant baby boomers. *Hosp Community Psychiatry* 45(6):586–596.

Robbers J, and Tyler V. 1999. *Tyler's Herbs of Choice—The Therapeutic Use of Phytomedicinals.* New York: Haworth Press.

CHAPTER 18—ARTHRITIS

Christensen B, et al. 1992. Acupuncture treatment of severe knee osteoarthritis: a long-term study. *Acta Anaesthesiol Scand* 36:519.

Ernst E. 1997. Acupuncture as a symptomatic treatment of osteoarthritis. A systematic review. *Scand J Rheumatol* 26(6):444–447.

Muller-Fassbender H, et al. 1994. Glucosamine sulfate compared to ibuprofen in osteoarthritis of the knee. *Osteoarthritis Cartilage* 2:61–69.

Rovati LC, et al. 1994. A large, randomized, placebo controlled, double-blind study of glucosamine sulfate vs piroxicam and vs their association, on the kinetics of the symptomatic effect in knee osteoarthritis. *Osteoarthritis Cartilage* 2:56.

CHAPTER 19—ASTHMA

Bucca C, et al. 1990. Effect of vitamin C on histamine bronchial responsiveness of patients with allergic rhinitis. *Ann Allergy* 65:311–314.

Collipp PJ, et al. 1975. Pyridoxine treatment of childhood bronchial asthma. *Ann Allergy* 35:93–97.

Dorsch W, et al. 1985. Antiasthmatic effects of onion extracts—detection of benzyl- and other isothiocyanates in mustard oils as antiasthmatic compounds of plant origin. *Euro J Pharmacol* 107:17–24.

Gore MM. 1982. Effect of yogic treatment on some pulmonary functions in asthmatics. *Yoga Mimamsa* 20:51–58.

Haury VG. 1940. Blood serum magnesium in bronchial asthma and its treatment by the administration of magnesium sulfate. *J Lab Clin Med* 26:340–344.

Lewith G, et al. 1996. Unconventional therapies in asthma: an overview. *Allergy* 51(11):761–769.

Panganamala RV, et al. 1982. The effects of vitamin E on arachidonic acid metabolism. *Ann NY Acad Sci* 393:376–391.

Simon SW. 1951. Vitamin B$_{12}$ therapy in allergy and chronic dermatoses. *J Allergy* 2:183–185.

Skobeloff EM, et al. 1989. Intravenous magnesium sulfate for the treatment of acute asthma in the emergency department. *JAMA* 262:1210–1213.

Vanderhoek J, et al. 1980. Inhibition of fatty acid lipoxygenases by onion and garlic oils inhibit platelet aggregation. *Biochem Pharmacol* 29:3169–3173.

CHAPTER 20—CANCER

Amkraut A. 1975. From the symbolic stimulus to the pathophysiological response: immune mechanism. *Int J Psychiatry Med* 5(4):541–563.

Bahnson CB. 1980. Stress and cancer: the state of the art. *Psychosomatics* 21(12):975.

Fawzy I, et al. 1993. Malignant melanoma: effects of an early structured psychiatric intervention, coping, and affective state on recurrence and survival 6 years later. *Arch Gen Psych* 47:720–735.

Greer S, et al. 1982. Psychological concommitants of cancer: current state of research. *Psychol Med* 12:567–568.

Lerner M. 1994. *Choices in Healing—Integrating the Best of Conventional and Complementary Approaches to Cancer*. Cambridge, MA: MIT Press.

Lerner M. 1999. *Choices in Healing—Integrating the Best of Conventional and Complementary Approaches to Cancer*. Presentation at Alternative Medicine: Implications for Clinical Practice and State of the Science Symposium. March. Boston: Harvard University.

Siegel BS. 1993. *How to Live Between Office Visits*. Hingham, MA: Wheeler Publishing.

Siegel BS. 1986. *Love, Medicine and Miracles: Lessons Learned about Self-Healing from a Surgeon's Experience with Exceptional Patients*.

Simonton OC, et al. 1978. *Getting Well Again: A Step-by-Step Guide to Overcoming Cancer for Patients and Their Families*. New York: Bantam.

Spiegel D, et al. 1989. Effect of psychosocial treatment on survival of patients with metastatic breast cancer. *Lancet* 2:888.

Watkins, A. 1977. *Mind-Body Medicine—A Clinician's Guide to Psychoneuroimmunology*. New York: Churchill Livingstone.

Wirth, S (ed). 1999. *Integrative Medicine—A Balanced Account of the Data*. Ukiah, CA: Boitumelo Publishing.

CHAPTER 21—CORONARY ARTERY DISEASE AND CONGESTIVE HEART FAILURE

The Alpha-Tocopherol, Beta Carotene Cancer Prevention Study Group. 1994. The effect of vitamin E and beta carotene on the incidence of lung cancer and other cancers in male smokers. *N Engl J Med* 330:1029–1035.

Baggio E, et al. 1994. Italian multicenter study on the safety and efficacy of coenzyme Q10 as adjunctive therapy in heart failure. CoQ10 Drug Surveillance Investigators. *Mol Aspects Med* 15:287–294.

Balz F. 1999. Antioxidant vitamins and heart disease. Presented at the 60th Annual Biology Colloquium. Oregon State University, February 25.

Barefoot J, et al. 1996. Symptoms of depression, acute myocardial infarction, and total mortality in a community sample. *Circulation* 93(11):1976–1980.

Benson H, 1996. *Timeless Healing: The Power and Biology of Belief.* New York: Simon & Schuster.

Blumenthal M (ed). 1998. *The Complete German Commission E Monographs— Therapeutic Guide to Herbal Medicines.* Boston, MA: Integrative Medicine Communications.

Brezinka V, et al. 1996. Psychosocial factors of coronary heart disease in women: a review. *Soc Sci Med* 42(10):1351–1365.

Cousins N. 1983. The healing heart. *Int J Cardiol* 3:57–65.

Dunn A, et al. 1999. Comparison of lifestyle and structured interventions to increase physical activity and cardiorespiratory fitness—a randomized trial. *JAMA* 281:327–334.

Frasure-Smith N, et al. 1993. Depression following myocardial infarction. Impact on 6-month survival. *JAMA* 270:1819–1825.

Friedman M, et al. 1959. Association of specific overt behavior pattern with blood and cardiovascular findings. *Am Heart J* 169:1286–1295.

Friedman M, et al. 1986. Alteration in type A behavior and its effect on cardiac recurrences in post-myocardial infarction patients: summary results of the recurrent coronary prevention project. *Am Heart J* 12:653.

Fukai T. 1993. Role of coronary vasospasm in the pathogenesis of myocardial infarction in patients with no significant coronary stenosis. *Am Heart J* 126(6):1305–1311.

Gottlieb SS, et al. 1990. Prognostic importance of serum magnesium concentration in patients with congestive heart failure. *J Am Coll Cardiol* 16:827–831.

Gottlieb S. 1989. Importance of magnesium in congestive heart failure. Am J Cardiol 63(14):39G–42G.

Greenwood DC, et al. 1996. Coronary heart disease: a review of the role of psychosocial stress and social support. *J Public Health Med* 18:221–231.

Hallfrisch J, et al. 1994. High plasma vitamin C on plasma lipids. *Am J Clin Nutr* 60:100–105.

Kostreski F. 1999. Ornish program to get national test. *Family Practice News* 29(21):1, 5.

Leslie D, et al. 1996. Is there a role for thiamine supplementation in the management of heart failure. *Am Heart J* 131:1248–1250.

Leuchtgens H. 1993. Crataegus special extract WS 1442 in NYHA II heart failure. A placebo controlled randomized double-blind study. *Fortschr Med* 111:352–354.

Mayou R, et al. 1994. Non-cardiac pain and benign palpitations in the cardiac clinic. *Br Heart J* 72:548–553.

Morisco B, et al. 1993. Effect of coenzyme Q10 in patients with congestive heart failure: a long-term multi-center randomized study. *Clin Investig* 71: 134–136.

Nixon P, et al. 1997. Ischemic heart disease: homeostasis and the heart. In Watkins A: *Mind-Body Medicine—A Clinician's Guide to Psychoneuroimmunology.* New York: Churchill Livingstone.

Ornish D, et al. 1983. Effects of stress management training and dietary changes in treating ischemic heart disease. *JAMA* 24:54–59.

Pace-Asciak CR, et al. 1996. Wines and grape juices as modulators of platelet aggregation in healthy human subjects. *Clin Chim Acta* 246(1-2):163–182.

Phelps S, et al. 1993. Garlic supplementation and lipoprotein oxidation susceptibility. *Lipids* 28:475.

Rapola J, et al. 1997. Randomized trial of alpha-tocopherol and beta-carotene supplements on incidence of major coronary events in men with previous myocardial infarction. *Lancet* 349(9067):1715–1720.

Rimm E. 1993. Vitamin E consumption and the risk of coronary heart disease in men. *N Engl J Med* 328:1450–1455.

Stampfer J, et al. 1993. Vitamin E consumption and the risk of coronary disease in women. *N Engl J Med* 328:1444–1448.

Tauchert M, et al. 1994. Effectiveness of the hawthorn extract LI 132 compared to ACE inhibitor Captopril. Multicentre double-blind study with 132 NYHA stage II. *MMW Munch Med Wochenschr* 136(suppl):S27–S33.

Warshafsky S, et al. 1995. Effect of garlic on total serum cholesterol: a meta-analysis. *Ann Intern Med* 119:599.

Wenneberg S, et al. 1997. Anger expression correlates with platelet aggregation. *Behav Med* 22(4):174–177.

Yusef S, et al. 2000. Vitamin E supplementation and cardiovascular events in high-risk patients. *N Engl J Med* 342:145–153.

CHAPTER 22—DIABETES

Engel ED, et al. 1981. Diabetes mellitus: impaired wound healing from zinc deficiency. *J Am Podiatr Med Assoc* 71:536–544.

Levin ER, et al. 1981. The influence of pyridoxine in diabetic peripheral neuropathy. *Diabetes Care* 4:606–609.

Paolisso G, et al. 1992. Daily magnesium supplements improve glucose handling in elderly subjects. *Am J Clin Nutr* 55:1161–1167.

Paolisso G, et al. 1993. Pharmacologic doses of vitamin E improve insulin action in healthy subjects and non-insulin-dependent diabetic patients. *Am J Clin Nutr* 57:650–656.

Ravina A, et al. 1995. Clinical use of the trace element chromium (III) in the treatment of diabetes mellitus. *J Trace Elem Exp Med* 8:183–190.

Sinclair AJ, et al. 1994. Low plasma ascorbate levels in patients with type 2 diabetes mellitus consuming adequate dietary vitamin C. *Diabetic Med* 11:893–898.

Vague P, et al. 1987. Nicotinamide may extend remission phase in insulin-dependent diabetes. *Lancet* 1:619–620.

CHAPTER 23—GASTROINTESTINAL PROBLEMS

Blumenthal M (ed). 1998. *The Complete German Commission E Monographs—Therapeutic Guide to Herbal Medicines.* Boston, MA: Integrative Medicine Communications.

Blumenthal, M, Goldberg A, and Brinckman, J. 2000. *Herbal Medicine—*

Expanded Commission E Monographs. Boston, MA: Integrative Medicine Communications. 257–261, 300–301.

Dew MJ, et al. 1984. Peppermint oil for the irritable bowel syndrome: a multi-center trial. *Br J Clin Pract* 38:394–398.

Hotz J, et al. 1994. Effectiveness of plantago seed husks in comparison with wheat bran on stool frequency and manifestations of irritable colon syndrome with constipation. *Med Klin* 89:645–651.

Liu J-H, et al. 1997. Enteric-coated peppermint-oil capsules in the treatment of irritable bowel syndrome: a prospective, randomized trial. *J Gastroenterol* 32:765–768.

Kassir Z. 1985. Endoscopic controlled trial of four drug regimens in the treatment of chronic duodenal ulceration. *Irish Med J* 78:153–156.

Murray M, and Pizzorno, J. 1998. *Encyclopedia of Natural Medicine.* Rocklin, CA: Prima Publishing.

Rees WD, et al. 1979. Treating irritable bowel syndrome with peppermint oil. *BMJ* 2(6194):835–836.

Robbers J, and Tyler V. 1999. *Tyler's Herbs of Choice—The Therapeutic Use of Phytomedicinals.* New York: Haworth Press.

CHAPTER 24—HEADACHE

Benson H, and Stuart E. 1992. *The Wellness Book, The Comprehensive Guide to Maintaining Health and Treating Stress-Related Illness.* New York: Simon & Schuster.

Field T, et al. 1997. Job stress reduction therapies. *Altern Ther Health Med* 3(4):54–56.

Mazzotta G, et al. 1996. Electromyographical ischemic test and intracellular and extracellular magnesium concentration in migraine and tension type headache patients. *Headache* 36:357–361.

Murray M, and Pizzorno J. 1998. *Encyclopedia of Natural Medicine,* ed 2. Rocklin, CA: Prima Publishing.

NIH Consensus Development Panel on Acupuncture 1998. *JAMA* 280:1518–1524.

Pizzorno J, and Murray M. 1999. *Textbook of Natural Medicine.* Edinburgh: Churchill Livingstone.

Robbers J, and Tyler V. 1999. *Tyler's Herbs of Choice—The Therapeutic Use of Phytomedicinals.* New York: Haworth Press.

Shellenberger R, et al. 1994. *Clinical Efficacy and Cost-effectiveness of Biofeedback Therapy.* Wheat Ridge, CO: Association for Applied Psychophysiology and Biofeedback.

Vutyananich T, et al. 1995. Pyridoxine for nausea and vomiting of pregnancy: a randomized, double-blind, placebo-controlled trial. *Am J Obstet Gynecol* 173:881–884.

CHAPTER 25—HYPERCHOLESTEROLEMIA

Brody J, and Flaste R. 1994. *Jane Brody's Good Seafood Cookbook: A Guide to Healthy Eating with More Than 200 Low-Fat Recipes.* New York: W.W. Norton & Co., Inc.

Frei B. 1991. Ascorbic acid protects lipids in human plasma and low-density lipoprotein against oxidative damage. *Am J Clin Nutr* 54(6 Suppl):1113S–1118S.

Head KA. 1996. Inositol hexaniacinate: a safer alternative to niacin. *Alt Med Rev* 1:176–184.

Hein HO, et al. 1996. Alcohol consumption, serum low-density lipoprotein cholesterol concentration, and risk of ischaemic heart disease: six year follow up in the Copenhagen male study. *BMJ* 312:736–741.

Hendriks HF, et al. 1994. Effect of moderate dose of alcohol with evening meal on fibrinolytic factors. *BMJ* 309:911–918.

Jain AK, et al. 1993. Can garlic reduce levels of serum lipids? A controlled clinical study. *Am J Med* 94:632–635.

Moosewood Collective. 1996. *Moosewood Restaurant Low-Fat Favorites.* New York: Random House.

Murray M. 1995. Lipid-lowering drugs vs. inositol hexaniacinate. *Am J Natural Med* 2:9–12.

Pizzorno J, and Murray M. 1999. *Textbook of Natural Medicine.* Edinburgh: Churchill Livingstone.

Rimm E. 1993. Vitamin E consumption and the risk of coronary heart disease in men. *N Engl J Med* 328:1450–1455.

Rimm E et al. 1996. Review of moderate alcohol consumption and reduced risk of coronary heart disease: is the effect due to beer, wine or spirits? *BMJ* 312:731–736.

Schlesinger S, and Earnest B. 1990. *The Low Cholesterol Olive Oil Cookbook—More Than 200 Recipes—The Most Delicious Ways to Eat Healthy Food.* New York: Random House.

Warshafsky RS, et al. 1993. Effect of garlic on total serum cholesterol. *Ann Intern Med* 119:599–605.

CHAPTER 26—HYPERTENSION

Appel LJ, et al. 1997. A clinical trial of the effects of dietary patterns on blood pressure. DASH Collaborative Research Group. *N Engl J Med* 336:1117–1124.

Digiesi V, et al. 1990. Effect of coenzyme Q10 on essential arterial hypertension. *Curr Ther Res* 47:841–845.

Hornsby L, et al. 1991. Ambulatory blood pressure monitoring in hypertension. *AFP* 43 (5):1631–1638.

Jacob RG, et al. 1991. Relaxation therapy for hypertension: design effects and treatment effects. *Ann Behav Med* 13:5–17.

Johnston DW, et al. 1993. Effect of stress management on blood pressure in mild primary hypertension. *BMJ* 306:963–966.

Kawano Y, et al. 1998. Effects of magnesium supplementation in hypertensive patients. *Hypertension* 32:260–265.

Langsjoen P, et al. 1994. Treatment of essential hypertension with coenzyme Q10 in essential hypertension. *Mol Aspects Med* 15(suppl):S257–S263.

Ness AR, et al. 1997. Vitamin C and blood pressure—an overview. *J Human Hypertens* 11:343–350.

Resnick LM. 1999. The role of dietary calcium in hypertension: a hierarchical review. *Am J Hypertens* 12:84–92.

Schneider RA, et al. 1995. A randomized controlled trial of stress reduction for hypertension in older African Americans. *Hypertension* 26:820–827.

Staessen J, et al. 1997. Antihypertensive treatment based on conventional or ambulatory blood pressure measurement. *JAMA* 278:1065–1072.

CHAPTER 27—MUSCULOSKELETAL PROBLEMS

Carey T, et al. 1995. The outcomes and costs of care for the acute low back pain among patients seen by primary care practitioners, chiropractors, and orthopedic surgeons. *N Engl J Med* 333:913–917.

Field T, et al. 1997. Job stress reduction therapies. *Altern Ther Health Med* 3(4):54–56.

Kanter M. 1998. Free radicals, exercise and antioxidant supplementation. *Proc Nutr Soc* 57:9–13.

Lininger S (ed), Wright J, Austin S, Brown D, Gaby A. 1999. *The Natural Pharmacy*. Rocklin, CA: Prima Publishing.

MacDonald A, et al. 1983. Superficial acupuncture in the relief of chronic low back pain. *Ann R Coll Surg Engl* 65:44–46.

Nespor K. 1989. Psychosomatics of back pain and the use of yoga. *Int J Psychosom* 36(1–4):72–78.

Pope MH, et al. 1994. A prospective randomized three-week trial of spinal manipulation, transcutaneous muscle stimulation, massage and corset in the treatment of subacute low back pain. *Spine* 19:2571–2577.

Schneider CJ. 1987. Cost-effectiveness of biofeedback and behavioral medicine treatments: a review of the literature. *Biofeedback Self Regul* 12(2):71–92.

Shekelle P, et al. 1997. Spinal manipulation for low back pain. *Ann Intern Med* 117(7):590–598.

Telles S, et al. 1997. Yoga for rehabilitation: an overview. *Indian J Med Sci* 51(4):123–127.

Thomas M, et al. 1994. Importance of modes of acupuncture in the treatment of chronic nociceptive low back pain. *Acta Anaesthesiol Scand* 38:63–69.

Weintraub, M. 1992. Alternative medical care: Shiatsu, Swedish muscle massage, and trigger point suppression in spinal pain syndrome. *Am J Pain Mgmt* 2(2):74–78.

CHAPTER 28—UPPER RESPIRATORY INFECTIONS

Blumenthal M (ed). 1998. *The Complete German Commission E Monographs— Therapeutic Guide to Herbal Medicines*. Boston: Integrative Medicine Communications.

Cohen S, et al. 1991. Psychological stress and susceptibility to the common cold. *N Engl J Med* 325:606–612.

Cohen S, et al. 1997. Negative life events, perceived stress, negative affect, and susceptibility to the common cold. *Br J Nutr* 77(1):59–72.

Cohen S, et al. 1997. Social ties and susceptibility to the common cold. *JAMA* 277: 1940–1944.

Dorn M, et al. 1997. Placebo-controlled, double-blind trial of *Echinacea pallida radix* in upper respiratory tract infections. *Comp Ther Med* 5:40–42.

Hemila H. 1992. Vitamin C and the common cold. *Br J Nutr* 67:3–16.

Hemila H, et al. 1995. Vitamin C and the common cold: a retrospective analysis of Chalmers' review. *J Am Coll Nutr* 14:116–123.

Holmes TH, et al. 1967. The social readjustment scale. *J Psychosom Res* 11:213–218.

Klein T. 1993. Stress and infections. *J Fla Med Assoc* 80(6):409–411.

Lewith G, et al. 1996. Unconventional therapies in asthma: an overview. *Allergy* 51(11):761–769.

McEwan BS, et al. 1993. Stress and the individual: mechanisms leading to disease. *Arch Intern Med* 153(2):93–101.

Mossad SB, et al. 1996. Zinc gluconate lozenges for treating the common cold: a randomized, double-blind, placebo-controlled study. *Ann Intern Med* 125:142–144.

Murray M, and Pizzorno J. 1998. *Encyclopedia of Natural Medicine.* Rocklin, CA: Prima Publishing.

Pizzorno J, and Murray M. 1999. *Textbook of Natural Medicine.* Edinburgh: Churchill Livingstone.

Sanchez A, et al. 1973. Role of sugars in human neutrophilic phagocytosis. *Am J Clin Nutr* 26:1180–1184.

Zarembo JE, et al. 1992. Zinc (II) in saliva: determination of concentrations produced by different formulations of zinc gluconate lozenges containing common excipients. *Pharm Sci* 81:128–130.

CHAPTER 29—URINARY TRACT INFECTIONS

Ofek I, et al. 1991. Anti-escherichia activity of cranberry and blueberry juices. *N Engl J Med* 324:599.

Sobota AE. 1984. Inhibition of bacterial adherence by cranberry juice: potential use for the treatment of urinary tract infections. *J Urology* 131:13–16.

Murray M, and Pizzorno J. 1998. *Encyclopedia of Natural Medicine.* Rocklin, CA: Prima Publishing.

Robbers J, and Tyler V. 1999. *Tyler's Herbs of Choice—The Therapeutic Use of Phytomedicinals.* New York: Haworth Press.

Index

Page numbers followed by f indicate figures; those followed by t indicate tables.

379